I0031619

Richard M. Billow's Selected Papers on Psychoanalysis and Group Process

This comprehensive volume presents Richard M. Billow's unique contributions to the theory and technique of psychotherapy, along with summaries and explications by the volume's editor, Tzachi Slonim.

Through their behavior, therapists define the clinical culture: how relationships are to be regarded and the depth to which narratives and exchanges may be considered. Known for his integration of Bion's metapsychology with contemporary psychoanalysis, Billow extends our understanding of "relational" to include the emotional relationships people have with individual and collective ideas, and the behaviors attached to these ideas. "Doing our work" (the title of the last section) involves the therapist's whole being, including cognitions, dreams, words, deeds, and very presence—mental and somatic. Drawing on Lacan, Billow suggests that therapeutic work ought to include a willingness to penetrate other minds with provocative, controversial ideas. His clinical vignettes portray a masterly clinician-in-action, describing his evolving feelings, thoughts, and assessments.

Billow's intimate knowledge of Bionian theory, coupled with his down-to-earth demeanour and clear writing, allows him to explicate and expand upon Bion's important contributions in a manner accessible to the novice and expert therapist alike. With one eye on therapeutic process, and the other on each participant including the therapist himself, Billow invites each of us to change our minds.

Tzachi Slonim, PhD, studied philosophy in the critical rationalist tradition before becoming a clinical psychologist. He maintains a private practice in New York City and is an adjunct professor at the Doctoral Programs in Clinical Psychology at the City University of New York and Pace University and at the Postdoctoral Program in Group Psychotherapy at Adelphi University.

Richard M. Billow, PhD, is a clinical psychologist and holds postdoctoral certificates in psychoanalysis and group psychotherapy. For many years he directed the Postgraduate Group Program at the Derner Institute, Adelphi University. He is a frequent contributor to psychoanalytic and group literature, and the author of *Relational Group Psychotherapy: From Basic Assumptions to Passion* (2003), *Resistance, Rebellion and Refusal: The 3 Rs* (2010), and *Developing Nuclear Ideas* (2016). He is a clinical professor in the Postdoctoral Program in Psychoanalysis and Psychotherapy at Adelphi, and practices in Great Neck, New York.

The New International Library of Group Analysis (NILGA)
Series Editor: Earl Hopper

Drawing on the seminal ideas of British, European and American group analysts, psychoanalysts, social psychologists, and social scientists, the books in this series focus on the study of small and large groups, organizations and other social systems, and on the study of the transpersonal and transgenerational sociality of human nature. NILGA books will be required reading for the members of professional organizations in the field of group analysis, psychoanalysis, and related social sciences. They will be indispensable for the "formation" of students of psychotherapy, whether they are mainly interested in clinical work with patients or in consultancy to teams and organizational clients within the private and public sectors.

Recent titles in the series include the following:

The Art and Science of Working Together
Practising Group Analysis in Teams and Organisations
Edited by Christine Thornton

Why Group Therapy Works and How to Do It
A Guide for Health and Social Care Professionals
By Christer Sandahl, Hjördis Nilsson Ahlin, Catharina Asklin-Westerdahl, Mats Björling, Anna Malmquist Saracino, Lena Wennlund, Ulf Åkerström and Ann Örhammar

The Portuguese School of Group Analysis
Towards a Unified and Integrated Approach to Theory Research and Clinical Work
Edited by Isaura Manso Neto and Margarida França

Richard M. Billow's Selected Papers on Psychoanalysis and Group Process
Changing Our Minds
Edited by Tzachi Slonim

Richard M. Billow's Selected Papers on Psychoanalysis and Group Process

Changing Our Minds

Edited by Tzachi Slonim

Routledge
Taylor & Francis Group

LONDON AND NEW YORK

First published 2021
by Routledge
2 Park Square, Milton Park, Abingdon, Oxon OX14 4RN

and by Routledge
52 Vanderbilt Avenue, New York, NY 10017

Routledge is an imprint of the Taylor & Francis Group, an informa business

© 2021 selection and editorial matter, Tzachi Slonim; individual chapters, Richard M. Billow

The right of Tzachi Slonim to be identified as the author of the editorial material, and of the authors for their individual chapters, has been asserted in accordance with sections 77 and 78 of the Copyright, Designs and Patents Act 1988.

All rights reserved. No part of this book may be reprinted or reproduced or utilised in any form or by any electronic, mechanical, or other means, now known or hereafter invented, including photocopying and recording, or in any information storage or retrieval system, without permission in writing from the publishers.

Trademark notice: Product or corporate names may be trademarks or registered trademarks, and are used only for identification and explanation without intent to infringe.

British Library Cataloguing-in-Publication Data
A catalogue record for this book is available from the British Library

Library of Congress Cataloging-in-Publication Data
Names: Billow, Richard M., 1943– author. | Slonim, Tzachi, editor.
Title: Richard M. Billow's selected papers on psychoanalysis and group process: changing our minds / edited by Tzachi Slonim.
Description: Milton Park, Abingdon, Oxon; New York, NY: Routledge, 2021. | Includes bibliographical references and index.
Identifiers: LCCN 2020045346 (print) | LCCN 2020045347 (ebook) | ISBN 9780367743352 (hardback) | ISBN 9780367743369 (paperback) | ISBN 9781003157304 (ebook)
Subjects: LCSH: Group psychotherapy. | Group psychoanalysis.
Classification: LCC RC488 .B4753 2021 (print) | LCC RC488 (ebook) | DDC 616.89/152—dc23
LC record available at https://lccn.loc.gov/2020045346
LC ebook record available at https://lccn.loc.gov/2020045347

ISBN: 978-0-367-74335-2 (hbk)
ISBN: 978-0-367-74336-9 (pbk)
ISBN: 978-1-003-15730-4 (ebk)

Typeset in Times New Roman
by codeMantra

Contents

Acknowledgments

I would like to thank, most of all, Richard Billow, for trusting me enough to edit this volume and encouraging me to be ruthless with my edits. In his initial email to me, he said he hoped this would be an edifying experience, and that it has.

Dr. Hilary Callan Curtis proofed the entire manuscript and alerted me to a range of linguistic and stylistic mistakes and inconsistencies. She did this admirably fast and with authority and a delightful wit.

My colleagues and friends Dr. Wayne Ayers and Frumi Stroli read some of my editor's notes and provided useful feedback and encouragement.

I am also grateful to my friends Drs. Elik Elhanan, Yuval Kremnitzer, and Dan Tsahor who served as an informal support group. They offered companionship, critical remarks, and creative ideas from their respective intellectual domains.

Finally, I would like to thank my wife Juliana May. Her support goes beyond the usual compliments one pays their partner and family in such acknowledgments (patient, encouraging, and so on). Her keen aesthetic sensibility and sharp compositional skills make her the kind of critical reader each writer or editor needs.

Tzachi Slonim

In preparing for publication, I envision the individuals and groups who people this volume—generations who have contributed so much to the pleasures and challenges of my professional life. I hear voices too, none louder than Charles Raps, Ph.D., the brilliant uber editor of all my publications. Other guiding spirits include the journal editors and anonymous peer reviewers of earlier versions of these chapters. Les Greene, Ph.D. and Dominick Grundy, Ph.D., successive editors from the International Journal of Group Psychotherapy have been prominent. Among the many other supportive figures I thank are Malcolm Pines, Ph.D. and Earl Hopper, Ph.D., the welcoming guardians of the Series, and my wife, Elyse, and family, upholders of love and good spirits. Dr. Slonim's strong editorial hand has passed over every page, along with the good works of our recently added grammarian, Dr. Hilary Callan Curtis.

Richard M. Billow

Permissions acknowledgments

From *The International Journal of Group Psychotherapy* © American Group Psychotherapy Association, www.agpa.org, reprinted by permission of Taylor & Francis Ltd, http://www.tandfonline.com on behalf of the American Group Psychotherapy Association.

Richard M. Billow (2019) Doing Our Work: Words, Deeds, and Presence, 69:1, 77–98. DOI: 10.1080/00207284.2018.1483197

Richard M. Billow (2016) Psychic Nodules and Therapeutic Impasses: Three Case Studies, 66:1, 1–19. DOI: 10.1080/00207284.2015.1089682

Richard M. Billow (Director) (2006) The Three R's of Group: Resistance, Rebellion, and Refusal, 56:3, 259–284. DOI: 10.1521/ijgp.2006.56.3.259

Richard M. Billow (2016) Reality Testing and Testing Reality in Group Treatment, 66:4, 551–570. DOI: 10.1080/00207284.2016.1176498

Richard M. Billow (2013) Developing the Nuclear Idea: Concept, Technique, and Process, 63:4, 544–570, DOI: 10.1521/ijgp.2013.63.4.544

Richard M. Billow (2003) Bonding in Group: The Therapist's Contribution, 53:1, 83–110. DOI: 10.1521/ijgp.53.1.83.42805

Richard M. Billow (2017) On the Origins of Clinical Interventions, 67:sup1, S24-S35. DOI: 10.1080/00207284.2016.1239935

Richard M. Billow (2018) On Deconstructive Interventions, 68:3, 355–375. DOI: 10.1080/00207284.2017.1413376

Richard M. Billow (2019) Witnessing: The Axis of Group, 69:1, 54–76. DOI: 10.1080/00207284.2018.1483196

Richard M. Billow (2019) Attention-Getting Mechanisms (AGMs): A Personal Journey, 69:4, 408–433, DOI: 10.1080/00207284.2019.1649984

Richard M. Billow (2010) Modes of Therapeutic Engagement Part I: Diplomacy and Integrity, 60:1, 1–28, DOI: 10.1521/ijgp.2010.60.1.1

Richard M Billow (2010) Models of Therapeutic Engagement Part II: Sincerity and Authenticity, 60:1, 29–58, DOI: 10.1521/ijgp.2010.60.1.29

Richard M. Billow (2012) It's All About "Me" (Behold the Leader), 62:4, 530–556, DOI: 10.1521/ijgp.2012.62.4.530

From *Contemporary Psychoanalysis* © William Alanson White Institute of Psychiatry, Psychoanalysis & Psychology and the William Alanson White Psychoanalytic Society, www.wawhite.org, reprinted by permission of Taylor & Francis Ltd, http://www.tandfonline.com on behalf of the William Alanson White Institute of Psychiatry, Psychoanalysis & Psychology and the William Alanson White Psychoanalytic Society.

Richard M. Billow (1999) Lhk the Basis of Emotion in Bion's Theory, 35:4, 629–646. DOI: 10.1080/00107530.1999.10746406

Richard M. Billow (2003) Relational Variations of the "Container-Contained", 39:1, 27–50. DOI: 10.1080/00107530.2003.10747198

From *The Psychoanalytic Quarterly* © The Psychoanalytic Quarterly, Inc., reprinted by permission of Taylor & Francis Ltd, http://www. tandfonline.com on behalf of The Psychoanalytic Quarterly, Inc.

Richard M. Billow (1999) An Intersubjective Approach to Entitlement, 68:3, 441–461. DOI: 10.1002/j.2167–4086.1999.tb00541.x

Richard M. Billow (2000) From Countertransference to "Passion", 69:1, 93–119. DOI: 10.1002/j.2167–4086.2000.tb00556.x

Richard M. Billow (2004) A Falsifying Adolescent, 73:4, 1041–1078. DOI: 10.1002/j.2167–4086.2004.tb00192.x

Permission has been granted by Guildford Publications for the following publication:

Billow, R. M. (2000). Self-disclosure and psychoanalytic meaning: A psychoanalytic fable. *Psychoanalytic Review*, 87 (1), 61–79.

Series editor's foreword

In the Epilogue to this selection of his published contributions to group analysis and psychoanalysis, Dr. Richard Billow concludes that his clinical interventions are precipitated by his personal experience of "stupidity," that is, his sense that he has not understood the communications of a group or even a single patient. Without wishing to debate the meaning of either stupidity or understanding, I am pleased to express my gratitude to Richard Billow for helping me acknowledge and accept my own scotoma and addicted understandings of clinical processes, as a first step towards interpersonal change in my clinical relationships and perhaps in my private life as well. These incisive and iconoclastic excursions and explorations of both that which is most familiar and that which is most far reaching in our professional field have been carefully and authentically edited by Dr. Tzachi Slonim, a colleague who has been supervised by Billow. I have the impression that this important book is in part the product of a challenging but appreciative dialogue that has developed between them, although in this case the conversations have not taken place in an atmosphere of dire mastery (Roustang, 1976). I am reminded of my own supervisory experiences with and continuous questioning of the founders of the Group Analytic Society and the Institute of Group Analysis, who were proud to acknowledge their hybrid identities as psychoanalysts and group analysts, and were increasingly aware of the basic ideas of sociology and social psychology.

Richard and his wife Elyse maintain their very full but separate practices in Great Neck, while enjoying the cultural life of New York and other gallery and museum-laden cities, where they deepen and broaden their knowledge and collection of art. Although now retired as Director of the Adelphi Program in Group Psychotherapy, which continues to have a dynamic cohort of postdoctoral students, Richard continues to teach, supervise, lecture, and demonstrate nationally and internationally, making good use of internet technology. I would be remiss if I did not mention that the Billow family, including their growing number of grandchildren, punctuate this busy schedule of work with a fully engaged life on the mountain slopes of the world, ranging from Utah to Japan to Argentina. Richard is aware that his triumph over mogul bumps is not without its costs.

Tzachi Slonim, the editor of this new selection, was born in Tel Katzir, a kibbutz in the north of Israel. He studied philosophy and specifically the philosophy of education in Israel, where he also studied group analysis, and participated in conflict resolution work. He was a member of Courage to Refuse, an organization of soldiers who would not serve in the occupied territories. Tzachi received his PhD in clinical psychology at City University of New York (CUNY). He is influenced by the "art making" of his wife Juliana May, whose aesthetic sensibilities and compositional skills he is pleased to acknowledge. They have two children, one of six years of age and one who is one year old, born during the gestation of this book. Living in Long Island City but working in private practice with individuals, couples, and groups in Manhattan, Tzachi teaches group therapy in the Clinical Psychology Program of CUNY and the postdoctoral program at Adelphi.

I am extremely reluctant to bridge the experience of a new reader of these papers with Dr Billow's experience of writing them, Dr Slonim's experience of editing them for publication in this book, and my own experience of considering them in some depth during the past few years as a friend, colleague, and editor of the New International Library of Group Analysis (NILGA). Nonetheless, I would like to draw attention to a few aspects of the project that have particular meaning for me. There can be no doubt that Billow has himself become a bridge to the work of Bion whose contributions that illuminate the darkest recesses of our personal minds remain split-off from those that illuminate the interpersonal and group processes which give rise to them and in which they are manifest. Somehow Billow succeeds in bringing together many of these insights and ideas, often in a casual almost unassuming manner.

Another aspect of the work is that there is an unconscious or at least unintended acknowledgment of the common place, insights embedded in the everyday language of the so-called man in the street—if not in the "citizen" of the United States. These insights hold and define features of persons and their interpersonal lives which have not been conceptualized and theorized in traditional depth psychology of any kind. For example, consider the concept of attention-getting mechanisms (AGMs) and their attendant disorders as a strategy for psychic survival. This is conceptualized and illustrated in ways that the essays on narcissism by many of our colleagues have been unable to capture. After reading this chapter, I was better able to communicate with a young professional singer who was deeply distressed by her inability to stabilize her vocal register, which we understood in terms of her need to shriek in pain while at the same time to narrate her family's story.

My experience of reading and in many instances re-reading the chapters of this book is characterized by a resonance of silent assent slightly distracted by the optimistic Americanization of the psychoanalytical project, with its implicit shift from the European pessimism of envy and the recognition of the inevitable tragedies of life. How unconsciously liberating, but how seemingly a-political!

I am impressed by the editorial work of Tzachi Slonim. This selection of contributions from one of our leading scholars and practitioners of psycho-analytic group psychotherapy should be read by colleagues and students alike both in America and elsewhere. They will appreciate Billow's loyalty to our founding fathers and mothers, as well as his willingness to move beyond them. Richard Billow remains a highly productive and creative enigma who is simultaneously both conservative and radical in his thinking, fully engaged in our collective and mutual project in its most existentialist sense.

Earl Hopper
Series Editor

Reference

Roustang, F. (1976). *Dire mastery: Discipleship from Freud to Lacan*. Baltimore, MD: The Johns Hopkins University Press.

Introduction

Changing our minds

Tzachi Slonim

I first heard of Billow from my colleagues at the Eastern Group Psychotherapy Society (EGPS), with a mixture of admiration and fear of the intensity of his groups and his direct, irreverent style. I was intrigued, decided that I wanted more, and began reading his series on *Relational Group Psychotherapy* (Billow, 2003b; 2010b; 2015). The texts, and especially Billow's integration of theory and clinical work, left a deep impression on me. Could he really be thinking and feeling all of that while paying attention to his patients? I was also struck by a genuine, familial-type fondness he and his patients felt for each other. That affection, it seemed, made it possible for them to be blunt and refreshingly honest. Just as impressive, for me, was Billow's commitment to his craft, like a veteran baseball player, never fully satisfied with his swing, who watches and rewatches his at-bats in the video room and seeks input from coaches and peers. I then reached out, asking him to be my supervisor. His answer was short and inviting, and we set up an initial consultation at his office in Great Neck. I told him about my admiration for his clinical acumen and said that I was envious. Ever the Kleinian, he responded with "Why not just good old-fashioned jealousy?"[1]

In editing this volume, condensing and revising a selection of previously published analytic and group journal articles, I aim to highlight what drew me to Billow's work—a clinician-in-action openly describing his thought processes and his assessment of his actions. This is not an easy task. Orwell (2008) once wrote that "autobiography is only to be trusted when it reveals something disgraceful" (p. 210), referring to the human tendency to (mis) represent oneself in a favorable light. In that spirit, Billow's anecdotes and vignettes, which constitute the heart of this book, are crafted as closely as possible to the experiences they represent, including the therapist's humanity and flaws.

Theoretically, Billow's work is located in a unique juncture, integrating Bionian metapsychology with contemporary relational psychoanalysis, with a dual focus on individual and group psychotherapy. Billow is known for his explication and synthesis of Bion's later work and its application to the group situation. After decades during which, especially in the United States, interest in Bion's group-related ideas has dwindled,[2] Billow has shown the clinical relevance of constructs such as bonding, the desire to know and be known, the container-contained, truth-seeking and falsity, the analyst's passion, and so forth.

In contrast to the group literature, Bion's work has garnered so much attention in psychoanalysis that Ogden (2011) has termed the past few decades the "Winnicott-Bion era of psychoanalysis" (p. 929). However, most Bionian scholars do not run groups, and therefore their understanding of Bion's group-related constructs (even when he is writing about individuals) remains conceptual. For Billow, as a committed group practitioner, the group is always in the room, even before patients join one of his groups, or after they leave. His firsthand knowledge of group dynamics and the intricacies of resistance, defensive maneuvers, and transference-countertransference permutations aid him in expanding perceived notions of Relationality, in the direction that Bion (1961) anticipated when he wrote that "no individual, however isolated in time and space, should be regarded as outside a group or lacking in manifestations of group psychology" (p. 169).

In addition to expanding Relationality from a two-person model to include groups, real and imagined, Billow's brand of Relationality is unique in its emphasis on the therapist's subjectivity and fallibility, the centrality of the search for emotional meaning, the awareness of the role of mutual falsity, and the therapist's active leadership. I now present an overview of the sections and flesh out some of these ideas. In the body of the book, I include an editor's note before each section, providing further detail about Billow's ideas and approach.

Book overview

Section I: It's all about "me"

Resonating with Racker's (1968) assertion that analysts are never wholly free of infantile neurosis, Billow writes how "in each of us there is a baby, easily distressed when wrenched away from our comfort zones of attachments" (Chapter 1). While making a general claim about the human condition, Billow's intended audience is therapists. Our need to love and be loved, know and be known, is ongoing and subject to inevitable disappointments. Like others, we are susceptible to feeling rebuffed, ignored, or unfairly treated by our patients, and to consequently retaliate. To avoid such therapeutic (and everyday relational) pitfalls, we must continually tend to our not-well-enough analyzed selves. Maintaining a Bionian stance which privileges truth and meaning-making as a source of emotional nourishment, Billow suggests what I will call "inter-spection," inviting mutual exploration, learning about how others experience us, and subsequently tolerating the often-painful truths we discover about ourselves.

Drawing on Lacan (1953/1977), Billow suggests that the therapist's "Me" include a willingness to penetrate other minds with provocative, controversial ideas. Over time, this symbolically aggressive function becomes part of the dyadic or group culture and does not reside in the therapist only. One of the most thought-provoking claims Billow makes is that *everything* that goes on in a treatment is impacted by patients' shifting perspectives of their therapist's subjectivity (Chapter 3). He expands on Freud's (1921) idea that groups cohere through identification with—and internalization of—their leader's values, and the Kleinian assertion that patients' communications always include transference implications. He diverges from these classical formulations by calling attention to the therapist's *actual* behaviors and attitudes and the realistic element of patients' perceptions regarding their therapist's character.

Section II: For the love of K

The Yiddish poet Anna Margolin's (2005) analogy of the truth's bitterness as an intoxicating wine that cannot be matched captures something about the thirst for emotional honesty and the pain it often exacts. For Billow, the search for truth is not primarily carried out by the uncovering of unconscious material. Rather, the search is ongoing, as thoughts are offered, contained, and made sense of by thinkers. In line with what philosopher of science Joseph Agassi (Agassi & Meidan, 2008) calls the greatest advance in 20th-century philosophy, Billow moves away from questions like *how do I learn* and *how do I know* towards questions like *how do we learn* and *how do we know.*

Psychological, or more accurately—relational, learning occurs as basic affects are allowed to develop and reach awareness. Billow's adaptation of Bion's theory of basic affects, with its shorthand LHK, suggests that the very intensity of Love and Hate in the therapeutic relationship, coupled with the desire to Know and be Known, fosters the emergence of new ideas about self and other (Chapter 5). Basic affects, welcomed, partially understood, and harnessed, create interpersonal and intrapsychic links, and form the building blocks of psychological growth. A supportive relational context, where our love (and hate) are conveyed, makes it more likely that all therapeutic participants will contain and be contained.

I would like, at this point, to highlight what I consider to be a significant difference between Billow and other relational writers, with regard to a central relational construct—enactments. Billow does not view enactments themselves as the crux of therapeutic action (see Atlas & Aron, 2018, for a description of that point of view). Rather, he sees enactments as inevitable processes wherein less sophisticated parts of the personality are mobilized (akin to Bion's basic assumptions). Growth and change occur as individuals struggle to acknowledge both the primitive and the sophisticated to integrate the "babyish" elements with the mature, reality-focused parts of the personality. This occurs not only through surrender to inevitable transference-countertransference enactments but also by subjecting them to analytic discipline—using Love and Hate to further Knowledge (meaning)—whenever possible.

Section III: Group process: moving towards K

Unlike Bion, who practiced group psychotherapy only a very short time and gave it up because of Klein's disapproval (Ganzarian, 1989), Billow's theory and practice evince decades-long commitment to the group modality, with a preference for combining with individual treatment (Billow, 2009). As I mentioned earlier, this leads to a culture where the group therapist is personally, and explicitly, involved with each patient. Whereas Bion (1961) viewed attention to individuals in a group as a form of the therapist's unconscious apology for the group's presence, Billow argues that it serves no useful purpose (and is in fact iatrogenic) to ignore the therapist's individual relationships with group patients and the valuable emotional information these relationships offer.

The emphasis on nonjudgmentally recognizing, and at times even "gratifying," patients' dependency needs was brought into the analytic mainstream by Kohut and his followers. Billow adapts these ideas to the group setting, departing from the early Bion (1961) who viewed the group's dependency on its leader as "some emotional survival [mechanism] operating uselessly in the group as archaism" (p. 39). Instead, he builds on the later Bion's (1970) theory of the container-contained, which maintains that symbiotic bonding is the foundation that allows for language-based meaning-making to occur. It is part of the therapist's job, then, to understand and actively respond to patients' bonding needs and fantasies (Chapter 8).

Bonding supports meaning-making, which in turn strengthens bonds. Yet much more is required from the therapist to establish and maintain a dynamic, growth-producing therapeutic environment. Chapter 9 describes how the therapist listens to, organizes, and responds to clinical data to move the participants (including oneself) into new emotional terrain. Influenced, of course, by the network of associations and other data derived from the clinical discourse, Billow does not merely follow the group's (or analysand's) lead. Utilizing his own subjective experience along with theoretical understanding, he offers his point of view, even if this means disrupting or changing the ongoing process.

Section IV: Impasses and opportunities

In one of his best-known contributions, *resistance, rebellion* and *refusal* in groups: the 3 *Rs*, Billow heeds Racker's (1968) call for "social reform" in the psychoanalytic situation by revising the saturated term *resistance*, traditionally defined as "everything in the words and actions of the analysand that obstructs his gaining access to his unconscious" (Laplanche & Pontalis, 1973, p. 394). Such a definition maintains a dated view of the analyst as an objective scientist who doesn't impact the field of investigation and the patient as the only one unaware of his or her unconscious motivations. Also, it does not account for "words and actions" that may constitute legitimate challenges to the therapist's way of working, or even to his or her personal shortcomings. To address this, Billow created a rubric of three Rs: *resistance*, *rebellion*, and *refusal* (Chapter 12). Resistance in the narrower sense calls attention to dreams, enactments, and other transference-countertransference phenomena that communicate, albeit in a symbolic or partially inchoate form, aspects of one's self to the other (in Bion's terms this is analogous to the container-contained process). Rebellion is a communication meant to alter the way the therapist or group is operating, and if given a fair shake need not lead to a destructive cycle. Refusal to engage in psychological exploration may signal that certain emotional materials seem too toxic to touch without the right gloves, or by the wrong person, while others may need to be left untouched, at least for a while. Each constellation, per Billow, is not necessarily anti-therapeutic and may help clarify something about individual psychologies, as well as about the state of the therapeutic relationships.

The first element of the "social reform," which Billow writes about, then, is an expansion of the possible meanings of what were traditionally termed "resistant behaviors." The second element is the understanding that therapists are just as likely to irrupt, dissociate (Chapter 13), falsify (Chapter 14), or tightly hold on to entitlements (Chapter 15). When (not if) we are impacted by "nodules" (involving paranoid-schizoid and depressed mental states), we are likely to derail therapeutic productivity. Thus, we need to continue to grow and mature through personal therapy, supervision, self-reflection, and openness to patients' feedback, as part of the Rackerian checks and balances.

Taken together, these two elements challenge the widespread notion that groups are inherently destructive (Agazarian, 2012; Freud, 1921; Nitsun, 1996) and relatively unimpacted by the person, attitudes, and behaviors of the therapist (Bion, 1961). Instead, Billow suggests that many manifestations of basic assumptions and anti-therapeutic behavior are avoidable or easily workable if the therapist is involved, is approachable, and maintains a willingness to learn and change.

Section V: Doing our work

Adam Smith, considered by many "the father of Capitalism," introduced the term "invisible hand" to refer to an imaginary force that regulates people's self-interest and results, without much intervention, in a well-running society. Similarly optimistic views have been used to describe the group's inherent ameliorative qualities. The Foulkesian group analytic tradition, for example, recommends that therapists "trust the group," believing that "the group will ultimately know how to treat itself" (Rappoport, 2017, p. 153). Billow, in contrast, does not see the group as inherently destructive or constructive, separate from its therapist's leadership. He argues that to advance therapeutic goals, and to forestall both destructiveness and stagnation, there is always work for the therapist to do: with himself, with each member, and with the group as a whole.

Part of that work, for Billow, is to mistrust unanimous agreements, neatly resolved problems, or unruffled encounters. Led by the therapist (not always, of course), participants in the clinical encounter raise doubts, criticize, distinguish between significant and insignificant problems, and press to have influence on others (Searles, 1979). Something needs to happen, Billow declares, to challenge unhelpful rituals and the urge for repetition. Rife with multiple layers of meaning, these emotional events have the potential to change individual psychologies (including the therapist's) and the way the dyad or group members relate to each other.

Doubt, collaboration, and evidence-defying feelings

To change minds, including our own, we require reminders of our tendency to overestimate how much we know about ourselves and others. We must accept the fact that friends, patients, colleagues, and therapists are more likely to notice our blemishes (and sometimes our strengths) than we are. Billow adds that we need others not only to alert us to our distortions but also to suggest alternative narratives or to witness and validate our experiences. When therapy is going well, each participant's contribution adds to the collaborative search for meaning.

Minds, however, do not easily change. A patient of mine once lamented that "some feelings just defy evidence," a statement poignantly conveying how difficult it is to integrate other points of view even if they seem reasonable and communicated in a friendly manner. Laing (1970) called these intransigent states of mind "knots" and admired their unique "formal elegance" (Nelson, 2011). While this book does not offer a master plan for untying such knots, it does tilt us towards an optimistic view wherein new psychic and relational realities can be tested and experienced.

Its complexity notwithstanding, Billow's approach is common-sensical and down-to-earth. More often than not, his patients call him Rich, and the lack of formality is intentional. He encourages therapists to abandon attempts to present as Bionian oracles or use overly clever symbolism. Though we are always also playing a role, it is counterproductive to amp up falsity by hiding behind therapeutic anonymity or disingenuous technical schticks. Ideally, he advises, we enter each session with a measure of humility, try to relax and be present, and approach the work as a poem, a piece of art, or a dream, whose meaning may only be incompletely discovered over the course of time.

Notes

1 Klein considered envy an impulse, operating from beginning in life, that seeks to spoil and take away something that others possess. Jealousy is considered less destructive and does not necessitate a desire to spoil or take away another's possession.
2 The latest edition of Yalom and Leszcz's (2005) *The Theory and Practice of Group Psychotherapy*, often referred to as the "bible" of group therapy, for example, mentions Bion once, inaccurately, and for less than a paragraph (in a 668-page book!).

Section I

It's all about "Me"

Editor's note

Observing one of the groups he was invited to "take" by the Tavistock Clinic, Bion (1961) noticed an intense preoccupation with his personality, interpersonal skills, and fitness for leadership. This focus on the leader, he noted, was characteristic of most groups. The premise of the first section of this book is similar—regardless of the therapist's theoretical orientation, level of activity, or attitudes about disclosure (among other factors), his or her (evolving) subjectivity continues to assert influence on almost every aspect of the therapeutic encounter.

Chapter 1 is based on a paper published in a special issue of the *International Journal of Group Psychotherapy (IJGP)* on the occasion of American Group Psychotherapy Association's (AGPA's) 75th anniversary. Dr. Joseph Shay assigned group therapists of different theoretical persuasions an exaggerated group vignette where a well-trained individual therapist—but a novice group therapist—fictitiously named Pat Newland, was unable to turn a struggling group of six members into a functional one. The purpose of the assignment was to compare and contrast different models of group therapy. To emphasize the therapist's subjectivity, Billow described a disturbing dream he had following the assignment and used different dream elements to illustrate his clinical thinking. One of the elements, *a disowned baby*, conveyed a troubling truth— that like our patients, we therapists rely on "babyish," developmentally early schemas of psychic organization, to think and defend against thinking. In this chapter, Billow reports that only after he was able to symbolically *retrieve* his troubled, disowned baby was he able to complete the assignment and tend to the troubled, imaginary members of Dr. Newland's group.

The ideas for Chapter 2 were originally developed for a conference on self-disclosure and mutuality in psychoanalysis and in response to papers by Aron (1999) and Jacobs (1999). Expanding on Aron's (1999) fictitious example of a young analyst who struggles to respond to his patient's request for old magazines from his waiting area and consults three supervisors of different orientations, Billow presents a fable where the same analyst consults yet another supervisor, suggestively named Supervisor B. The fable illustrates two inconvenient truths. First, try as he or she may, the analyst/

supervisor cannot avoid self-disclosing. But, when the analyst/supervisor taps into what is personally and affectively salient, he or she is less likely to come across as a detached representative of the traumatically inaccessible parent from childhood. In Billow's fable, the supervisor was mainly interested in the fact that the analyst consulted FOUR supervisors in order to finally make the "right" decision, as if that were a possibility. This aspect of the supervisory hour (wanting to do the "right" thing) seemed rife with personal meaning for patient, analyst, and supervisor, and highlighted an important, superegoish, aspect of their relationships to each other and to themselves. Using his subjective experience, the supervisor introduced an idea for all to consider, think through, and feel.

The third chapter in this section is evocatively titled "It's all about 'Me'". Here Billow both follows and departs from Bion's way of "taking" groups. Conceptually, Billow maintains the emphasis on authority, stating that the leader's relationship with each and every member—and with the group-as-a-whole—is closely observed by the entire membership and continue to be a prerequisite for meaningful psychological work. His down-to-earth, intentionally responsive style of intervention, however, is quite different from Bion's (1961) oracular style, which emphasized the infantile desire to be led: "Either the desire for a leader is some emotional survival operating uselessly in the group as archaism, or else there is some awareness of a situation, which we have not defined, which demands the presence of such a person" (p. 39). In contrast, Billow suggests that each member legitimately seeks a special relationship with the leader.

Closing this section is a chapter that tackles the challenges of working with therapists as patients or students. While it may seem unkind or at least unintuitive to criticize our therapist patients for being too helpful or "empathic," Billow discusses why this is necessary, at least for him and his personality. Psychoanalysts are wary of the idea that human beings are, or should be, "gentle creatures who want to be loved" (Freud, 1930, p. 111). Some, like Freud, emphasize patricide as the defining desire of the male subject, while others, like Kristeva, view matricide as the *sine qua non* of our individuation (Nelson, 2011). While ever skeptical of both myths, we attempt to make sense of our aggressive impulses and incorporate them into a broader and fuller sense of self. In this chapter, Billow considers how his words, deeds, and presence help group members own these less charitable aspects of themselves and begin to be a little less "helpful."

The first four chapters introduce the reader to Billow's style through his spirited clinical examples and his often ironic and self-referential prose. His use of hyperbolic terms such as "prepostmodern" and "post dichotomous," for example, pokes fun at relational jargon to which he is also susceptible. The chapters demonstrate that the art of psychotherapy, and writing about psychotherapy, need not be narrowly utilitarian or hyper-serious and may even be, at times, poetic, aesthetically pleasing, and enjoyable.

Chapter 1

On the origin of clinical intervention

My agreeable response to Dr. Shay's invitation[1] took a sudden and unpleasurable turn in reading the clinical situation. Aversion towards the whole group: a bunch of disgruntled individuals paired with "Pat," a struggling, ineffective therapist.

All of us therapists share the fantasy that the group will do our work—or at least some of it—and it is not unreasonable to expect that group members be useful. I suspected that these (imaginary) patients were thrown together because their (imaginary) individual therapists did not know what else to do. And now, along with the (imaginary) group leader, I was thrown in with them.

Dr. Shay's exaggerated clinical example intended to make it easier. It offered us six characters in search of a leader. Too much for a novice group therapist, and too little for me to work with, and I did not want to. The catchphrase, "Why can't they just get along," rattled my thinking, and I realized that the platitude virtually echoed Dr. Newland's parting message to the group: take turns, be helpful. With only partial success, I put the group out of mind for several weeks.

And then, this disturbing dream:

> My wife and I are raising our four children.[2] My wife suggests we think about giving away the youngest, perhaps eight months old, to a young Southern family. I am surprised, but only mildly, and with some relief, arrange a drop off to their home. Their two children, who I discover are about seven and nine years old, are very excited and so happy to have a little girl plaything.
>
> About a day later I am back in New York and at a meeting of some sort. I recount the details of my recent trip to a friend or colleague. He too registers only mild surprise by the thought and now reality of giving away our baby, which surprises me, and I mull it over uncomfortably.
>
> Now I am perturbed: What were we thinking? How could we do that? After an anxious pause that in dream time felt like an hour, I resolve to

retrieve the baby. I wonder how difficult this might be legally for us, and emotionally for the disappointed family. I wake up with these questions, along with a disturbing urgency.

The dream stayed with me throughout the day, and longer. Although it was not difficult to make immediate sense, I could not put the dream away. Taking ownership of the dream made me feel ashamed for being out of touch and hurtful, in a moral stupor that I distributed to my maternally oriented wife—who better than a mate to be the target of projection?—and later to an unidentified friend.

I reminded myself to stop indulging in painful depressive ruminations, an old, apparently enjoyable tendency. I had to get on with retrieving this project and forgive myself for wishing to abandon it. Over time, thoughts began to generate; disjointed as they were, they gradually supplied sufficient confidence and mental order to concentrate and commit.

Why my self-disclosure?

My aversive responses, conscious, unconscious, and dissociated, impact my conceptualizations, and for that reason among others, they are clinically relevant. A basic premise of the relational approach is that psychoanalytic data are mutually generated by the therapeutic participants, co-determined by conscious and unconscious organizing activities, in reciprocally interacting subjective worlds (Stolorow, 1997).

All players—including imaginary ones of this clinical example—influence how we therapists think (and do not think), comport ourselves, relate to our groups, and therefore how they relate to us. It follows that the group therapist's psychology, and the members' experience of the therapist's psychology, *should* be a focal center of the therapist's clinical interest.

I have declared, somewhat facetiously and for emphasis, that it is "all about 'Me'" (see Chapter 3). Not myself, especially, of course. "Me"—the therapist's working self—functions variably and inconsistently; it is professional and yet personal, mature and immature, healthy and neurotic (Racker, 1968). And always: regulated by the emotional state of the relational matrix.

In my opinion, no therapist is a "seer," "mystic" (Bion, 1970), "analyzing instrument" (Lipin, 1992), or "telephone receiver" (Freud, 1912). The therapist's unconscious conflicts, character structure, and misunderstandings lead to inevitable iatrogenic resistances; however, they also provide vehicles for learning and transmitting intersubjective information (Boesky, 2000). Contemplating one's evolving mental relationship to the group, and its influence on the group, brings layers of meaning to the clinical situation, however conceptualized.

The dream connects me to the assignment

I had not merely put off but had attempted to wall myself off from the troublesome group. I could not think about the group in a meaningful way, or even not think about it, until I dreamed it back into conscious experience (Ogden, 2003).

What the dream revealed described a course of mental action and potential clinical behavior: resentment, isolation, and refusal, and then guilt, curiosity, and concern. The dream had purpose to reconnect me to Dr. Shay's assignment of addressing the evolution of my thinking.

> [I resolved] to retrieve the baby. I wonder how difficult this might be legally for us, and emotionally for the disappointed family. I wake up with these questions, along with a sense of disturbing urgency.

I took five elements out of the dream that I decided would direct this chapter (other elements were possible too): *a disowned baby, retrieval, legal difficulty, emotional difficulty*, and *a sense of disturbing urgency*. Without illusions of clinical precision, or need to evidence mechanisms of projective and introjective identification (which I take for granted), I assumed that these elements had or could have relevance to the predicament of Dr. Newland and the struggling group.

A disowned baby

In each of us there is a baby, easily distressed when wrenched away from our comfort zones of attachments. Whatever the benign actualities of the referral processes, in psychic reality, the members of this imaginary group felt abandoned by their individual therapists, thrust into to a strange situation, and hated—exiled from all that was or could be good. Distrustful, aggrieved, and envious, these self-centered people were alienated from themselves, from others, and from the idea and reality of group.

I had to face an aggregation of contact-shunning individuals (Hopper, 2001), each encased within a self-protective shell of refusal (Billow, 2007). The very thought of the group disturbed my equilibrium and I turned away.

I had attempted to banish the group. Dr. Pat self-vanished, hid behind the proverbial blank screen of classical individual and group technique. Allegiance to vestigial ideas of neutrality and anonymity produced an emotionally detached therapist, devoid of personality.

Dissociated, suppressed, and enacted baby thoughts and feelings—terror, anger, and hatred, as well as longing, hurt, curiosity, and joy—need to be gathered up in the here-and-now group situation and connected to ongoing process. In the lifeless group under discussion, the vitalizing baby had revealed itself only by being disowned by us all.

Retrieval

In all individuals, "two different categories of mental activity" coexist, and it is the "painful bringing together of the primitive and the sophisticated that is the essence of the developmental conflict" (Bion, 1961, pp. 159, 172).

All individuals and all groups rely on primitive—meaning developmentally early—preverbal schemas of psychic organization to think, communicate, and group, and to defend against these processes. To function with "sophistication," that is, with clinical intuition, empathy, and accuracy, the therapist must embrace the "developmental conflict" and eradicate as much as one can, not anxieties, resistances, wishes, and fears, but their repression (Racker, 1968). The developmental conflict—to remain a baby or to *also* be mature—cannot be banished or hidden from. We rely on others to help us think about what we cannot bear alone.

Freud (1921) concluded that we are "horde animals," for no matter the protestation, individuals seek groups, and groups seek leaders. We are inherently groupish. The pull to group is irresistible, and pulling away leaves one that much more socially preoccupied, although unsatisfactorily. Shunning the group, I succeeded in joining it, only after my "baby" reemerged.

Legal difficulty

The therapist has access to legitimate and illegitimate modes of leadership. The illegitimate may hide under a stiff rubric of "correct" technique (Jacobs, 2001), while the legitimate extends to the unconventional, to humor, linguistic play, affective openness, challenge, and confrontation.

To preserve a well-working group, or attend to the difficulties of this ineffective one, the leader wears "two faces," being constructive and deconstructive (Billow, 2005). To establish trust and secure relationships, the therapist defines boundaries of participation, addresses the needs of each person, and closely monitors and often directs group process. However, he or she must also challenge characterological boundaries, falsities, and social collusions that obstruct or preclude emotional learning. Without such leadership, a group—whether in formation or ongoing—is more likely to be marked by conventionality, stalemate, and submission to and rebellion against authority.

Ideally, what the therapist says, and how it is said, should represent personal risk and open the way for mutual discovery. In a relatively new group with an unfamiliar therapist, the members may not immediately understand the intended meanings of some of the leader's interventions, but the discourse goals must be perceived as ethical: caring and helpful. Incongruities and discontinuities should be interesting, relevant, and sufficiently safe to be enjoyable and stimulate curiosity.

Emotional difficulty

Retrieval entails painful loss (to the split off Southern self) and gain (an integrated "United States"). What an individual discovers and the group reveals may feel "not nice," judged as immature and irrational (which is, indeed, what it often is), socially inappropriate and personally embarrassing.

Therapy is an act of symbolic aggression, interfering, challenging, and undermining beliefs, values, and relationships, and even a sense of self. Therefore, individuals remain in conflict over developing emotional truth, since it causes anxiety and pain. All group members (including the therapist) struggle with a limited ability and willingness to pursue the infinite potentials of the meaning-making process. We tend to wall off that which is unpleasant, unknown, or confusing.

Dr. Shay presented us with a difficult group situation— troubled patients "expelled" or "exported" from their individual therapies, "aliens" in a "new land" of group therapy with an unskilled therapist. However, no matter the group and the sophistication of the leader, the self of the therapist also remains troubled[3] and must be attended to before, during, and after interventions are made to others.

A sense of disturbing urgency

Experience does not roll out smoothly. Each paper (and each group) needs time and mental freedom to unfold. However, papers do not write themselves nor do groups flourish without active, ongoing leadership. A group in early stages of formation has urgent purpose. While a group comes together and depends on combinations of emotional linkages, member-therapist bonds usually are primary. Member-member and member-entire group bonds follow.

Early on, but in all stages of group life, the group therapist needs to pursue that which is painfully immediate and most meaningful. At the same time, he or she must shield others from that which is immediate, but too painful to become meaningful. In situations of high stress and aggressive charge, such as this group, the therapist must function as a lightning rod, diverting unbearable affects and antagonisms away from the group and towards him- or herself, providing the ground for safety—easing angry and alienated members back into their own functional minds.

The variety and flexibility of the therapist's activity, internal and interpersonal, exposes the qualities of the therapist's care and establishes the therapist's authenticity. Through his or her behavior, the leader or therapist defines the working group culture: how group relationships and experiences are to be regarded and the depth to which narratives and exchanges may be considered.

I present an alternative reality to illustrate urgent responsiveness.

Relationally revising the group interaction[4]

THERAPIST: Hello. Anyone want to begin today?

ANGELA: Why can't you just let us start the way we want to start? We'll begin if we want to begin.

THERAPIST (UNPERTURBED AND AMUSED): Well, Angela has begun!

DIANNE: I'm happy to begin.

THERAPIST: Whoa…. no reaction to Angela? She's begun, and not so happily.

DIANE [IGNORING THERAPIST]: This weekend, I didn't want to work on my dissertation so I went to a party and had too much to drink.

THERAPIST [EVENTUALLY BREAKING]: Don't we have dissertation work to do right here? You [Diane] don't want to do it!

DIANNE [IGNORING THE METAPHORIC PLAY]: I was talking about *my* dissertation and going off with this guy and I wound up in a lot of trouble.

THERAPIST [SHADING THE MEANING OF "TROUBLE"]: That's why I want you to slow down and stay focused on your work here, so you won't be so troubled.

DIANNE: Well I am feeling "troubled" by you, just like being controlled by the dissertation committee, who I hate! But I think you are trying to help me to take control.

ANGELA: Well, I don't like it. It's like before when you asked us to begin.
Therapist responds with wordless agreement, as if to say I understand what you don't like and how you feel.

DIANNE: Don't you see Pat is trying to help you too. You're always criticizing Pat.

ANGELA: You're always defending Pat.

ANOTHER: How does that help to get Angela angry at Dr. Pat? Or Dianne? I'm confused.

BETTY: There is a lot of arguing in here and I'm not sure what the purpose is.

THERAPIST: Are you angry at me too, Betty?

BETTY: No, I just don't think I'm getting anything out of this group.

THERAPIST: That sounds like anger. You are saying, "I don't agree with how you play and I am going to take my marbles and go home." Even though it is pretty lonely at home. The purpose here is to learn about how you feel and how others feel about you.

BETTY: Well, I'm annoyed at you.

THERAPIST (BIG SMILE): I like that a lot better!

NED (TO DR. PAT): I like how you are standing up to criticism. I was able to get back to working on my novel because I stopped worrying about the criticism the readers had made of my writing.

ANGELA: I wish I could let criticism roll off my back.

WILL: You said it!

DIANE: What do you mean, Will?

WILL: I'll pass, but thanks.

OTTO: Criticism is very hard for me too.

NED: Not for me. People who criticize are often just jealous so I'm not going to let it get to me.

THERAPIST: Mmm. Is Ned talking about us? Are we a jealous group?

Silence; the group seems mystified.

Several members move to other subjects, which Dr. Pat soon connects to "Ned's idea of jealousy."

Members pick up the ideational thread. Like Ned, they focus on being the target of jealousy, freely dispersing criticism and blame to outside forces.

THERAPIST (*WITH IRONIC EXAGGERATION*): So much comfort with anger and frustration! A good way to express your own jealousy!

The session is ending—no opportunity to further contextualize jealousy within the group. The members had gone deeper in their exploration of psychic reality and that had satisfied the therapist. A nuclear idea had emerged, a unifying theme with personal resonance (Billow, 2016). Even for the leader who realized that jealousy of "better" groups and experienced group leaders had contributed to the therapist's disaffection. Dr. Pat felt gratitude towards Ned and the whole group for this disinhibiting insight, which would be useful in future sessions.

Conclusion

No one said that running groups is easy, or that it should be. To organize a group and make it transformative, the leader must be both "woman" enough to establish preverbal bonding and "man" enough to enter in and fascinate with language (Billow, 2013a; Harper & Rowan, 1999; Lacan, 1977/1953).

An essential aspect of the professional/personal "Me" involves, then, existing in one's own mind as a complex, procreative partner to each person (and to the group-family) and exposing this self in words and behavior. If the leader feels or is "de-skilled" by the group, he or she is effectively neutered or castrated and cannot successfully carry out the dual symbolic role.

I used my own experience in responding to Dr. Shay's assignment to illustrate key relational principles. The first is the emphasis on intersubjectivity, that is, on relationships, internal and external, and their dynamic, life-supporting qualities. The second is a rejection of the classical model of the healthy analyst and neurotic patient or group. Those we treat and we ourselves have transferences and other perplexing, often unconsciously motivated emotional and cognitive responses. Therapeutic relationships are reconceived in terms of co-constructed or mutually inspired interactions that are worthy of understanding rather than evaluated in terms of pathology.

Third, psychoanalytic purification (Freud, 1912), resulting in ideal equanimity, detachment, and clinical objectivity, is an impossibility. Moreover, such a posture constrains us from accessing and creatively utilizing our own subjective experience in connecting to others. Rather than aiming at a false "professional" stance, we need to possess and convey a warm, human presence.

Finally, as therapists, we are subject to compelling social forces, remain embedded in them, and enter group representing deeply rooted identifications, perspectives, and reality beliefs based on ethnic, national, and political affiliations, economic status, gender, sexual orientation, race, age, and so forth.

I suspect that all theories, formulations, and case presentations, such as my imaginative revision, are in some ways retrofitted or aligned to the personality of the formularizer. Therapists of all persuasions bring foundational concepts to clinical work, which provides structure and direction—shifting mindsets that lead to certain paths and potentialities but may foreclose others. Ideally, we allow ourselves passage to other places by other thinkers, particularly by our group members. If the therapist is emotionally open and creative, new mental pathways may be tested.

Notes

1 Dr. Shay's (2017) invitation to illustrate Billow's approach to group therapy is further described in the editor's note to Section I.
2 In actuality, we have three adult children. I gave birth to a fourth child because apparently, even in a dream, I could not bear to part with one of our own. Likely, too, the child was the assignment itself.
3 The analyst's "internal and external dependencies, anxieties, and pathological defenses...[respond] to every event of the analytic situation" (Racker, 1968, p. 132).
4 The original group vignette can be found in Shay (2017).

Chapter 2

Self-disclosure and psychoanalytic meaning

Feeling helpless and cutoff from a patient, the analyst Jacobs (1993) disclosed something of his emotional experience:

> I told Mr. D that I thought I knew from my own feelings of the moment what, as a child, he must have experienced trying to make contact with a father who was utterly unreachable. I said that when he went into one of his periods of withdrawal, as he was doing now, I felt myself completely cut off from him, as though a wall of iron had come between us... He had become, I said, the father sitting in darkness, the father who, in his hurt and anger, shut out the world.
>
> (p. 244)

Jacobs (1993) found that

> this new way of speaking, intense and personal, in turn, had a powerful effect on Mr. D. ... Somehow my words pierced that shell. Altering his defenses, they worked on my patient in a way that scores of interpretations similar in content had not.
>
> (p. 20)

The patient also acknowledged the success of Jacobs's communication: "I heard what you've said before, but you seemed to be speaking words—something abstract and analytic, not felt and genuine" (p. 19).

So often when we speak, our listeners hear only words, which do not accomplish their purpose of establishing meaning. Our intervention seems correct and our timing in synch, yet the patient is left untouched. We may justify our technique by concluding that the patient is too resistant. However, it is possible that we fail to convey sufficient emotion to the patient. It is likely that all analysts unintentionally function at times like the traumatizing father in the case example. Our words, rather than making contact, make patients feel that we are utterly unreachable. We then attempt to address this situation, most often by using words.

In forgoing protective anonymity (Renik, 1995) and revealing authentic pain, Jacobs also personified aspects of the patient's complex identifications. Jacobs's words metaphorically equated him to the patient-immersed-in-pain. In his verbal action (Greenberg, 1996), Jacobs symbolically enacted the wished-for father-analyst responding with sorrow and understanding for the pain he had caused and now must repair.

A number of contemporary psychoanalysts have concluded that by embracing a technique of self-disclosure, the patient may feel the analyst's emotion, without which an authentic analysis is impossible. To illustrate certain complexities and ironies relating to the topic, I present a fable in which a young analytic candidate encounters a self-disclosing supervisor. I then consider the relationship of self-disclosure to language, to growth of the analytic participants, and to "truth."

Emotional co-participation and "inner experience": a psychoanalytic fable

To illustrate the beneficial effects of awareness of subjectivity on theory and clinical choice, Aron (1999) presented an imaginary exercise in which he took a male analyst, "A," to three different supervisors. The analyst had a specific problem: his female patient requested some of the accumulated, out-of-date magazines from his waiting room to utilize in her work as a teacher of disabled children. The three supervisors had different theoretical orientations and several styles of supervision as well. Supervisors X and Y were classically Freudian and self-psychologically oriented, respectively, and gave conflicting advice. However, they were both patient-centered in their supervisory approach and maintained a didactic, explanatory style with the supervisee. Supervisor X suggested that the patient was acting out in the transference, seeking symbolic gifts from her analyst/father. He recommended not to accede to the request but to analyze its meaning in terms of the immediate context of the analysis. Supervisor Y made the opposite recommendation. The supervisor felt that in acceding to the request for the magazines the analyst would be gratifying a legitimate need for a therapeutic object relationship.

Supervisor Z was interested in understanding the relational matrix rather than promulgating any particular theory. In further contrast to the other supervisors, Supervisor Z was therapist-centered, not patient-centered. Supervisor Z did not give specific advice regarding the request for magazines. Rather, following the Socratic method, Supervisor Z investigated the subjectivity of Analyst A in relationship to A's theories and to his clinical choices. For example, Supervisor Z asked how Analyst A felt about giving and receiving gifts. What would it be like for him to say no to the patient or to say yes? Would A have made a similar request of his analyst, and how would the analyst have responded? Through Supervisor Z's sensitive yet persistent questioning, Analyst A became aware of subjective experiences that influenced his theory and technique.

I thought it would be interesting to extend Aron's exercise and consider how the process might work with a supervisor who shared as well as encouraged emotional participation in the supervisory exchange. An intentionally self-revealing supervisor may bring to the fore aspects of the supervisee's experience not necessarily available through a didactic or Socratic method. The hypothesis, of course, is that expanding the supervisee's experience—and awareness of the experience—with the supervisor may provide a salutary domino effect on the supervisee's relationship with the patient.

I now depart from the usual discursive format to present a fable. I take the reader on a brief imaginative excursion to the "inner experiences" of a supervisory dyad. I bring Aron's Analyst A to still another supervisor; let us call him Supervisor B. We journey into the mutually regulating subjectivities of Analyst A and Supervisor B. Joining them somewhere in the middle of the initial consultation, we first follow Analyst A's interior monologue.

Inner experiences of Analyst A

Supervisor B seems fascinated that I have now consulted four supervisors. He seems more fascinated with this knowledge than with my case. He hasn't seemed particularly interested in the patient or in her request for the magazines. I finally asked him forthrightly what he thought of the conflicting recommendations of Supervisors X and Y. I also shared my countertransference realizations discovered with Supervisor Z. Supervisor B said he thought everything the other supervisors said made good sense and that I seemed to have learned a lot.

An uncomfortable silence ensued, which I attempted to end by agreeing with him. I said that with all the good supervision from our institute, I indeed could make sense of what the patient's request for the magazines might mean for her and for me. But, I continued encouragingly, I was sure Dr. B would have something interesting to say too.

I was kind of anxious, but I think Supervisor B got irritated. He said because I thought the issue of the magazines was so important, pursue the issue with her, but realize that the pursuit—or lack of pursuit—reveals something about who I am and what I am interested in. My verbal activity might be as important in her experience as my clarifications, interpretations, provision, or deprivation of the magazines.

I suddenly realized that I was not really sure if, and why, the patient's request for the magazines was important to me, even though, after all my supervision, I understood that the magazines had many meanings to the patient and to me! Maybe it wasn't important to me, but should be important because the patient, whether she knew it or not, had challenged the analytic frame. I was proud of myself for not having acted out my anxiety and confusion with the patient. I had followed the analytic dictum "When in doubt, shut up." I said to Supervisor B that it was a good thing, then, that I had preserved my neutrality and didn't impinge on the patient's transitional space. Supervisor B said that my "quote neutrality"—not answering the question the patient asked but waiting for a post-supervisory session—may have as much of an impinging effect as anything else. That stung and I defended myself. I told Supervisor B what I had said to the patient:

> You know, your request for the magazines may seem casual and without much meaning, but everything that takes place here has meaning, meaning that sometimes emerges as we leave time for reflection. Let us take some time and come back to your question in another session if you wish.

Supervisor B said that my response was skillful, sensitive, and empathic. He said I sounded just like a real analyst. That was nice to hear. So why wasn't I feeling any better? Something in his answer didn't seem sincere. Was he putting me on? I wasn't going to take it from him. I said, most diplomatically, for I'm still in analytic training and have to watch myself,

> I like what you are saying to me, that I was empathic and all, but maybe it is the way you say it, or maybe I'm getting paranoid from all these supervisors, but I don't think you really mean what you said about my response being so good.

Supervisor B said he didn't think I really meant what *I* said to the patient. I was not authentic, just analytic, and he didn't say my response was *good*, just that it was skillful, sensitive, and empathic. Just! What does he want from me? Supervisor B realized from my expression that I was not pleased. He said that by now I realized that *he* wasn't that skillful, sensitive, and empathic. He said that maybe being skillful, sensitive, and empathic isn't the whole story. Maybe the patient felt that my response was skillful, sensitive, and empathic, but that she felt perplexed and angry anyway. For now, she was deprived of the magazines, deprived of the answer to her question as to whether or not she could have them, and deprived of understanding what the analyst *really* was saying, meaning, and feeling. Perhaps he thought she was bad, bad for asking, bad for being spontaneous, and bad for not free-associating. Perhaps he was mad, and did not like her anymore, and was hiding behind his analytic words. Supervisor B suggested that the patient may have a difficult time telling me about her feelings because I am so skillful, sensitive, and empathic. What I referred to as "holding," he called my "Trojan horse gift of 'space.'" According to him, if I did not confuse and mystify the patient, or make her feel bad, scared, and mad, I might have done something even worse.

I might have made the patient P feel soothed, grateful, indebted, obligated, and too guilty even to think about her true feelings. The patient may be developing a theory that she also should be skillful, sensitive, and empathic. Then we both would be "analytic." We would not, however, be talking about what we both felt was emotionally meaningful.

Now *I* was really perplexed and angry. "Can't I do anything right?" I said. B seemed to enjoy my question and responded by saying, "No, I couldn't do anything right." Whatever I do or don't do reveals something about me, and I can't be sure what I'm really feeling and really meaning when I do it; furthermore, the patient may interpret something very different from what I intended. If I give her the magazines, I am enacting something; if I don't give her the magazines, I am enacting something; if I suggest that we wait and discuss things further, I am enacting something. Everything I do and do not do may have many emotional meanings for me and for the patient, and these meanings may not begin to reveal themselves to us until I do what I do and the patient does what she does. And once we began to discuss the possible meanings, the open-ended discussion itself may be particularly meaningful.

Supervisor B said that both the patient and I wanted to be "right." After all, the patient had a similar question. She asked if it was "all right" to take the magazines. Supervisor B suggested that there might be some "parallel process" (Gediman & Wolkenfeld, 1980) going on such that the patient wanted me to assure her that she was doing something right, and that I wanted reassurance that I was doing something right.

B suggested that he did not want to give me assurance. He said that he and I enacted different theories with each other and were in conflict. He said I had a theory of right *versus* wrong. He had the postmodern, post-dichotomous, relational theory of right *and* wrong: there is little that we do that is "all right," but not being all right does not necessarily make us all wrong, either. If I understand this theory correctly, being all right is all wrong, because this makes me the "one who knows," the arbiter of reality (Levenson, 1996, p. 242). Being wrong is right. My anxious, stumbling, "irrational, emotional involvement" may contribute to a successful clinical psychoanalysis (Renik, 1996, p. 392). Supervisor B wondered if the patient also had an unenlightened, prepostmodern theory, that her theory of right *or* wrong might be an important dimension in her suffering. When Supervisor B observed that his theory of right *and* wrong was making me suffer during the supervisory hour, I had to acknowledge that there is something painful in his approach. Is B a relationalist? According to what I read (Aron, 1996), relationalists follow the principle of sharing their thinking and self-disclosing aspects of their subjectivity. I think he is doing that, at least. He likes me but sort of hates me, too. I guess it is equally obvious that I have such feelings towards him.

I thought I knew who I was and what I was doing after Supervisors X, Y, and Z, but now I'm not sure of what I think or what I feel. What really is meaningful to me emotionally? Maybe this is a good thing not to be sure. Maybe this is a good and bad thing. Uh-oh, I'm beginning to sound like him.

We leave Analyst A in this questionable state of affairs and move now to the interior monologue of Supervisor B.

Inner experiences of Supervisor B

All along, during this supervisory hour, Supervisor B was flooded with thoughts, feelings, and memories. How foolish to think that it could ever be otherwise. Could an analyst be completely free of painful and pleasant personal associations relating to the past, present, and future (Jacobs, 1993)? If the analyst were to function in a manner resembling Freud's (1912) telephone receiver metaphor, the analyst would be listening on a party line. So many voices interfering with clear reception, all talking at once: parents, significant others, analysts, supervisors, good and bad objects of all sorts.

Supervisor B was listening to these voices as he was listening to Analyst A. He felt cared for and caring, but also annoyed and impatient. The disparate inner and outer events of the supervisory hour pulled together into a moment of what James Joyce called an "epiphany," and Bion called the "selected fact." B realized that all these voices had similar, comforting, yet also irritating messages. Some voices told him he *better* behave, and others told him *how* to better behave. This was the issue the patient had presented to Analyst A: Was it "all right" for her to behave in a certain way? How should *he* behave? was the question Analyst A brought to his four supervisors. B considered how he was behaving. Not very well. He was dominating the supervisee. Perhaps Analyst A wished to be dominated, and his patient wanted domination as well. The patient asked Analyst A to dominate, and Analyst A asked Supervisors X, Y, Z, and B. Who was regulating whom, the sadist or the masochist?

Supervisor B thought he liked this Analyst A and the patient. But he did not like their dominating superegos. Perhaps a battle of control was being waged within each of the participants, as well as between them. Supervisor B enacted the currently dissociated aspects of the supervisee and the patient that rebelled against the mythic "patriarchical order of the superego" (Racker, 1968, p. 132). The patient and Analyst A submitted to it and attempted also to create a patriarch in an other: the patient in her analyst, A in his supervisors. Who was going to be king? A manic rebelling ego as represented by Supervisor B, or a persecuting, conforming superego as represented by the patient and Analyst A?

Supervisor B became concerned for Analyst A, and for himself as well. He experienced that particularly Kleinian form of compassion related to productive guilt and depression. He worried about his own behavior, which he now recognized had aspects of unresolved adolescent and preadolescent rebelliousness. He questioned whether Analyst A received something good from B's not entirely tongue-in-cheek deconstruction of A's "analytic attitude." Supervisor B then realized how much he, himself, was like the patient and Analyst A. He, too, expressed aspects of the superego myth of being "all right."

We leave Supervisor B in the privacy of his self-analysis and return to further consideration of self-disclosure in relationship to the analyst's language and opportunity to promulgate mutual growth.

Language, self-disclosure, and mutual growth

The above fable suggests that self-disclosure may foster emotional meaning and lead to growth and change. Ogden (1997) recently described a number of qualities of the analyst's use of words relevant to this purpose. He recommended that the analyst strive to maintain a tension between using language in a "crisp and clarifying manner" and aspire to a "particular form of evocative, sometimes maddening, almost always disturbing, vagueness." (p. 11). By "vagueness," I understand Ogden to suggest that the analyst's communications need to call attention to their quality of being symbolic and multileveled. Thus, he wrote that "it is essential that the analyst's language embody the tension of forever being in the process of struggling to generate meaning while at every step casting doubt on the meanings 'arrived at' or 'clarified'" (p. 12).

Ogden does not, however, concentrate specifically on countertransference or the analyst's emotional experience, including subjective responses to his or her own communications. In my opinion, the analyst's words—their form as well as content—must be evocative personally as well as to the patient or supervisee. In extending Aron's (1999) fictitious example, I tried to illustrate how the clinician may utilize language "to upset (unsettle, decenter, disturb, perturb) the given" (Ogden, 1997, p. 12).

If the analyst/supervisor is a "surgeon" (Freud, 1912), he or she operates with dirty hands. I am borrowing Sartre's metaphor to suggest that, no matter how well analyzed, we remain "guilty" for not being "objective," for being unaware of many levels of symbolic meaning and intent. Supervisor B, in verbally committing himself to his own emotional experience, disturbed his own "givens" along with Analyst A's. Nothing in the exchange or in the interior monologues resolved in being "all right." Both parties left the supervisory interaction with unresolved feelings and thoughts that necessitated productive working-over in their conscious and unconscious inner lives. Each continued private dialogue with the other.

Conclusion: self-disclosure and "truth"

I wrote a paper (Billow, 1997) in which I presented case material involving a supervisee and her patients, the supervisee and her supervisor, and the parallel processes between clinical situations. I gave the supervisee a draft of the

paper. She reported positive feelings, but also anger. "Was I creating a doc-
ument or a docudrama?" she asked. She was referring to that low art form
that is neither documentary nor drama, neither truth nor fiction. "My patient
did not say that," she complained regarding one exchange I had detailed. Referring to another: "You got that patient down right, but not my part." She
insisted that some of the comments I reported making to her in supervision
I had not in fact made. Maybe I thought I made them, but I did not, and of
some of the comments I had made, she claimed I did not say them nearly as
well as I did on the written page. Why can't I be as clear when I am with her!
Finally, she commented that in supervision I always seem so sure of myself,
I do not seem to be uptight about patients or about issues that arise between
us in supervision. But in the paper, I share my doubts and insecurities. Who
is the real me, how honest am I with her, how do I really work in therapy?

I should clarify that her anger was in the context of a friendly relationship in which we both felt safe to express a variety of feelings towards each
other and our work. I appreciated her remarks, not the least for dramatically demonstrating to me the distance that may exist between the clinician's
beliefs about the emotional meaning revealed in his or her self-disclosures
and the patient's or supervisee's experience.

Where is fact, where is fable? Bion (1974) spoke to this issue when he wrote,
in evaluating presentations by other analysts:

> You are not obliged to say whether you regard the scientific papers as
> works of fiction or not. But you can form some opinion of the kind of
> fiction that those particular analysts write, or the kind of reality which
> they describe.
>
> (p. 185)

My self-disclosures give some idea of how I think and feel, how I think
I think and feel, and how I would like others to believe I think and feel.
Perhaps we need to put a "Surgeon General's Warning" on all clinical con-
tributions, certainly not just those intending self-disclosure:

> The analyst's communications contain aspects of infantile as well as
> dissociated inner experience. Gross commissions and omissions are
> to be expected, involving conscious and unconsciousness censorship,
> relating to the analyst's emotional, cognitive, and psycho-linguistic
> limitations, shame and guilt, fear of embarrassment, humiliation and
> ostracism, fear of the unknown, and fear of loss of livelihood. In clinical
> reports, any similarity to persons living or dead depends on the narra-
> tive talents of the analyst and the imaginative talents of the receiver.
> Your construction of meaning may be unstable, subject to further pro-
> cessing by waking and dream thoughts, and deleterious to the health of
> preformed opinions.

The analyst's communications, then, reveal evolving emotional experience, including emotional resistance to emotional experience (Bion, 1977). At their best, the analyst's words convey what Ezra Pound defined as the successful poetic image: "That which presents an intellectual and emotional complex in an instant of time" (cited in Wellek & Warren, 1956, p. 18). By "image," Pound did not mean specifically a pictorial representation, but a potent verbal formulation which evokes an emotionally meaningful response. Thus, self-disclosure—intentional or otherwise—may be understood as an evocation of the analyst's intellectual and emotional experience in an instant of time. It is not, of course, the complex experience itself. Nor is it the only experience the analyst is having. As with any human communication, truth remains ambiguous, meaning incomplete and evolving; its success is limited.

Chapter 3

It's all about "Me"

When I declare "It's all about 'Me'," I am asserting two broad principles:

1   Every intervention the therapist makes (including silence) is filtered through his or her subjectivity, of which the therapist has imperfect knowledge. Given the leader's importance to what occurs and does not occur in the group, the therapist needs to keep a "third ear" acutely attuned to "Me."

    And then, there is the old joke: "Well, enough of 'Me'. Let's hear about you. What do *you* think of me?" We have limited access to our unconscious, our character, and our reactivity, so we need to hear about "Me" from other group members. The members respond directly and indirectly, through what they say and do not say, via symbolic derivatives (metaphors, dreams, jokes, scapegoating, basic assumptions), and by participating in individual, subgroup, and group resistances, rebellions, and refusals (see Chapter 12 for an elaboration of the "three Rs").

2   The members' shifting perceptions of who the therapist is impact everything that takes place in group. We have just met as reader and writer. Although existing in different time and space, we are linked in a relationship, defined in part by our mutual "desire to know" (Bion, 1970), and reconfigured as you confront "Me."

I illustrate the above principles by providing a clinical example of it not working the way I believed and wanted, until the group's interventions. Something about "Me" emerged unexpected; it occurred in the course of a day's conference I offered during an annual American Group Psychotherapy Association (AGPA) meeting.

Clinical example: talkers and non-talkers

I asked the attendees—about 30—how they would like to spend the day and what they wanted to accomplish. This process allowed me to present myself, make eye-to-eye contact with each individual, and for the whole group to bear witness to the ideas presented. Not everyone took the opportunity to talk, of course, but there was general agreement that I would present some didactic material that would address some of the members' questions and interests, do a "fishbowl" demonstration group in the morning, spend the afternoon conducting a full-group process experience, and end with a return to concepts and a debriefing.

The morning's interactions confirmed my impression that this was a lively, interactive group with some large personalities dispersed through the wide range in age and clinical training. But as we resumed after lunch, I realized that some of the attendees had spoken minimally or not at all. I had tried to involve them, such as inviting participation with a welcoming smile, picking up on body language, and "bridging" (Ormont, 1992) by having one member "translate" another's feelings about a third member's feelings.

Now I addressed their lack of verbal participation specifically: "You will get more from this afternoon's meeting if you say something. Even one comment gives you a new sense of the group." The room remained quiet. Then I said, "It's okay even if you grunt or groan." My humorous intervention met with some success.

"I've been wanting to talk, but I've been afraid. Thanks for noticing." The member then filled in some biographical data, as did several others who followed. Some of the active members made appreciative and encouraging gestures, but the process ran out of emotional steam, and the group turned to other interactions.

Still, I felt dissatisfied and curious, and near midpoint in the afternoon I said, "There seem to be two groups here—the talkers and the nontalkers." That drew the group's eyes to the verbally nonparticipating and then I felt anxious about scapegoating them by applying peer pressure.

Someone came forward: "In my family, I was always very quiet. At home, I let my mother speak for me until I left for college."

"Who reminds you of your mother?" I asked. My purpose was to encourage more individual participation and member-to-member involvement and also to introduce transference analysis and intrapsychic exploration in the group setting.

"I don't know… maybe anybody who dared to speak."

I had found a useful angle to extend participation: who reminded someone of whom and why, and how did it feel. I was feeling relaxed and successful, until an attendee broached what seemed like a change of direction: "If I were running this group, I'd want to know what I did to cause the 'two groups'".

I felt embarrassed, as if accused of not practicing what I preach about considering the impact of "Me," but the comment was delivered respectfully and I answered in the same way.

"What do you think I did to cause subgrouping?"

"You like people who talk."

Several members came to my rescue: "Well, he was faced with a new group, of course he wanted people to talk." "He tried to bring people in, he's doing it now, [and to the person who posed the challenge], you tried too."

But I thought the comment deserved a fuller consideration and, in thinking about it, I felt inspiration in the question I had posed a few moments earlier: the topic of family relations and intragroup transferences. I shared an insight that felt sudden and intense: "Well, I was the first born in my family, and I maintained my position by doing a lot of talking."

In conducting groups, I do not make a habit of intentionally self-revealing, but here saw no reason to be evasive. Now other people—including some of the formerly quiet—pressed to talk, and I kept further introspections to myself. "This is my first workshop as a member. I did not know what to expect. I never heard of you but I liked the topic [the '3 Rs']. Since I'm going to start working with drug addicts next month, I thought I better learn about refusing. I'm learning a lot anyway. Am I resisting, rebelling, or refusing? I don't know yet."

"I'm here because my professor is here, and [humorously] she threatened to flunk us if we didn't come. She didn't say we had to 'talk'. Yes, me too, we read your papers in her class. They were real good, although I can't say I understood them or this group [laughter]."

I reflected that it takes courage for the students and teachers to mix it up in this group setting, with expanded boundaries and rules of exchange.

A woman spoke up: "I must come out of the closet. I'm the 'mean' teacher. I've been so impressed by your writings, Dr. Billow, that I guess I feel intimidated." I lightened the atmosphere by saying that other people must be a lot less impressed because they seem comfortable calling me "Richard" and challenging me to think about what I've been doing.

More people took chances with themselves in reflecting on the "two groups":

"I was the 'golden boy' in my family. Talking, but not talking too much. I want to be the golden boy in your group. Just me. [humorously] Am I being it now?"

"I was the second fiddle. I feel like that here, and that's why I haven't revealed myself. I have to think about my responsibility. You welcomed me, several times."

"I was my parents' 'joy', their 'ray of sunshine'. [and with irony] See how I always smile and am seen and not heard."

A young man volunteered: "Maybe I've been Cinderella here, waiting to be invited to the ball. I need to man up, I got my own balls."

We turned to the professor self-described as "mean," who seemed to be crying: "In my family, I was the oldest, and my job was to take care of my siblings, as they arrived, one by one. But I liked it. My parents weren't close,

I was afraid of my father and my mother wasn't very warm either. I wanted to have my students here. [turning to them] I felt you would make me feel safe and secure. Thanks for coming ... You all get an 'A'," she said, smiling between visible tears.

One of the members who had tried to shield me from criticism joined in: "I had to protect my mother. She has 'issues' and gets depressed. When you blamed Richard for creating the 'two groups', I worried that he would fall apart. I'm always worried that my patients are going to fall apart, and then my psychotherapy group that I run. I see that not happening here."

With some sadness, we drew the group process to a close. During the debriefing and evaluation, one of the members complimented me for the day, but wondered: "Could you have gotten the same results if you had stayed out ... and not worked so hard?"

Discussion

"Me": a fratricidal leader

> Cain said to his brother Abel, "Let's go out to the field." And while they were in the field, Cain attacked his brother Abel and killed him.
>
> (Genesis 4: 8)

> It snowed last year too: I made a snowman and my brother knocked it down and I knocked my brother down and then we had tea.
>
> (Thomas, 1954, p. 12)

To illustrate the effect of intersubjective factors on group formation and process, I share some personal thoughts. Freud (1921, pp. 120–121) traced the development of our inclination to group (gregariousness) to the reaction against the initial envy and aggression an older child experiences to the arrival of a younger sibling—who now is a rival for the leader's (i.e., the father's) attention. Whereas this hypothesis does not seem universally applicable, it may partially explain my own interest in groups and my style of leadership.

I could easily justify my technical approach to the silent members: after all, people unfold at different times, and not always verbally. And besides, some of them had asked questions at the workshop's beginning—and I kept in mind and addressed the questions throughout the morning. But I came to realize that projection, envy, rivalry, guilt, and reparation were among the emotional elements I utilized—for better and worse—in conducting the workshop.

As we know, silent members and subgroups exert power, and may even hold a group hostage (Billow, 2012), demanding special attention by their very quietness. In terms of my psychology, of which I was not conscious at the time, such individuals represented my younger brother.

I felt envious of the attention he received, and interested in him too. His emotional unavailability was irritating and intriguing, and both stimulated and frustrated my curiosity. I provoked him to respond, teasing, wrestling, and socking him when necessary, which was often.

In my reflective, adult consciousness, I know (and probably knew as a child) that he wished to isolate himself from any unpleasant intensity of our family. Selective withdrawal seemed to be beyond my emotional capabilities. In my ongoing unconsciousness, he was (and is) a rivalrous model of a "better" type of individual, self-contained and without need.

In the group, the quiet members entered my unconsciousness as rivals too, competing with the talkative ones, which included me, for my attention (as father–leader) and for the group's attention (my "parents").

I could easily express curiosity, fight, and embrace the talkative ones. Whether they were friendly or hostile, I knew who they were, and I "liked" them. In terms of infantile narcissism, they were reflections of "Me." I resented the quiet ones, the "better than us," who deigned not to participate in the intensity of our group. Caught between deciding to kill or love the quiet ones, I tried both.

The group reveals "Me" before I find myself

Self-disclosure is inevitable and continuous in any human interaction. Even classically oriented psychoanalysts, such as Ralph Greenson (1967), have acknowledged that as therapists,

> everything we do or say, or don't do or say, from the décor of our office, the magazines in the waiting room, the way we open the door, greet the patient, make interpretations, keep silent, and end the hour, reveals something about our real self and not only our professional self.
>
> (p. 91)

Some writers have argued that because the therapist cannot help being self-disclosing, why not consider the opportunity to make explicit that which reveals oneself to be emotionally involved? Relational therapists reserve the option to gradually and purposefully reveal aspects of themselves, in an attempt to model openness, to propel patients to deal more realistically with the nature and basis of their beliefs, to encourage mutual exploration of interactional dynamics, and to take responsibility for their actions and effects on the other (e.g., Jacobs, 1999; Searles, 1979).

The lines between intentional and unintentional self-disclosure are ambiguous and fluctuating. The therapist's behaviors may range from spontaneous exclamation to measured revelation, from those that are seemingly consciously determined to those unconsciously enacted. Levels of meaning, revealed by subtleties in timing, tone, and cadence, may contradict what is verbally spoken (Chused, 1992; McLaughlin, 1991).

When the group therapist utilizes him- or herself in an open, spontaneous manner, the therapist may be producing more obvious disclosures, or different types of disclosures, than those that also occur in traditional individual or group technique.

One issue to consider in taking or avoiding the opportunity for self-disclosure is whether it serves to open or close things up, a question that may be answered only retrospectively, and even then without certainty that another way may not have been better (Aron, 1996; Greenberg, 1995).

Group members see a therapist-in-action, responding to intense group, subgroup, and dyadic situations. The perspectives are multiple, and members may not be in agreement with each other, and much less with the therapist. Still, the therapist learns about "Me" by attending to these various perspectives: listening to the members' expressions in feelings, fantasies, symbols (e.g., metaphors, jokes, dreams), thoughts, behavioral reactions, and reflecting on how he or she impacts the group culture (e.g., in co-creating the "two groups").

We may directly invite members to share their opinions. I question my work, often asking members what they think I am doing and why. Also, could they or I have done it differently, and better? I respect that I do not have full command of how I feel and respond; I cannot and do not want to be a "blank screen."

Signs that I "like people who talk" were many and obvious to certain members and not all of them are evident to me at this time. I am now more acutely aware of the possible differences in enthusiasm in which I invite, meet, and sustain the gaze of various group members, and also more aware of their visual and bodily reactions to me. My "liking" was co-regulated, encouraged by some (the talkers), and held in abeyance by others (the non-talkers).

In the development of human attachment, a prolonged period of mutual "eye love" (Beebe & Stern, 1977) between mother and infant occurs, involving not only the visual sense but also touch, sound, and movement (exteroception-interoception). In this "dance," each partner enjoyably takes into account and makes moment-by-moment adjustments in response to the other's shifts in behaviors.

So, who did what to "cause the two groups?" It was not me alone who decided whom I "danced" with and when. The therapist cannot expect to be aware and in control of all, or even of many, of the group members' varied and variable transferences to the leader, other members, and the group situation itself.

Like the mother, the therapist needs to maintain relaxed but intense interest, empowering the members to seek and avoid engagement without anxiously "chasing" after them. I believe that even with my inevitable clinical and personal shortcomings, my behaviors of "liking" were sufficiently well distributed to propel bonding, mutual recognition, and the development of the group's identity.

In being (selectively) self-revealing, I took responsibility for "Me"—acknowledging and expanding on the group member's insight regarding my contribution in "sucking" (Horowitz, 1983) members into their respective roles. This seemed to encourage members to take responsibility for their "Me-s" too: discovering in their respective psychologies and personal histories the emotional equipment for the part they played and their influence on others. In our group, the technical decision seemed to have facilitated greater openness among members and furthered the development of group autonomy and cohesiveness.

Emotional co-participation: loving, hating, and being curious in the group

To drive change and stimulate creative growth, the therapist needs to provide an ongoing sense of security, but also must encourage a breaking down of pre-established and safe emotional attitudes. Leadership entails aiding the group and its members to tolerate, communicate, and eventually integrate a wide range of emerging, contradictory, and intense feelings.

Hypothetically, our emotions derive from basic affects, drives, or instincts involved in Loving (attachment or bonding), expressing frustration-aggression (Hating), and exercising curiosity (Knowing) (Bion's shorthand of LHK will be the focus of Chapter 5). While these affects are basic, they do not operate in pure form. Like everyone else, it is difficult for the therapist to "know" what he or she feels, or "really feels." Feelings hide behind their opposites, and defense mechanisms of denial, dissociation, reaction formation, and projection are to be expected, particularly in situations of anxiety and conflict.

In the group under discussion, one simple sentence jarred me out of any complacent fantasy of being in full command of how I felt and what I was doing. "You like people who talk." My "not nice" feelings were exposed, and I felt guilty, personally and professionally deficient. For the group member was implying that I did not like people who did not talk (H) and did not embrace them with full curiosity (K). The communication had a ring of truth, and "suffering" the meaning-making process provided access to my love and compassion (L) towards these same members, my brother, and myself as well.

I had believed I was working with professional ease and competence, eliciting involvement from a significant segment of the attendees. I do not think too many observers would disagree with this perspective. But other perspectives jarred me out of any tendency to rest secure in my relative comfort zone: "You like people who talk"; "If I were running this group, I'd want to know what I did to cause the 'two groups'"; "Could you have gotten the same results if you had stayed out?"

I cannot say I found these remarks to be pleasant—but they were on point and deserved to be respected as legitimate responses to "Me" and my impact, and not prematurely interpreted as "transference," "resistance," an expression of a *basic assumption*, and so forth. In terms of my functioning as a clinician, I had to re-evaluate my feelings, technical actions, and even my very way of "being."

As therapists become aware of avoided feelings, they are gradually able to exert more control over their expression and to participate more fully. I did not wish to banish my negative feelings towards the non-talkers, but I wanted to know where they came from and how they affected my group relationships. Then I would be able to use a fuller array of feelings, with greater clinical acumen.

Activity level of the relational group therapist

Of all the comments, questions, and criticisms directed to me during our six-hour group, one rankles my retrospections: "Could you have gotten the same results if you had stayed out… and not worked so hard?" I heard my mother's voice behind the questioner: "Why can't you behave like your brother!" "Who was this questioner?" I wondered. "A junior colleague or a critical competitor? A friend, or a foe?" Given my emotional involvement with my family of origin, I could not be sure of the accuracy of my judgment, then or now.

As much as I hated the comment and the commentator, I took it and him as sincerely curious, and I respectfully replied that my way of working was something he and other people could think about. I did not wish to intellectually reduce the experience and provide premature closure. Besides, a didactic rationale would have felt defensive. But here I will offer my point of view, which puts the "Me," the group therapist's experience, as a center of action.

The major group theorists have described groups as organic entities, evolving through stages, rebounding from one defensive position to another in accordance with developmental conflicts consequent to group membership. According to their theories, successful groups depend on the therapist's effective performance in pretherapy tasks such as patient selection, composition, and preparation, and in negotiating the novice group through its formative stages of boundary formation, structuring, resistance, and goal direction. It follows that the mature group more often treats itself, coming to appreciate the therapist as a consultant rather than as the continuing mesmerizer of transference.

Foulkes wrote that the group therapist "does not step down but lets the group, in steps and stages, bring him down to earth … [the group] replaces the leader's authority" (Foulkes & Anthony, 1964, p. 61). Along this line of thinking, Yalom (1995) presented the maxim:

> Unlike the individual therapist, the group therapist does not have to be the axle of therapy. In part, you are midwife to the group: you must set a therapeutic process in motion and take care not to interfere with that process by insisting on your centrality.
>
> (p. 216)

In my opinion, while the classic contributions in theory and in descriptive phenomenology are fundamentals of every group therapist's thinking and practice, the emphasis on member-inspired dynamics seriously underplays the enduring role of the therapist, most particularly, the authority of the therapist's evolving psychology on what occurs and does not occur in group.

The therapist remains the figure of inspiration, and the most important member of any group, no matter its focus or duration. Our amiable, sincere, and patient efforts to reach the group count for a lot, and we fumble and are forgiven for our fumbling more than we know. No school of thought owns exclusive or automatic rights to empathy, or to understanding of the self and others. And, in our striving for depth, clinicians of all theoretical persuasions may miss what is timely and most relevant.

We may think about the question, "Could you have gotten the same results if...?" without concluding that there is one way, or a best way. Each group therapist plays his or her own music, as well as capturing a particular version of the music of others. While some notes resound forcefully, others remain faint, distant, or unheard, waiting for the occasion of their development along with other players from within and outside the group.

While I do not rush to make judgments and form conclusions, I value the interpretative mode in group as well as in individual analysis, which may be addressed to the group-as-a-whole, subgroups, or individuals. I believe that there are no clear demarcations between interpretation and other forms of interventions. As do most contemporary therapists, I keep in mind the members and the group's developmental and ongoing needs, and accept the legitimacy of noninterpretative activity involved in symbolic play and certain other forms of enactments. A group therapist's respectful silence or brief appreciative acknowledgment in the face of an apprehensive member's challenge may be a powerful, even decisive intervention. Conversely, verbal formulations that reach into the realm of unconscious phenomena, involving constellations of fantasy, desire, anxiety, character, and defense, rightly may be valued for their effort and concern as much as for their acuity and depth.

When I am confused or unsure, which is often, I may seek clarity from other group members, although I do not necessarily agree with or follow their guidelines. In the group under discussion, I asked for help and achieved insight, which inspired me to develop the thoughts in this chapter. Also, I received several jolts of pain; their effects linger.

Concluding remarks

The therapist's subjectivity—the complex of basic affects, feelings, thoughts, and fantasies, many of which remain out of awareness—affects how we comport ourselves, how we relate to our groups, and how they relate to us. Using myself as an example, I have illustrated how unresolved Oedipal and sibling dynamics were involved in my perceptions, theory, and technique—perhaps in every micro-action and interaction that comprised the group experience.

The variety and flexibility of the therapist's activity, internal and inter-personal, exposes the qualities of the therapist's care and establishes the therapist's authenticity. Through his or her behavior, the group therapist defines the working group culture: how group relationships and experiences are to be regarded, and the emotional depth to which exchanges may be considered.

All psychoanalytic psychotherapy is grounded on Freud's belief that the understanding of others is based on self-understanding. However, self-understanding is an evolving, affective process, stimulating strong and often painful emotions that influence and are influenced by others. Self-awareness remains tentative and uncertain, and is revised according to the shifting currents of present-day reality. Inspection, introspection, retrospection, and the longevity and stability of a group—these factors do not vouchsafe objectivity or inoculate therapists from the tendency to rationalize who we are, how we feel, and what we are doing.

We cannot be sure of all the factors that drove the process of the group under discussion, the accuracy of my evaluations of the interactional dynamics, or even the emotional realities that I have described. The therapist cannot neatly separate self from others and from the group at large. Emotional reality is not a concrete, unchanging something, from which truth can be derived with certainly or finality, but an ever-incomplete process of becoming. The group therapist and member's communications are intersubjectively constructed; their intent and effect remain highly personal, and no final, or even fully objective, assessment is possible.

Whatever the therapist is attending to, he or she is also reflecting upon and revealing oneself, influencing other members in this process. Contemplating one's evolving mental relationship to the group, and its influence on the group, brings layers of meaning to the here-and-now clinical situation, however conceptualized. All benefit from a group therapist unequivocally involved in "Me," in personal discovery and growth.

Chapter 4

Working with therapists in group

It doesn't seem kind or generous to call people out for being wise, gentle, empathic, or helpful. Yet, as a leader in groups with other mental health professionals, I find myself struggling against humane tendencies to be therapeutic in just that way and to participate in a manner appropriate, yet suitable, to my personality. Ideally, the group provides the opportunity for all members to escape confined mindsets and find their own voice, but as we know, groups breed conformity and seek a leader to follow. Given their professional histories and identifications, therapists may enter group with an idealized leader in mind or a composite of the valued individuals they have read, worked with, or who have guided them. It is inevitable to disappoint, even if that leader they had in mind is me.

I cannot say that I have resolved this dilemma, both personal and professional, regarding how to do the work, even after 45 years of educating and treating therapists. But I can share some thoughts and give the reader a sense of what I experience and tend to do.

I describe a frequent situation: let's say that this one is from an extended workshop in which I functioned as invited presenter, but the circumstance could occur in any experiential encounter blessed with therapists. Though I crafted this vignette with purposeful vagueness, I am aware that therapists with whom I have worked might nonetheless see themselves in my imaginings.

The session

It took only a few minutes before I developed a fantasy of having entered a reunion from a summer camp that I had not attended. I felt and expected the typical tensions in beginning a session—some awkward silences, shy approaches, and affectionate or deferential references to the leader. Instead, I found a groundswell of civility, friendliness, mutual interest, and resonance. Who could not be touched by the warmth and concern (although none directed at me)? Perhaps this is what Yalom, Foulkes, and so many other theorists talk about—the group does the work; psychotherapy by the group. But this quickly? Even though I knew better, I questioned the very principles that I have written about—that a group keeps one eye on the leader, and that, to some extent, everything that takes place relates to the leader's person and symbolic representations (see Chapter 3).

Frankly, I do not enjoy spectator sports and would rather play. That, plus an intermittent loyalty to my beliefs, now waning, led me to join in, professing doubts about my function in a group of such caring individuals. I considered my commentary a whole-group interpretation, albeit submerged and implied. I'm not sure if it had the intended effect of bringing some awareness to our experiential field, but the mood shifted. Someone broke the brief silence with a dream:

> I'm on a bus and said I want to get off, maybe it's going in the wrong direction. I'm not sure. I never ride on buses. I think I did (exit) and felt relieved.

"Rich can't do anything right," someone volunteered with relish. "You're holding all our feelings of fear and distrust." "Not feeling contained on the group bus." "I admire your courage in exposing yourself with a dream, you must be feeling safe enough, contained enough." "You're dreaming of us, I feel complimented." "You're not thinking of leaving, are you?" "I can join you in not wanting to leave, but to go off in my own direction." "I might have stayed on, not trusting myself." "I'd go for the ride too; I like that you didn't." The dreamer did not elaborate other than express a few words and gestures of appreciation.

I was at a familiar threshold, what Faimberg (2005) referred to as the essential countertransference position: "the meeting point of intrasubjectivity, intersubjectivity, and metapsychology" (p. 49). It is a difficult juncture, an unclear horizon of psychological problems, mine and I assume others' too. There was a lot going on here, more than I or anybody else could process or fully come to understand. Still, there were clues in the dream and in the group's discourse. And in order to access these clues, I had to locate "me."

I try to stay attuned to my emotional state and what it might mean—benevolent, irritable, curious, calm, a dynamic amalgamation of too much and not enough. What symptoms was I feeling and how did they relate to the countertransference three-factor meeting point? Since it connects with intersubjectivity and with metapsychological formulations, intrasubjective discovery (which interests me greatly) might provide some clarity to what was occurring and what could occur.

The dream was apt—too apt and too useful in spurring the members' so-called "free floating discussion" (Foulkes, 1964/2018), and too successful in winning the group's uncritical approval. It would have sounded overly reproachful to note that no one had tolerated the anxiety of making psychic space for the dreamer or to remark on the dreamer's blatant culpability in not taking space: the flat delivery, incuriosity, and passive response both to the dream and to the group's comments. I decided to intervene first with the dreamer who never rides on buses and discover for myself how that feels.

"Have you ever felt you were part of a group?" I asked dubiously, unconvinced that dreamer was even connected to the dream or to the other members. The dreamer obligingly reeled off a history of affiliations: school, church, and community. I just stared, as if to say, "you can't be this literal."

"I had a good family, everyone seemed to get along, although I can't say we were close. It didn't bother me at the time, not now either, although I couldn't separate easily. Didn't go away to college; my siblings did; I felt jealous and resentful at missing that experience. In my dream, I went my own way. Thanks for giving me a chance to get something for myself."

"Mmm, how much of something? Is it your way if you dreamt that someone drove you to dream it?"

"Like you?"

No reply seemed necessary and I addressed the group: "You stayed on board, making helpful comments. Is that what you wanted to do, or what the driver directed? Did anyone get something for oneself?"

Certainly, my remonstrations did not cure members from going along with what they surmised I wanted them to do; still, a sobering conversation followed. Several people declared that they could not stop being helpful, resentfully so, to mates, patients, parents, siblings, and affiliations, and began to explore why. We entered a new phase when one member straightforwardly confronted another: "I keep an eye on you. I'm concerned that you're not satisfied and are going to say you're leaving. I would feel terrible. It's not your fault I feel burdened."

"Why so sure?" I intervened, and was amiably ignored.

Discussion

As I confessed at the outset, I struggle with how to participate appropriately yet authentically in groups. I was in a conflict between submission and assertion, desiring to be embraced by this idealized family, yet be truthful in ways that would not unduly upset its members, or me. Given what I perceived, there was reason to assume that the members were in a similar dilemma and that they contributed to mine.

I witnessed a group of individuals depending on empathy and clinical wisdom to rebound off each other—a type of mutual projective control—their very compassion shielding fears of exposure, humiliation, and worse. The members shared a contagious fantasy (albeit based on the reality of texts, cultural institutions, and professional training and affiliations) of how groups are supposed to be and how members are supposed to behave (Caper, 1997).

Whenever a group convenes, the leader should be warm and hospitable, but not overstay a welcoming process by being too friendly, too sensitive, or too empathic, qualities that are symptomatic and represent a contribution to the pool of paranoid and depressive anxieties. Therapists must possess "a certain amount of cruelty" and not be "too nice," Carl Jung declared (Atlas & Aron, 2018, p. 117). Cruelty is necessary to relate to the destructive, life-constricting forces implanted in our personalities.

A certain amount of cruelty does not preclude being caring; in actuality, it more authentically conveys it. However, the leader's communications cannot just be directed at the group, which is too cruel, depriving each member's legitimate desire for a unique connection to the leader (and the leader's longing as well). The leader *does* develop a distinct relationship with each person, why not be forthright, something that we want from all members? When member–leader connections are acknowledged and explored, candid member–member bonds are more likely to emerge.

In the workshop, as with any intersubjective encounter (mental as well as actual), shadows of figures lurk, reflections of vertical and horizontal relationships of varying developmental periods. Some are friendly; others less so, infiltrating with messages that drive and shape the individual's thoughts and actions. They are enigmatic (Laplanche, 1999), unconsciously transmitted and transcribed; moreover, the messages are disowned by the messengers who would be horrified to know of their possible primal intents.[1]

To avoid naïve historiography, the therapist must get close, feeling in body, affect, and reverie the disavowed symbiotic, sexual, masochistic, aggressive, fratricidal, patricidal, matricidal, and cannibalistic urges that cluster at the nucleus of the here-and-now. The clouded lens of the countertransference position reveals, then, our usable clinical truths: inklings of the primary messengers, obtrusive messages, and the re-transcribed replays underlying self-narration, discourse, and enaction. Arguably, all families, groups, and cultures seduce and enjoin their members to be helpful, to get along and go along. No wonder we remain discontent (Freud, 1930), burdened, "not close," alienated from each other and from ourselves. The best we can do as a helpful leader is not try to act like one and help individuals and not try to act like helpful group members.

Note

1 Freud (1905, p. 223):

> A mother would probably be horrified if she were made aware that all her marks of caring [derived from her own sexual life] were rousing her child's sexual instinct and preparing for its later intensity....She is only fulfilling her task in teaching the child to love.

Section II

For the love of K

Editor's note

My patient Jonathan, an intelligent and professionally successful man in his late 30s, had an ice-cold relationship with his severely depressed, physically unkempt father. During one of his visits, he saw his father characteristically sitting on the couch in worn-out jocks, his genitals on display, with food remains everywhere. When the father asked a seemingly innocent question about his whereabouts, Jonathan's rage turned violent and he smashed the father's bowl on the floor. In supervision, I mentioned how I framed Jonathan's outburst as a result of *pent-up anger* and how we had discussed his *rage-a-holic* tendencies. Billow responded by saying, "Well that's another theory isn't it?" and later suggested that I say to Jonathan (regarding his father) something along the lines of "he's very hard to love." The refocusing on thwarted love opened up surprising new avenues in the treatment. Over the next few months, Jonathan got in touch with the pain of not having the relationship he longed for (L) with his father and at certain moments was even able to feel concern (K) for him.

This section focuses on a central aspect of Billow's clinical theorizing—the importance of knowing and being known, and the process of attaining emotional/psychological knowledge. Though "thinking" has been snubbed in many therapeutic circles, often with devaluing terms such as "detached" and "intellectualized," the following chapters demonstrate that it would be unwise to buy too heavily into this narrow depiction. In fact, the human urge to communicate, to seek others and to be in contact with them, is predicated on one's capacity for—and love of—genuine emotional thinking.

In Chapter 5, Billow reviews Bion's shorthand of LHK (Loving, Hating, and Knowing) and demonstrates how these constructs can aid in practically understanding, reorienting one towards meaningful intrapsychic and inter-subjective links. The experience of—and interest in—one's love and hate, especially towards significant others (past, present, and future, real as well as imagined), can contribute to a lessening of the split between affect and ideas (Atlas & Aron, 2018; Freud, 1894). And while Billow warns that this process is often avoided, dreaded, and feared, I believe he would agree with Foucault (2001) that "the truth gives beatitude to the subject" and that "in the truth, and in access to the truth, there is something that fulfills the subject himself, which fulfills or transfigures his very being" (p. 16).

As therapists, our interest (K) in our patients and ourselves, and in finding new "truths," is often, thankfully, charged with "analytic libido," a quality that inspired the title for this section— "For the love of K." In Chapter 6, Billow focuses on a related construct—the analyst's "passion," which he defines as "an ongoing process of integrating and utilizing one's most basic and important affects...a process which is intense but does not involve suggestion of *unnecessary* violence." While this definition of passion is somewhat different than its use throughout the history of ideas, it does situate "analytic passion" in conflict with "analytic prudence," a stance which to some extent is shared by classical analysts and contemporary Winnicottians. The British analyst Adam Phillips, for example, considers the patient's ability to speak freely a radical act, but prescribes that the analyst "freely listen" (in Bollas, 2011, p. viii). In contrast, analytic discipline, according to Billow, entails being authentic, taking risks, feeling, and making meaning. Here Billow continues the tradition of one of his therapeutic heroes, Harold Searles, who considered inauthenticity "degrading to the essential uniqueness and emotional profundity of any human being" (Searles, 1968–1969, p. 698).

An additional, equally important process necessary for the achievement of K is containment. In Chapter 7, Billow demonstrates how containment, with its three variants (commensal, symbiotic, and parasitic), operates in the clinical encounter. As Bion (1970) noted, our fear of mental pain often leads us to avoid "suffering" meaning. We do this through a host of defensive operations, but if we are lucky, others can help us transform pain by "applying words to wounds" (Goldman, 2017, p. 101). This variant of containment is termed "commensal," where language is used to organize and explain conscious and unconscious experience. However, as we know all too well, words do not always reach their intended recipient. One's level of dysregulation, the relational context, and the accuracy of the words all play a role in whether commensal containment is possible or desired. At other times, reassuring, symbiotic communications may be called for, providing the foundation for later, more sophisticated linguistic meaning-making. Finally, the chapter deals with parasitic attacks on meaning-making. Bion (1959) hypothesized that these "attacks on linking" were due to an "implicit hatred of emotion and the need to avoid awareness of it" (p. 310). In addition to clarifying Bion's often cryptic constructs, this chapter also emphasizes that at different moments (and sometimes simultaneously), patients, analysts, and supervisors pull for commensal, symbiotic, or parasitic containment.

Chapter 5

LHK[1]: Bion's basic affects

While Bion's work continues to inspire contemporary psychoanalysis, his ideas on human emotion have received less attention and are not as well known. This chapter focuses on the three basic affects he posited: the urge to love, the urge to hate, and the urge to seek knowledge (particularly emotional knowledge), notated, respectively, as "L," "H," and "K." These are primitive psychic stimuli—the constitutional or instinctual givens—which the individual brings to his or her experience. Within the analytic situation, the analyst may observe how both patient and analyst struggle with these affects as they emerge, often vaguely at first, and without coherence, and are later transformed by mental functioning into symbols, nameable feelings, and thoughts.

Ongoing binocular emotional thinking

Psychoanalysts, beginning with Freud, have been concerned with the relationship between affects and ideas. Freud (1915) had established that only ideas can be repressed and made unconscious, and characteristically paid less attention to unconscious affective experience. To some extent, affects must be allowed to reach consciousness. Otherwise, they risk alienation from ideas—a common feature in all psychopathology.

Although Bion did not refer to Freud's formulation, he considered it essential for affects to develop such that they can be experienced and responded to (not necessarily consciously), and contribute to the growth of thinking. According to Bion's theory, "thinking" refers to an ongoing transformation of emotional experience by unconsciousness as well as consciousness. The systems conscious and unconscious together provide a "binocular" or correlative perspective on affects as they emerge and on reality as it is experienced (Bion, 1962, p. 53).

LHK foreshadowed in Bion's theory of group process

In *Experiences in Groups*, Bion (1961) described three types of basic affective states (basic assumptions) that predominated groups. When a group failed to progress, it was because of the suppression of emotion: "emotion being an essential part of the basic assumptions. The tension thus produced appears to the individual as an intensification of emotion" while the individual "feels as if his intellectual capacity were being reduced" (pp. 174–175). The group's "dis-ease" (Bion's pun) was diagnosed by a failure of activation, identification, and meaningful interplay among the underlying basic affects.

Three basic affects: "plus" or "minus"

Like Freud and Klein, Bion mythologized conflictual polarities in mental life. At various times, Freud wrote of basic conflicts between the pleasure and reality principles, and between the life and death instincts; Klein focused on the struggle between love and hate; and Bion described conflicting motives for thinking and for not thinking. A deep tension exists between a basic need for knowledge (particularly knowledge of emotional experience) and the human tendency to avoid meaning, because emotional knowledge so often brings painful realizations. "Disease" arises when the individual "decides" (unconsciously as much as consciously) not to develop emotional meaning. In this situation, affects are prevented from developing. Unconscious (particularly dream experience and "reverie") as well as conscious meaning becomes impoverished. The underlying affects must be reclaimed from their "frozen" states of suppression and dissociation, to be thought about and brought into an unfolding process of meaning-making.

Bion believed that the urge to find meaning in an object relational world is as basic as love and hate and thus gave the K drive overarching status. L and H are self-contained, but K represents not only a general curiosity drive but can involve L and H in its content. Further, K is necessary to derive meaning from L and H. It is the quality of one's thinking about affects—the movement of K over the fields L and H—that almost defines the quality of one's humanness, by rendering personal action comprehensible to oneself and others. The type of emotional thinking that links or meaningfully integrates the affects represents the aim Freud (1938) defined of Eros: "to establish ever greater unities and to preserve them thus, in short, to bind together" (p. 148).

Though he posited a strong urge to create links, Bion also highlighted a human tendency to undo them, akin to what Freud described as the aim of the aggressive instinct: "to undo connections and so to destroy things" (p. 148). "Things" may be understood as "mental things" or "emotional meaning." Bion relegated to a "psychotic part of the personality" (not necessarily clinically psychotic, of course) that evades or modifies emotional experience. This hypothetical suborganization defends against emotional experience by attacking the mental linking processes by which we come to know and integrate our thoughts and feelings, when such integration threatens to bring mental pain. The "anti-ego" or minus (−K) part of the personality defends against innate tendencies to develop and integrate the basic affects, providing minus versions: −L, −H, and −K.

"Pre-monitory" anxiety relating to LHK

Drawing on Platonic and Kantian epistemology, Bion posited that the human being has an inborn knowledge of its emotional needs, that is, of L, H, and K. Precursory knowledge of psychic reality exists from the beginning of life and continues to assert influence in the form of "pre-conceptions," related to precursory thoughts, and "pre-monitions," related to precursory manifestations of L, H, and K.

"Pre-monitory" affective expressions of the drives of L, H, and K are "released" to *inform*, as the individual applies reason to experience. Because they express the earliest levels of experience and are need-dominated, the emotional information they convey may be judged as infantile, contradictory, and repugnant. Hence, primal affects, as they begin to emerge, often are accompanied by pre-monitory anxiety, a state of warning and dread, and may be disavowed and left without further development. In this situation, affects remain, in Freud's (1915) words, "a potential beginning which is prevented from developing" (p. 178).

Pre-monitory anxiety relates not to any vague or unformulated affectual arousal, of which the human being is capable of an infinite variety. Rather, the anxiety refers to dawning awareness of particular, hypothetical affects that are activated, but defended against in the immediacy of here-and-now experience. The affects themselves thus exist as pre-monitions, anxiety-laden potentials. Until these potentials cohere, they are not available to participate in meaning-making. The individual remains deprived of the necessary emotional information to make adequate "mental sense" and understand ongoing experience.

Pre-monitory anxiety and suffering L, H, and K

Bion (1963) facetiously but pointedly observed that in clinical practice, when an emotion is obvious, it is usually painfully obvious. Psychoanalytic treatment is not about cure but about transforming the experience of obvious pain to enlarge the capacity to "suffer" meaning. Thus, to avoid unnecessary pain, by meaningfully utilizing one's emotional life, one must develop a capacity of openness to the development of a full range of affects that may not be obvious. I am referring here to the derivatives of L, H, and K, those which have been anxiously disowned and "prevented from developing."

To illustrate the value of suffering the meaning-making process over obvious pain, compare the mourning experience to the clinical syndrome of depression. The depressed person is preoccupied with obvious sadness, but stultifies and deteriorates mentally. The self and its objects, rather than being utilized for their capacity to generate thought, are worn down and rejected. This treatment applies particularly to the departed one, who is introjected, only to be killed off rather than truly cared for (Freud, 1917a). Intrapsychic and interpersonal growth and development are foreclosed, along with the emotions themselves.

The mourner, by contrast, endures the sense of persecution and depression that accompanies symbolically representing and integrating the painful drives emerging in the context of separation and loss. Thus, with pre-monitory anxiety, a warning of impending guilt, a mourner may experience premonitions of anger (H) towards the departed loved one. Also provoking guilt is the incipient revival of love towards oneself, and the wish to persevere (L). Integration alternates with disintegration, as repressed, suppressed, or dissociated anxiety-laden feelings towards the self and other cohere, evoke attention and curiosity (K). Memories of the departed one may arouse sudden happiness, which then recedes, followed by confusion, frightening premonitions of catastrophe (Eigen, 1985), anger, and renewed realization of loss and sorrow.

The mourner suffers, binding together through mental representations—conscious as well as unconscious thoughts, fantasies, and narratives—ambivalent and painful affects. Others remain appreciated and are utilized in the mourning process. In symbolizing and representing primitive, even psychotic-like emotional experience, the mourner deepens meaningful psychic ties to the lost object, now regained internally, and returns, enhanced and with gratitude, to the world of living (Klein, 1935, 1940).

To emphasize the point, clinical depression following loss is painful because new meanings are precluded. True mourning is an experience of painful meaning, which leads to a richer, fuller life.

Clinical example: pre-monitory anxiety and halting of L, H, and K

A 40-year-old physician entered treatment to address professional and family difficulties. He felt he was stymied in his career and was short-tempered and often mentally absent at home. He reported that he became a doctor because "My parents thought it would be a good idea. Nothing really appealed to me. I didn't know what I wanted to be when I grew up. I'm still waiting." A crisis erupted when his troubled, late-adolescent son had a paranoid outburst, ending in a physical fight with his father and placement in a mental hospital.

It was not until the next day that the father broke into tears.

> At first, I felt numb. I began to have all sorts of worries, and then they stopped and I just cried. I don't know what I was feeling, maybe guilt for hitting my son. I hate to think of him feeling so bad, maybe sorry for myself and where I am in my life, I spend a lot of time living numb, or springing into anger, like a cold-blooded animal. I get too angry and don't know what to do about it. I wish you would be like a hospital psychiatrist, medicate me and tell me what to do.

The patient experienced "bursts" of unintegrated affects of love or of hate but seemed unable to understand himself. His affects, however, were "all there," awaiting his attempts to develop them. Without their development, he felt "numb" or "cold-blooded," less than human. He remained emotionally immature and cognitively handicapped in coping with human relations of a nonmedical nature.

His parents' message had been that his family was "special," and he conformed by being a well-behaved child and adolescent, a star in the classroom and on the playing fields. In treatment, he soon realized that he had maintained an idealized version of his family, and that there had actually been prominent marital and family tensions that he had camouflaged by conforming to the considerable pressure to perform and achieve. Indeed, he remembered consciously refusing to respond to certain inner urgings that had to do with ambivalent and rebellious feelings towards the parents whom he had adored and obeyed. These urgings, premonitions of primal affects, he had refused to think about, really, to "feel" about. The price of his repudiation had been an inner sense of fear, foreboding, and guilt. Something bad was inside him, which he feared could and would "break out," harming those he loved. Now he understood his obvious and painful lack of satisfaction in all his achievements, and why he had often been sad and anxious, even during his supposedly happy childhood.

Thus, as we worked together, he developed an understanding of the dynamics behind his avoidance of emotionality. He began to "think," meaning here not mere *mentation*, with which this ruminative man had expertise. Rather, he became psychologically minded. He could tolerate the premonitory anxiety that accompanied the emergence of his affects, allowing them to cohere. His thoughts came to have emotional meaning to him and contributed to an assertive commitment to reality.

The patient reported that his vague, haunting "moodiness" seemed to dissipate, as he developed what he described as a new type of self-control: he could feel unpleasing affects without numbing himself or springing into action. Although he had to live through painful moments of emotional realizations, the progressive trust in his emotional knowledge formed the basis of much-improved, at times joyful, intrapsychic and interpersonal functioning.

Clinical example from group therapy

A distinguished and rather intellectualized woman, also the senior member of a long-standing group, volunteered that she divided the therapy into good sessions, in which she understood and could empathize with others, and bad sessions, in which she became "out of it." In these latter sessions, she would lose the focus, did not catch on the way others did, and felt bad for and about herself.

> And then I worry that you [the group therapist] are going to ask me what
> I am feeling, and I don't know what I am feeling. I am feeling nothing. I
> get so frustrated and angry at myself. The group is so important to me,
> I look forward to it all week.

Her obvious pain produced sympathy, but little interaction.

I suggested that although she might feel that the group was important to
her, she did not seem to be important to the group, given their lack of emotional response. The members strenuously protested my intervention and
described their admiration for her. At this point in her work, she understood
that their very admiration was an aspect of the problem. "All my life people
have put me on a pedestal. Now they 'admire' me for being in therapy 'at
my advanced age.' But I don't feel they really know me and don't want to."
I replied that she might be right, perhaps people would not want to know
her, but that we could not test this idea until she exposed who she really
is. The group could not know her until she accessed and expressed her
feelings. As long as she remained "elevated," that is, "above" her feelings
and idealized by others, she could not participate in the emotional give-
and-take of group life.

It was my conception that she decided to become "out of it" whenever
prompted and made anxious by emerging primal emotion. In not developing her love, hate, and (emotional) curiosity, she could be "admirable," but
not otherwise emotionally meaningful to herself or others. I encouraged her
to consider that she may have strong feelings towards the group (including
me) for insufficiently caring.

She tentatively began to express hurt and angry affects, and then discovered that she was curious where they would take her. She expected the group
to return anger with anger or to feel guilty for hurting her. Instead, they
cheered her on, with a genuine delight that she came to share. Eventually,
her thoughts began to express a new level of emotional meaning, personal
and relevant to her growth and to the growth of others. She actually became
more thoughtful, but less intellectualized, and rarely complained of being
"out of it."

Minus (−) LHK

Without the development of primal emotion, the individual, rather than informed of the personal meaning of experience, becomes *misinformed*. Individuals may also be misled by the intensification of whatever thoughts or
emotions are available, as in the earlier example about the physician whose
emerging affects felt painfully overwhelming.

To avoid emotional experience, the individual may halt or even "reverse"
the developmental trajectory of cohering primal affects. The activated but
unrealized affects persist, preformulated or unintegrated with each other,

fated for denial, dissociation, projection, and perverse transformations. Further, those affects that are consciously accessible tend to be exaggerated, misinforming by their very obviousness and intensity. Thus, by their absence or overwhelming presence, the primary affects serve a negative ("minus") function in terms of advancing learning by experience. The next set of examples illustrates the clinical utility of applying Bion's "minus" sign, the shorthand for the negative transformation of the three basic affects.

Clinical examples of −L, −H, and −K

1   A patient, a morbidly obese woman, became furious with me when I did not support her without reservations. Her mother had harshly criticized her in front of her children. She felt humiliated and took comfort in reporting that even the children found their grandmother to be hateful. She wanted and expected such comfort from me. But while feeling supportive, I found the whole situation, involving three generations, curious and worthy of further exploration. My response frustrated the patient. Everyone should hate her mother, why didn't I? She did not deserve a drop of sympathy or understanding. The analytic alliance of several years threatened to deteriorate quickly. Leaving treatment began to make sense to the patient, which scared her, for she suspected that something was wrong in her thinking.

I inquired: "Where is the love between us?"

The patient claimed that I had betrayed love, and that there was not any. The patient felt all alone, without a loving mother or mother-substitute in the analyst. No wonder she turned to food for comfort. I suggested that the patient's obvious "eating disorder" was really a "loving disorder." She couldn't keep love inside her. Without the nutritious emotion of love (L), her anger remained undigestible or unreasonable (−H). But needing love, she binged on its junky substitutes (−L), greedily pursuing supplies from the refrigerator and from those colluding with her rigid opinions. She needed to think about love, to retrieve the affect from the psychotic part of her personality and tolerate its coherence with her too-obvious hatred.

2   A graduate student came to her analytic hour quite upset by a dream involving her elderly father. "He had wet himself. I felt so bad for him, even in the dream, and bad that I would do this to him in the dream." She knew that she loved her difficult and harsh father and knew that she had gone to sleep with mixed feelings, set off by a difficult interview with her thesis chairman. Her angry feelings, expressed in dream imagery, were all too depressing to think about, even in the dream. She felt dreadful. "What was wrong with her?" she asked tearfully. Why did she keep on having such bad dreams? Why was she so evil towards those she loved?

By preoccupying herself with these ruminative questions, she could moderate, or even forestall, our working with her mixed emotional responses—her love (L) and concern (K), as well as her anger (H)—and finding where they would take us. Thoughts about dream affects made her anxious, and she had "decided" not to think about them. This seemed to be preferable to "leakage," as in a stream of associations that would link her to these premonitions, that is, certain basic affectual reactions she anxiously realized she had attempted to suppress rather than allow to develop.

I offered that thinking evil (H) and being evil (−H) were not identical. Further, thinking evil towards those she loved could be appreciated as a starting point, were she to remain curious about herself. Attending to her mixed affects, although initially anxiety-arousing, did not necessarily keep things more depressing, I suggested. Naming the unnameable might relieve dread. Remaining dubious about these ideas served to preserve her mentality to disassemble (−K) her otherwise quite functional curiosity (K).

3   A man with many borderline features quickly established a habit of asking me questions, such as "What do you think, Rich?" "What would you do?" "You think so?" At the end of a session, he typically launched into a new topic he felt pressing and needing resolution. He insisted that I was being unfair and arrogant if I did not say something to help him along until the next session. My calling attention to his behavior, and what I took to be his underlying motivation, only gave him a headache, he claimed. He departed with another unanswered question: "Is therapy making things worse?" The patient's demanding "need-to-know" frustrated his innate capacity to function psychoanalytically and impeded his growth and development. "K" crystallized prematurely, as a distracting symptom, an intolerable "ache" to understand and to be understood (−K). The cause of the patient's pain was, in part, the unavoidably frustrating nature of reaching insight, which he did not want to tolerate. Because I subjected him to the reality of the learning process, rather than "solving" (or dissolving) the necessity of learning, I became personified as a spitefully withholding analyst (−H), one who had no good reason to hurt him.

An obvious affect may be experienced as too exciting as well as too painful to be maintained in thought and may press for immediate discharge through action. Bion (1965, p. 141) referred to such affects as "hyperbolic," dominating and rivalrous in relationship to other affects, thoughts, and thinkers.

4   A young man announced to his parents and friends that he was gay. He made this decision because he had intensely sexual feelings towards men, which he had acted upon. He also had enjoyed several long-standing sexual and loving relationships with women, during which

time he felt little interest in men and "terrific" about himself and the meaning he was building into his life. He wished that he did not have the capacity to feel sexually towards men, but that he did, "proved" to him that he was homosexual.

In consultation, it seemed clear to me that he preferred to be in a relationship with a woman. However, the intensity of his sexual affectual responses towards men—whenever he felt such stirrings—made him disbelieve that he could live an authentic "straight" life. In the initial stages of therapy, the intensity of what he took to be unreasonable "lust" (−L) he felt towards men served to distract him from his difficulties in experiencing and working through his fear of and ambivalence towards (L and H) women and undermined motivation to think about and experiment with (K) heterosexual relationships.

The analyst's task: finding the "key" affect

Bion (1962) thought it technically effective for the analyst to appreciate the complexity of the patient's emotional experience of the session, but limit the description to the interplay among the primal affects participating in the emotional experience. The analyst's task is to choose a dominant or "key" affect of the session, one which then also imparts a key to the value of the other affectual components (pp. 44–45). The choice is not a record of the emotional experience of the session itself, but it is the best of the analyst's belief, a "true reflection of his feelings" (p. 45). Bion attached "great importance to the choice of L, H, or K" (p. 46) and advised the analyst to tailor his or her remarks according to what he or she believed to be the prevailing affectual tone of the session.[2] He did not think the choice was difficult for the trained analyst.

Case example: finding the "key" affect

The analysand, a college professor, well read in the psychoanalytic literature, reported the following dream:

> We were really "grooving," exchanging ideas. You were excited. There was antiaircraft firing going off in the background. Like our bombing Iraq. [An aspect of the day residue.] It made me nervous, but I tried not to pay attention to it.

The patient then said: "I don't want you to think that this dream is 'homo.'" I asked what he meant. "You know, the phallic imagery with the antiaircraft guns. Your being 'excited.' It must have to do with yesterday's session."

He had, in fact, expressed ideas that piqued my interest and curiosity, and we had engaged in a dialogue that seemed enjoyable to us both. I conveyed this impression of the prior session, and then asked, with doubt, if he had experienced our exchanges as sexual. He said that he had not, but I probably had. I had the "evidence" in the dream, and if not in the dream, in his associations to the dream. I would say that he was projecting the idea of his being "homo" and attributing the idea to me. He would have to spend the session dealing with psychoanalytic theories of the Oedipus complex.

We agreed that the prior session had seemed different and special: a genuine give-and-take. But now, its pleasure was gone, and he felt hopeless that any enjoyable intimacy between us could turn out well. Powerful men are very competitive; they have to show that they know more and put him down. When he is open and vulnerable, he gets "fucked."

Yesterday, the key to the session had been K. The patient had been exercising and developing his urge to know in the context of our emotional relationship. The current version of yesterday's session was −L. In terms of the patient's felt experience, I, rather than he, was the "homo." That is, he feared that I would gather in and use knowledge with the perverse intent to penetrate him with hardened, preformulated interpretations. He had every reason to be depressed and afraid of getting close to me.

I asked him if we had the freedom to look at the dream freshly. He said "go ahead," with a resigned sigh. Despite his felt certainty of my interpretation, which would emphasize an "L" oedipal dimension, my choice of the key to the present session was "H." I suggested that the antiaircraft fire was his anger—his own latent and dreaded aggression—which he had been attempting to keep in the background, or "in the closet," as we worked together. Apparently, he was coming to a different decision, one that was making him "nervous." He was beginning to get "fired up" emotionally. In the dream imagery, and in his frank dialogue in the current session, he was beginning to develop and utilize an essential emotional part of himself (H) in his relationship with me, confronting what he suspected (even in his dream) to be my unwarranted interpretations.

He associated to his father, who was constantly "up his ass," disturbing their relationship with his impulsive emotionality. The father demanded too much closeness (−L). He could be invasively curious (−K) about his son's private life and too angry (−H) when he felt thwarted or disappointed. Thus, he began to articulate his anger at his father, an anger he knew he had, but had tried not to attend to.

The patient was developing a formerly undeveloped affect in his own mind (in awake and dream thinking) to utilize in a here-and-now relationship with an authority figure. Our dialogue included the essential element of passion (Billow, 2000). All three of the patient's affects became constructively engaged as we worked together (L), applying reason (K) to the patient's experience: his fantasies, fears, and risks involved in his urge to hate me (H).

Further case discussion and conclusion: the analyst's LHK

I believe my "excitement" in the prior session had been a balanced expression and integration of L of K, and not a countertransference enactment reflecting a complementary identification (Racker, 1968), that is, an identification with his introject, the "overexcited father." The patient's dream ideas, and his associations to my anticipated interpretations, informed us of a different opinion. He could not trust my capacity to contain and develop primal affects.

It was my job to trust myself, although also to remain receptive to the patient's opinion. To unnecessarily suppress my spontaneity and enjoyment of the work would reflect a concordant identification (Racker, 1968) with the part of the patient that feared LHK. He unduly dreaded the consequences of responding to my affects, and developing his own, but I should not.

The analyst must utilize his or her own primal affects in reaching the interpretation, but not use the communication for countertransference conveyance, that is, "as a vehicle for transmission of some aspect of L or H" (Bion, 1965, p. 61). In addition, K must be exercised with patience and restraint. There should be no "irritable reaching after fact and reason" (Keats, in Bion, 1970, p. 125). The analyst must rein in "memory and desire," the urge to know and to apply knowledge, particularly when the urge involves an intolerance of not-knowing and not-doing. But at the same time, our urge to know about emotional experience may be enjoyed, and not only suffered, as we live through the meaning-making process with our patients.

Note

1 Loving, Hating, and Knowing
2 Bion (1961) earlier had advised the group leader to be aware of the prominent basic assumption: "The work-group function is always in evidence within one, and only one, basic assumption" (p. 154).

Chapter 6

From countertransference to passion

In a panel of the American Psychoanalytic Association, Friedman declared, "In today's world countertransference is God, and Heinrich Racker is its prophet" (Kelly, 1997, p. 1253). I put forth Bion as another "prophet" of this relational reformation. Like Racker, Bion held that the analyst's emotional participation—which he came to call "passion"—was a central organizer of meaning in the analytic interaction. However, Bion's thinking extended past countertransference, and his work contributes to establishing an emotional phenomenology of the analyst's subjectivity and a method which helps differentiate countertransference reactions and enactments from fuller emotional participation.

While Bion attempted to systematize the theory and practice of psychoanalysis, as well as introduce a metapsychological theory of thinking, he was not a systematic writer. His ideas concerning "passion" are dispersed among his major works and were never fully developed and integrated. In this chapter, I will disembed and articulate some of his important concepts which apply to the analyst's "passion" and its clinical utilization. I include a case example which, in extrapolating from Bion's ideas, reflects my personality and integrates aspects of contemporary relational theory.

Bion's conception of countertransference

Bion's ideas relating to emotional participation developed well in advance of theories of intersubjectivity, perspectivism, and co-constructionism (e.g., Gabbard, 1997; Gill, 1994), but they are remarkably contemporary. Over 50 years ago, Bion demonstrated the relational convention (see Aron, 1996) of the analyst's utilizing, at times self-disclosing, inner experience in the interpretation:

> It becomes clear to me that I am, in some sense, the focus of attention in the group. Furthermore, I am aware of feeling uneasily that I am expected to do something. At this point I confide my anxieties to the group, remarking that, however mistaken my attitude might be, I feel just this.
>
> (Bion, 1961, pp. 30, 45–46)

Bion was one of Klein's followers who modified the classical view of counter-transference as an emotional problem of the analyst's, necessarily represent-ing the analyst's conflicts and resistances, and an impediment to treatment. Countertransference was also the vehicle by which the analyst could come to understand the patient's emotions, conflicts, and resistances, expressed in fantasies, affects, and behaviors encompassing projective identifications. In his influential early work, Bion (1961, 1967b) showed how this special type of countertransference, based on projective identification, could be utilized constructively and serve as a basis for interpretation:

> The analyst feels he is being manipulated so as to be playing a part, no matter how difficult to recognize, in somebody else's phantasy. The experience consists of two closely related phases: in the first there is a feeling that whatever else one has done, one has certainly not given the correct interpretation; in the second there is a sense of being a particu-lar kind of person in a particular emotional situation. I believe [that the] ability to shake oneself out of the numbing feeling of reality that is a concomitant of this state is the prime requisite of the analyst.
>
> (1961, p. 149)

Countertransference thus represents an opportunity, an emotional problem to be solved, provided the analyst can achieve the psychological separation from the patient and from his or her own immediate emotional experience, which seems real and objectively justified by the situation (Bleandonu, 1994).

Passion defined

As elaborated in Chapter 5, Bion posited three primary affects, or dimen-sions of emotional experience, based on constitutional or instinctive drives: to love, to hate, and to seek knowledge (notated as L, H, and K). These primal feelings exist as constitutional potentials that are "released" by expe-rience. Primal affects (LHK) are the underlying invariants which the analyst as well as the patient brings to each and every psychoanalytic encounter, especially to one's thinking within the encounter.

Bion (1963) defined passion as "the component derived from L, H, and K. I mean the term to represent an emotion experienced with intensity and warmth though without any suggestion of violence" (pp. 12–13). Whereas Bion refers here to passion as a "component," and elsewhere as an "ele-ment," I believe the term "process" better conveys his meaning. I conceive of "passion" as on ongoing process of integrating and utilizing one's most basic affects.

As the analyst applies him- or herself to the psychoanalytic situation, a fresh coherence and integration of LHK may be reached and sustained. Pas-sion establishes and invigorates the links within and between the analyst's internal and external object-relational world, thereby nourishing our capacity to communicate to patients with intimacy and "warmth."

Bion (1963) wrote that "passion is evidence that two minds are linked" (p. 13). Linkage may be in one direction, and not complementary. And, although stimulated by sense experience, passion is not physical or dependent on the senses. For instance, two minds may be linked intimately when they are separated by time and space, just as one may link one's mind to Shakespeare's or Mozart's or Freud's. An analyst may be passionately involved with a patient who resists passion. The reverse is true as well, since a patient's passion may not be reciprocated by the analyst.

Passion notifies the self that it is experiencing experience, rather than merely "thinking about" or "reacting to" experience. The analyst achieves heightened emotional awareness of the self, the links, the other, and the relationship.

Powers of deduction

Bion (1963) assigned the notation "R" (reason) "to represent a function that is intended to serve the passions... by leading to their dominance in the world of reality" (p. 4). Along with a personal analysis, knowledge of psychoanalytic theory may expand capacity for this category of introspection and empathy.

The analyst uses "R" to consider such questions as: What denied feelings might be contributing to my (and/or the other's) anxiety, symptom, hallucination, etc.? What am I (and/or the patient) feeling, fearing feeling, dreading not feeling? "R" deduces elements which are conspicuous in their absence. For example, an analyst in empathic attunement with a patient may reason that there are disruptive feelings which are not being felt in the dyad. The analyst may "search and find" the repressed or dissociated emotional moments of fear, fragmentation, and aloneness which should be a part of every analytic session (Bion, 1974).

Containing and reverie

Bion suggested that symbols and thoughts, since they establish emotional meaning and thus contain anxiety, serve a function once provided by the mother. When the patient cannot develop emotional meaning, the analyst must provide the containing function. In this situation, the patient projects raw, that is, unmentalized, emotional experience into the receptive analyst. Even if the patient "refuses" to project and withdraws, the analyst may come to understand and bring meaning to this situation by making inferences (R) and utilizing his or her own internal processes. Utilizing primary processes—the capacity to free-associate, imagine, and dream—and secondary processes, the analyst gathers and deciphers the patient's disowned emotionality. The analyst gradually represents (re-presents) them to the analysand, transformed into words.

In reverie, the receiving individual utilizes dreamlike and irrational aspects of one's mind in order to understand and further develop the unformulated thoughts and feelings of another, and of one's own (Bion, 1962; de Bianchedi, 1997). Reverie is a necessary condition for intuition and empathy.

Containing is a two-way communicative process. The infant quickly becomes a container, utilizing reverie to receive and interpret the mother's thoughts and feelings, only some of which she herself may understand. An analogous process exists in the consultation room.

Containing also asserts a separate point of view, committing the analyst to, but also removing him or her from the intermediate, "transitional," or "third" (Ogden, 1994) zone of self and other. As an intrapsychic event, as well as an intersubjective construction (Ogden, 1997), containing evokes subjectivity, without an implication of pure objectivity. The analyst filters through a personalistic lens, and in representing the interaction, the analyst emotionally participates with unique individuality.

Negative capability and catastrophe

Bion adopted Keats's term "negative capability" to describe the mental discipline required of negative realization, which in turn is prerequisite to passion. In eschewing memory and desire, "any irritable reaching after fact and reason" (Keats, in Bion, 1970, p. 125), the analyst puts aside known subjective experience—the analyst's own as well as the patient's—in favor of what is not known. The analyst must ignore coherence so that he is confronted by the incoherence and experiences incomprehension of what is presented to him. His own analysis should have made it possible for him to tolerate this emotional experience although it involves feelings of doubt and perhaps even persecution. This state must endure, possibly for a short period, but probably longer, until a new coherence emerges (Bion, 1965, p. 102).

The process may be dreaded as "catastrophic"; often, old meaning must crumble before new meaning is built. Insight is not achieved solely by the incremental buildup of manageable experience. Analytic discipline involves coping with episodes of meaninglessness (the "beta elements"), alternating with the turbulent process of containment (which will be further elaborated in Chapter 7) and emotional thinking (e.g., Eigen, 1985). And there are consequences which cannot be foreseen or necessarily desired. Passion may bring forth an unpredictable "change of heart" (Maizels, 1996), fresh and not necessarily pleasurable attitudes, feelings, and inclinations to self and other.

Emotional disclosure differentiated from passion

Bion put faith in the well-analyzed ability to think and not be unduly controlled by patients' projections and provocations. By maintaining patience and an open mind, the analyst can maintain sufficient contact with his or her unconscious to function with the "balanced outlook" (Bion, 1967b, p. 104)—if not inner emotional equanimity—that Freud (1912) described as ideal. At the same time, Bion believed that the analyst, like other human beings, rarely lives up to this ideal (he included himself). We have to make "the best of a bad job" (Bion, 1979): thinking with a mind in conflict with its task.

Case example: the impasse—undeveloped emotions

The patient was a man about my age. We shared many similarities of education, interests, and accomplishments, although he was in a different professional field. The analysis had lasted many years, and we had developed an affectionate and easy relationship, except that periodically, in response to an intervention, he would erupt. These enactments all followed a similar pattern. I had hurt him, and he protested vociferously, subjecting me to a thoroughly unflattering character analysis.

And then, to show the difference between me and what he believed he had every right to expect, he paraphrased my intervention. He spoke with sensitive restraint and intelligence. His cultured voice, comfortable with public speaking, sounded far preferable to mine, often studded with slang and more than the occasional obscenity. Clearly, there was much to admire in his well-modulated version of me, and I found myself fantasizing that somebody else should become his analyst, perhaps he himself, and that he should become mine as well.

I felt bad and often wondered at these times how he could stand working with me. Yet it seemed rarely to be in his conscious mind (or in his dreams or associations, as far as I could discover) to consider ending the relationship and finding another analyst. He sometimes hated how I spoke, but he did not hate me. And what about my hatred of him—which I knew I must feel, given my fantasy of trading places and my belief in the accuracy of his complaints about my tendencies to be harsh and judgmental, which I have heard before. I confess I took some relief when he assured me that I did not hate him. I was not a cold or malicious person, but I could get oblivious and insensitive. I really had to change my attitude, he explained, and take a better look at how I expressed myself.

There seemed to be no way to talk us out of these situations. He was angry, that was obvious, and would not tolerate any "analysis." We were both aware that our interaction played out traumatic aspects of his relationship with his mother. I was supposed to help him work through them, not subject him to endless repetitions.

Equally obvious (at least to me) was my sorrow for hurting him and my guilt for possibly acting out. I never quite believed that I was as bad as he asserted, and occasionally floated the hypothesis that he had trouble with what I was saying, not how I was saying it. But I could not be absolutely sure. Since there was some truth in everything he said about my character, I thought I would be unduly defensive if I argued further or justified myself.

I felt that I had no choice other than to apologize for unintentionally hurting him and to acknowledge that I would think about my attitudes and untherapeutic tendencies. Then, testing if we could move forward again, I rephrased my prior insights, as carefully as I could. He seemed to appreciate the reparative sequence; our relationship was reclaimed and we ended the session in our usual harmony, one which I no longer trusted.

A change in my attitude

I had diagnosed our transference-countertransference impasse according to Bion's theory. We had pleasure, we had pain, but we had no passion. We got along very well, or not at all. These alternations made sense to him, for they were based on my behavior, he insisted, not on a transference to a mother whom he "knew all about." I could not bring out fresh love, hate, or even a fresh thought to his consideration of his relationship to me or to her.

Similarly, the patient's romantic relationships deteriorated into disappointing stalemates. He eventually withdrew from each of the women he loved. With them and with me, he could not tolerate and develop his ambivalent feelings, remain curious about them, and apply them in a way to further meaning in an affectionate relationship. The primal affects of L, H, and K stultified. As in his relationships with women, our manifest affects, our hatred as well as love, had outlived their useful informative function. We knew about these alternating and repetitive aspects of our experience all too well. In these moments, we were "stale mates," starving for the "release" of primal affects to foster the growth of meaning.

I attempted to approach certain subjects self-consciously, making sure not to use sarcasm or irony, and asking his permission before being blunt with my opinion. I did not always succeed, however, and from time to time I would offend him and be subjected to a tongue-lashing such as I have just described. On one occasion, I discovered that I had lost all appetite for our usual dialogue. I did not want to hear his criticisms and ruminate about how and what I had done or not done. I aborted the customary back-and-forth and eventual rephrasing of my intervention with the following:

"I said what I said the way I said it. I like it well enough, and it will have to stand, even if you could say it better."

"Now I can't work. You ruined the session," he remonstrated.

I could be so unconscious, so stubborn and superior. He had not seen my arrogant disregard in a long while and assumed that I had learned something from our work. Apparently I had given him lip service. I really did not understand how I affected him and did not even care. I had become a big "minus," a parasitic container, destructively drawing in his positive affects to feed my negative ones. Yes, he was quite aware of a transference dimension. But that I was so much like his imperious mother—and should know better—increased his justifiable fury.

The session ended on this unsatisfactory note, leaving me shaken and concerned about the next session, and the whole course of treatment. I was uncertain of what I was doing and where I was going, and worried about the possible harm I was doing to both of us. I knew that the patient was not in treatment with a perfectly analyzed therapist. Relational theorists have emphasized that this would not be desirable, even if possible (e.g., Aron, 1996; Renik, 1996). Yes, I could be all that he had accused me of, but was I really being unfriendly? Or, could he not appreciate that what he experienced as a negative affect could contribute positively to our relationship (Winnicott, 1949)? I felt I needed to be less "nice," just when he felt I needed to be nicer.

Still, I was troubled by the realization that I might be enacting hate towards him. I questioned whether my change in attitude represented success in utilizing this primal affect, in its state of only vague coherence, to understand and communicate my understanding, and not to act out my relationship to the patient and the situation between us.

I had to inspect my communications, my private as well as public dialogue, to see what I was really feeling, saying, and doing. The analyst must utilize his or her own primal feelings in reaching the interpretation, but not use the communication for countertransference conveyance, that is, "as a vehicle for transmission of some aspect of L or H" (Bion, 1965, p. 61). As far as I was aware, my motive in making the intervention was not to enact the transference-countertransference, to develop a more confrontational style with the patient, or to otherwise dramatize the situation. I had some confidence that my communications were good and appropriate; thus, we differed greatly in our opinions as to whether an apology or change in delivery was required.

I was surprised when, in the following hour, the patient made no reference to what had occurred and proceeded without further recrimination. We returned to our affectionate and respectful relationship until the next incident. This pattern continued: he became hurt and indignant, and I expressed little enthusiasm for apologizing or responding to his efforts to educate me. He remonstrated unsuccessfully, left unhappily, and returned without referring to the incident.

Inviting the patient to change his attitude

I began to inquire about his lack of follow-up to what he experienced as my egregious behavior. Such interventions only served to arouse his anger. "You again!" was the implication in his tone. "Haven't you learned anything?" At this point in our work, we still could not talk thoughtfully about what he experienced as the negative aspects of my emotional participation. I was being insistent and self-justifying. I was taunting him, exhibiting and making him deal with problems that were clearly mine, and not his or ours.

He was becoming resigned to putting up with me and would like simply to avoid rather than deal with the outbreaks of the uneducable, bad me. I felt I could not allow us this option. Certainly, I could not go back to the old way, which felt safe and known. It was all too passionless: my clumsy and arrogant disregard, his smooth righteousness. I had to trust that my persistence in raising the subject of our distressful interactions was reasonable and caring, and not motivated primarily by the unconscious pathological trends of which he accused me.

However, while I wanted to discuss these interactions, I was disinclined to budge from my view of them or effortfully explain myself. It was unlikely that he was entirely right about us and I was entirely wrong, I contended. But he would have to make his own decision. Even if the worst-case scenario were true and he had found an exact replica of his stubborn, self-justifying mother, he need not become a replica as well. An opportunity existed for him to respond differently, even if I would not.

The patient was of two minds regarding this line of intervention. He found it appealing that he could be, and should be, a better person than the dictators in his life (his mother and me). Yet he also found me infuriatingly clever, as if, with full awareness, I was using my mind to rationalize my behavior, to outwit him. I was torturing him, he decried, "brainwashing" him.

Typically, his response prompted another round of my self-doubt. When he analyzed my character pathology, he emphasized a dimension of my self-experience of which I was vaguely aware, and which had a ring of dreaded truth. For as I have indicated, I, too, worried over my verbal formulations, and self-consciously examined, along with the words themselves, subtleties in timing, tone, and cadence, to discover any dissociated hostile emotional intent, any motive to outpower (Billow, 1999).

Now when he would mention it, I guiltily could bring forth a desire to outwit him, even to torture him, for I felt he had tortured and brainwashed me. And at these times, I felt that I was doing so. Hence, when the patient criticized me for being like his tormentor-mother, he had captured and magnified an aspect of my self-experience. Was I caught up in the patient's fantasy, acting out his bad-mother introject? Or, was I properly exercising my primal affects, fulfilling the arduous job requirements of our profession?

Passion in the interpretation

A good intervention is an emotional experience for the analyst as well as for the patient. The analyst must unconsciously "decide" not to evade developing his or her own primitive fantasies and feelings, so that he or she (in reverie as well as "R") may achieve knowledge of what is being felt and not felt in the relationship. Empathy requires the analyst feeling the primal affects of that aspect of the patient's self to which attention is drawn. In effect, the analyst "becomes" the person of an interpretation (Bion, 1965, p. 164).

At the same time, the analyst feels the horror and resistance to that very becoming and is liable to reject the part of him- or herself motivated to think about, much less make, the interpretation.

I knew in my "gut" how it felt to be him. I had contained (unconsciously as well as consciously) those projected emotional elements of which the patient was only partially aware, and I was working them over myself. He had identified with an imperious mother who acted narcissistically injured when another person (her son) diverted from her felt needs. In asserting his autonomy by reacting against her, he chose her torturous weapons of defense: self-righteous indignation and moral condemnation. He could not tolerate his mother's behavior without protesting, but in his protest, aligned with her. He had difficulty separating from her (and from me) to develop his own way of thinking and feeling.

And apparently, in regard to our impasse, I had had similar difficulty in separating from him. I had been victim to the "numbing reality" Bion described: the feeling of being trapped in another's fantasy, of not giving and being unable to give the proper interpretation, and of being a particular kind of (sadistic and guilty) person in this emotional situation.

Like the patient, I was now of two minds. I felt and understood something of the interplay of the patient's projections with my concordant and complementary identifications (Racker, 1968). That is, I was aware that I could easily identify with his victimized self and experience him as the bad mother. I monitored my wishes to masochistically submit to the patient's sadism, or to sadistically rebel by becoming the mother and treating him harshly. I knew I could not continue to bend over backwards out of fear that he would otherwise connect his "bad mother" to me. Still, I dreaded becoming that sadistic person of the transference and felt—despite my intellectual understanding to the contrary—that I was being sadistic, unfair, even wrongheaded in raising his consciousness by bringing to the fore this view of me.

While all this was going on inside me and between us, I tried mentally to let go. Achieving passion requires moments of "mindlessness," in which feelings as well as thoughts and fantasies need to be suspended or negated. I had to bear being with him and bear being without him. Removing myself from the proverbial frying pan of "memory and desire" (Bion, 1967a), I landed in the fire of my isolation.

I was on my own and suffered loneliness, confusion, and worse, premonitions of personal and professional catastrophe. I could not be sure that I was committed to an evolving, independent point of view, rather than being stubborn and arrogant, megalomaniacal, or even crazy. I was without the patient, without the comfort of our painfully as well as pleasurably familiar transference-countertransference, and without the approving presence of my psychoanalytic ancestry: the theorists, teachers, colleagues, and patients, past and present, who bolster one's established point of view. The absence of these ongoing relationships intensified feelings of persecution and depression. And I dreaded the reemergence of my primal affects, for I did not know where they would take me or us. The relationship had undergone "catastrophic change," and there could be no going back.

There is, paradoxically, relief in "passion," relief in the analyst's tolerating the evolution of emotional meaning. My feeling of "becoming" the patient (and the patient's mother) was only part of the story. My pain and confusion, my very isolation from the patient and from being the authoritative "professional," contributed to the feeling that I was not being the person of the interpretation. I was a person feeling feelings and making sense of them as best I could. In being myself, I felt analytically disciplined.

Indeed, I felt intensely ambivalent about my patient and the predicament I was in. Ambivalence would seem essential to working through transference-countertransference (Bird, 1972). However, I believe I allowed my ambivalence to evolve such to be able to speak caringly and knowledgeably from an integrated subjectivity. In constructing my thoughts about him and our situation, and in formulating the intervention, I was experiencing hate, but also maintaining emotional linkages based on love and knowledge-seeking. That is, I loved and hated him, knew something about the how and why of these feelings, and was curious to learn more. Some of these feelings had to do primarily with him and his projected object relations, benign as well as pathological. These were relatively easy to understand and to interpret. Some were personal to me and my object relations, including those participating in my "infantile neurosis" aroused by the patient's transference and by the analytic situation itself (Racker, 1968). These were my responsibilities to know about, analyze, and not act out. Finally, some feelings evolved from the suffering of my passion: from thinking and not thinking about our emotional situation. Ideally, these are the feelings which the analyst attempts to integrate and make available to the patient, in silences as well as in verbal interventions.

Passion's effect

The patient signaled what I understood to be a significant change in his attitude when he offhandedly acknowledged that, in the past, he had been "ferocious" with me. I pressed on: And now? Only when I deserved it, he replied, with a humor that I did not share. But did I really deserve it? I continued, not expecting, or receiving, a satisfying response to my rhetorical question.

With time, the patient has become more tolerant of my referring to our irruptions and of pursuing a serious dialogue, as long as I do not "dwell" on the topic and deter us from what he considers to be more important business. Subsequent conversations have confirmed that, for the first time in our work, he is struggling with the possibility that perhaps I am not so bad when being bad, and that he has options other than to evade or "cure" me.

To different degrees, then, we both have become comfortable with the idea that, even when he experiences me at my hateful worst, I may be linking to him with interest and caring.

Further, he is beginning to realize what it is about him (rather than about me) which keeps him from relating differently. Modifying his intolerant attitude towards me has made it easier for him to consider his own difficulties with "passion." He has come to accept the hypothesis that his hatred of hatred—his fear and consequent ferocious intolerance of thinking about and integrating that emotion—has made it difficult for him to be different, with me and with the women he has sought to love.

We cannot be sure of the "causes" for the apparent changes in both our attitudes, of the accuracy of the interactional dynamics I have described, or even of the reality of my passion. The analyst can never be fully aware of his or her own feelings or of the patient's. Such awareness would assume knowledge of a verifiable, objective reality. The analyst can only speak of how he or she feels about what he or she feels, utilizing the primal affects to sustain the basis of signification. And the analyst's opinion may not represent the best assessment. Another person, such as the reader or the patient, may have a view of reality which is equal or better.[1] Since meaning develops over time, we may arrive at "second opinions." The passion of today's interpretation may come to be realized tomorrow as yesterday's enactment (see Renik, 1996, p. 392).

Conclusion: transforming pain into passion

Bion argued that psychoanalytic treatment is not about cure but about transforming obvious pain into the richer capacity to "suffer" meaning. This entails tolerating the emergence of the full range of primal affects—L, H, and K—and the concomitant persecution, depression, anxiety, and dread. However, the patient has come to treatment to be relieved from pain. He or she initially may display little toleration for increasing the range of felt feelings or for understanding and integrating them.

In psychoanalytic work, it is often left to the analyst to suffer mental pain. Grotstein (1995) contended that "the analyst's actual trial suffering of the patient's pains as his or her own *is* the transference, from the patient to the analyst" (p. 483, his emphasis). I have suggested that the analyst's "trial-yet-real suffering" (Grotstein, 1995, p. 483) involves tolerating the painful emergence of one's own primal affects. In essence, the analyst's activity of discovery and development of his or her own passion buffers the analyst from reactions to the patient's emotions and being taken over by them. The active processing of personal experience connects the analyst to, and separates the analyst from, the patient (and from the analyst's self in relation to the patient).

In the case I described, my fear of unconsciously enacting my hatred functioned as a suppressor of my creative emotional participation, as I initially treated the patient's demandingness with kid gloves. I had set the stage for repetitive experiences of transference-countertransference. I had to develop the confidence to be myself, trusting that in "releasing" my hatred, I was maintaining an outlook balanced by the participation of love and curiosity as well. The patient could continue to experience me as primarily hateful, but he needed me to maintain and express a separate opinion. In developing the confidence to think for myself and by myself, I could express passion.

In the clinical situation, the patient exists as a real person, a transference figure, and ideally a versatile mental object of the analyst. In the latter role, the patient provides a medium of growth in which the analyst converts his or her own pain into meaningful suffering. In this situation, the patient stands for the analyst's original object of passion, the mother who is present and absent, loved, hated, recognized but never fully known. The analyst needs to achieve a state of mind in which he or she has the "moral freedom" (Racker, 1968) to think, and hence to develop and exercise passion. When engaged passionately, the analyst may confidently "feel anything," if not "say anything." The analyst is not hampered by rigid transferences to inner or outer objects which obstruct formulating and, if appropriate, expressing feelings and thoughts in the form of interpretative opinions.

Paradoxically, while passion represents the deepest level of meaning in intimate relations (Meltzer, 1978), the attainment of passion disturbs conventional notions of intimacy. While passion integrates the primal affects with warmth and "without any suggestion of violence," the emotional process—the breakups and breakdowns of what is known and subjectively felt—may feel catastrophic. And, rightfully, the consequences of passion may be dreaded. For, while passion offers new possibilities and new beginnings, established links to patients, as well as to oneself, are altered in often unexpected ways.

Bion might have better defined "passion" as referring to an emotional process which is intense and which does not involve a suggestion of *unnecessary* violence. Applying reason to one's emotional experiences, and applying emotion to one's reasoning, disorients and reorients the thinker—to the past, present, and future, to the self and the other. Self-knowledge brings forth the primacy of self-integration over repression and splitting; hence, self-knowledge brings some inner peace and social harmony to our inherent as well as induced conflicts. "Passion" enlarges the capacity for ever greater levels of emotional turbulence, existential risk, and creative disharmony.

Note

1   Predating contemporary relational theories, Bion (1970) acknowledged an interactive or co-constructive element in the analyst's opinion: "The interpretation is an actual event in an evolution of 0 [the psychoanalytic experience] that is common to analyst and analysand."

Chapter 7

Relational variations of the container-contained

Thinking, according to Bion, is a primary emotional need and matures in the context of social communication. He formulated the essential process of how thinking and communicating mutually develop in terms of a model of "container-contained." The model draws attention to how we hear and think about another's communication, how we convey our experience back, and how this communicative interplay impacts the participants and the immediate future of the relationship.

The container-contained illuminates symbol formation, human development, internal and external object relations, and learning from (and resisting) emotional experience, and includes three variants: *commensal*, *symbiotic*, and *parasitic* interactions (Bion, 1970). The extended model of the container-contained offers a way of listening, processing, and formulating that can be helpful in doing, supervising, or reflecting on all types of clinical interactions. It is also helpful in framing how the therapist and patient interact at preverbal levels.

In this chapter, I utilize the model in recounting my thinking and clinical behavior while supervising an analyst.

The clinical problem, as presented

"I'm pissed at Mary. She's threatening to quit group. What should I do? I'm seeing her tomorrow. Hi, how are you?"

The speaker is an analyst, whom we will call Dr. A, and I am her supervisor of 11 months. Mary is a patient of Dr. A in a weekly group and also in twice-weekly individual psychoanalytic sessions.

In a recent group session, John had confronted Mary, which led to a heated exchange. In Dr. A's opinion, Mary gave as good as she got, but Mary felt hurt and withdrew for the rest of the session. She missed the next group, after leaving a message on Dr. A's answering machine that she had to attend a church function that was much more important. In the intervening individual session, Mary reported: "I have another church meeting to go to on group night. Besides, I'm thinking of leaving group. The church treats me better."

Although the patient had questioned the value of group and had threatened to terminate on other occasions during the past five years, this was the first time she had upped the ante by actually missing a session, and she seemed intent on missing another one.

Dr. A reported that she had remained neutral and, in her words, "above the fray" during the altercation between the two group members, which was but briefly responded to by others. In the individual session, the analyst had explored the patient's associations, which were rather concretely linked to her state of affairs in group. She had reminded the patient that they had been here before, cautioned against precipitous behavior, and encouraged her to deal with her anger and hurt in the group. These interventions and subsequent interpretations had failed to influence the patient. And now, Dr. A would have to report Mary's absence to the other group members. She feared being blamed for not intervening between the two members in a timely or adequate fashion. She would lose face and have more damage to control. Other patients would want to leave, the group would disband, and her individual analytic practice would be in shambles. Dr. A had, of course, attempted to withhold these anxious feelings and fantasies in her individual work, and not direct them at her patients.

I listened sympathetically and made a few theoretical remarks to establish that we saw the clinical situation similarly and that perhaps, in time, the patient might as well. I did not believe I was particularly useful, and I had no urgent desire to be useful. As far as I was aware, my prominent emotional state was one of unfulfilled interest or curiosity.

I now knew some "facts" of the clinical exchanges among analyst, patient, and group. But I did not have a good sense of what the clinician was really saying emotionally and what the patient and group were hearing. I was not sure what the analyst was asking for when she said "what should I do?", what she needed, and what I was willing, and able, to give. From my point of view, the necessity was to think: to learn about ourselves, our relationship, and, of course, the patient, other members of the group, and the ongoing individual and group psychotherapy processes. To avoid—as much as possible—a "situation in which two inarticulate personalities are unable to release themselves from the bondage of inarticulation" (Bion, 1970, p. 15), Dr. A and I would have to "think."

The container-contained and its three relational variations

Dr. A's opening comments, that she was "pissed" at Mary and what should she do about Mary's threat to leave group, and her anticipation of blame and abandonment, provided a wealth of emotional data. The analyst's communications had many levels of unarticulated emotional meaning and released in me feelings of my own. In making sense of my experience of being with the supervisee, Bion's relational morphology of the container-contained had come to mind:

> The individual cannot contain the impulses proper to a pair and the pair cannot contain the impulses proper to a group. The psycho-analytic problem is the problem of growth and its harmonious resolution in the relationship between the container and the contained, repeated in individual, pair, and finally group (intra and extra psychically).
>
> (Bion, 1970, pp. 15–16)

This compressed passage pertains specifically to the inherent problems in human communication and the importance of others in supporting the individual's drive to think and develop meaning. The container-contained represents the transformatory process of the mind—one mind or many minds—reaching emotional awareness. It is a model of emotional learning that develops and is sustained in interaction with others. Force is exerted in both directions; to some extent, the container and the contained mutually determine each other.

In human development, container-contained processes initially are *symbiotic*, based on early infant-[m]other projective–introjective exchanges. The infant's symbolic "sojourn in the breast" (Bion, 1962, p. 183) makes manageable the child's need to understand itself and others, placing the need—and its satisfaction—in the relational context. The normally empathic [m]other gathers in (introjects), deciphers, and communicates back to the infant aspects of its psychic experience beyond its current cognitive and emotional capabilities. By containing the infant's primitive feelings, and interesting the infant in them, the receptive [m]other fosters the development of a "normal part" (Bion's terminology) of the infant's personality that concerns itself with psychic quality.

To an increasing degree, the child becomes able to contain feelings while in the [m]other's absence, and to transform them into images and rudimentary prototypes of sophisticated thought. These internal containers develop that which previously was split off and/or projected. In other words, symbols and thoughts now serve the functions to transform preverbal emotional meaning, functions once provided primarily by the other. The developing child gradually comes to tolerate and process its own emotional experience, developing a rudimentary consciousness of self and other. The child has formed an internal model of a thinking couple. Independent thinking has begun, as *commensal* relations are established with one's own mind and the minds of others.

However, as we know, psychic development and functioning does not at all times proceed smoothly. Thinking and relating may easily regress to the dependent level of symbiotic communicating. More pathological is the *parasitic* variation, in which severe blockages develop between the container and

the contained. Because of traumatic early failures in infant–caretaker relationships, the individual (or the traumatized part of the personality) comes
to experience containing and being contained as untrustworthy, painful,
and dangerous. When parasitic dynamics prevail, the container-contained
represents a hostile and destructive process. Thinking—and thinkers—
must be avoided or attacked.

The clinical problem, in terms of the three variations of the container-contained

I felt that we had not got at the analyst's presenting problem, which involved
some disturbance in the container-contained. It seemed apparent that the
disturbance existed on many levels: in Dr. A, in Mary, in their relationship,
and in Mary and Dr. A's relationships to the group. Most likely, a disturbance also existed in Dr. A's relationship to me. For didactic purposes, I
framed our dialogue through Bion's tripartite model of container-contained
to the supervisee, and now to the reader, in the order commensal, symbiotic,
parasitic. I emphasize that all three relational levels happen at once, and the
therapist has to attend mentally to all three levels at once.

Commensal relations

In commensal relationships, "two objects share a third to the advantage of
all three." The participants create and share the "analytic third" (Ogden,
1994), the dialogic emotional relationship that becomes the primary subject of mutual interest. Language functions as container, used to organize
and explain conscious and unconscious emotional experience, and language
also exists as the contained, a mode of experience.

Assuming that we were in, or could easily shift to, commensal relating,
I treated as evocative metaphor and as unexplored fantasy the supervisee's
description of her internal state ("pissed"), her entreaty ("What should I
do?"), and her anticipation of blame and group dissolution. I did not respond symbiotically, such as by trying to be reassuring, or even "helpful."
Calling attention to our relationship instead, I agreed, sardonically, that
we ought to "do" something to relieve the analyst's state of mind. And, to
underline how unhelpful I was at doing, I noted that nothing the analyst did
with her patient—neither her interpretations nor her entreaties—or I was
doing with her, accomplished this goal.

The analyst responded indirectly to my rueful comments by reminding
us that the group had heated up since she had been in supervision, and
she liked the liveliness. But she did not like feeling that emotions were
getting out of control. She was referring to her patient, and to the fighting
in group, but also communicating that she did not like the sense that her
emotions were getting out of control. I wondered playfully whether she

ever felt her supervisor was out of control, and whether, at present, she even liked him.

She smiled conspiratorially. "I know you want me to be very 'bad,' and my patients to be bad too." And then, quite seriously: "My mother didn't tolerate anybody being out of control, and when I feel I might be, I freeze up with anxiety and fear, and try to 'get it right' by being very good. This is how my mother wanted me to be."

In freezing up her not nice emotions, the analyst had attempted to suppress and deny her sense of internal badness, that is, her own bad feelings, fantasies, and thoughts, and possibility of bad behavior. By inviting a dialogue, and not freezing these aspects of her subjectivity, she offered us emotional ideas. These we could develop commensally within the supervisee–supervisor relationship and apply to a nesting of clinical and personal situations. Our relationship existed as a shared, dynamic structure, growing in emotional flexibility and abstraction, while remaining linked to our ongoing, lived-out present, and was thus commensal.

If she were to "do" what the supervision experience hopefully modeled, she would have to find her own way to establish the commensal pattern of relationships. The patient, Mary, had threatened to terminate group but not individual work. This suggested an unanalyzed split in the patient's mind between a bad group therapist and a good analyst. The split also existed in the therapist's mind, but she was attempting to address the split in the supervision. Did other members find their group therapist to be bad? And how so? These investigative questions are emotional ideas that may be presented to the patient and group, to be contained for mutual consideration. But to present difficult ideas to others, the analyst must first be willing to think and feel about them.

That is, to maintain commensal relations, the clinician must be in and not above the fray. Containing—putting into words transformations of the patient's conflictual feelings, thoughts, and fantasies—brings to the fore aspects of the history and current state of the analyst's own conflicts. In this example, by sharing painful inner experience, the supervisee was willing to be in the fray with me. To meet her commensally as the clinical supervisor, I also had to be in the fray. This meant achieving (relative) comfort with the inner experience of my own "badness" and being willing to re-evoke and think about my badness with the supervisee. With this accomplished, I could then help the supervisee become more comfortable containing the idea of "badness," hers, mine, her patients', such that she could think about and share the idea within her clinical practice.

Commensally based relations are characterized by this important dimension of self-analysis, a willingness to feel, think about, and, if appropriate, put into the dialogue, that which otherwise would not be shared openly, but suppressed or acted out.

There are times, of course, when the patient or group is not ready or not willing to tolerate the internal and interpersonal processes of feeling, thinking, and sharing conflictual experience, or allow the therapist to do so. In contrast, words are valued as vehicles to express need and to have needs met. This brings us to the symbiotic dimension of the container-contained.

Symbiotic relations

In symbiotic relations, "one depends on another to mutual advantage." Symbiotic interactions are characterized by projective identifications that evoke enactments in which one individual comes to feel contained by another. Language is employed for irrational or pre-rational uses, via mechanisms of introjection and projection, for interpersonal connection and not valued primarily for their semantic content. For example, a patient may store (i.e., introject), the analyst's words, deriving a sense of connection and comfort from the very act of being spoken to. The individual also may discharge (i.e., project), affectual need through the release of words, successfully establishing contact and influence, via vocal intonation and emphasis, verbal repetition, and so forth.

Mature dialogue, in which semantic meaning participates fully, rests on the relational bed of such pre-articulate, projective–introjective exchanges. These exchanges are "emotionally rewarding...[establishing] a sense of being in contact...a primitive form of communication that provides a foundation on which, ultimately, verbal communication depends" (Bion, 1967b, p. 92).

To maintain empathic contact, the therapist must invite such communications, without making demands on the other to be consistent, intellectually articulate, or morally "correct." In this example, the patient, Mary, felt "badness" emerging in the therapeutic relationships and alerted the therapist by her words and behavior. Dr. A, perhaps to a lesser degree than Mary, had difficulty containing "badness," accepting and thinking about bad feelings, without external support. And, parallel to the patient, the analyst was signaling the clinical other (me) to do something about these feelings, making them less bad, such that Dr. A could accept and think about them herself.

To think commensally, and to help the other move from a symbiotic to commensal level, the receiver needs to be in contact with goodness and badness, while maintaining the love of one's own inner objects. From this position of inner security, the receiver can more easily evaluate that which the other is projecting and also what the other dreads to project and therefore to reveal.

It was not clear how anxious the patient was, how serious her threats were, or what she needed from her therapist or group to foster a dialogue. To think about these clinical issues, the analyst would have to place herself in the transferential-countertransferential vortex of the total situation, momentarily becoming the patient with bad feelings, as well as the patient's bad object. She would have to engage her own basic affects in the process of understanding, allowing these affects to develop into fantasies, thoughts, wishes, and fears that could appear, to the mature mind, to be primitive, immoral, unprofessional—"not nice." Dr. A had not done this, but responded "analytically." From this point of view, the analyst's analytic attitudes, her neutrality, limit setting, admonitions to return to group, insight-oriented interventions, and so forth, served as actions taken to relieve the analyst's anxiety about "badness," to avoid thinking about badness, and not to contain the patient's.

In the supervisory session, I served as the symbiotic other who welcomed basic affects, including what was "not nice," particularly about me. Symbolically, I took in her piss, accepting with good humor, caring, and commensally based understanding, her sense of badness about the whole clinical situation, consisting of her patient, the group, herself, and me. Unburdening and placing in me to develop, modify, and return what she could not emotionally process by herself, she could resume thinking.

"I haven't let Mary play out her anger, the way you're doing with me," the analyst volunteered, "but I think I'm ready to now. I'll bite the bullet. We'll see what will happen." I had confidence that she would return to the individual and group work communicating an increased toleration for emotional experience.

We may appreciate how containing on the symbiotic level requires far more than passive "holding," in which the therapist construes the task as supplying warmth and security until the patient indicates readiness for psychoanalytic dialogue. Symbiotic processing requires the analyst to think actively about—and to respond strategically to—intense emotional reactions that are ambiguously communicated. And consequently, the analyst's counter-reactions must also be understood.

The analyst attempts to accommodate to the individual's symbiotic needs, longings, and fears, without mindlessly submitting to or prematurely interpreting them. Accommodations may be subtle, communicated by bodily and tonal responses as much as by overt action or actual dialogue, and may be directed towards unexpressed rather than expressed wishes. The analyst must differentiate between expressions of genuine needs for contact and regressive exaggerations or defensive minimization of needs, and between fantasies involved in seeking symbiotic relatedness and pathologically entitled actions employed to gratify such wishes. In many instances, the dynamics and behavior of entitlement may be fruitfully—if not always immediately—interpreted (Billow, 1999).

Therapy at the symbiotic relational level depends on a trust that the therapist earns by establishing a balance between accommodation to and interpretation of symbiotic communications. Containing may involve limit-setting and other boundary-maintaining procedures, confrontation, verbal reframing, clarification, and interpretation. While the symbiotic communicator may not fully understand or care to understand the meaning expressed in such interventions, he or she is sensitive to the caring contained in them.

Hence, interventions must be delivered and experienced benevolently, their essential purpose being to establish "a sense of contact" with an area of the projector's personality that has insufficiently mastered self-containment. Patience, timing, and tact are particularly important in establishing and maintaining emotional contact on this relational level. Once intrapsychic and interpersonal containment is established or reestablished, individuals more easily may receive and reciprocate commensal communications.

The lines between various levels of a communication, such as affective and semantic meaning, or symbiotic and commensal interactions, are ambiguous and fluctuating, and may function in useful tension with each other. We must keep in mind that all communications, even those promoting insight, have overt and subtle performative features. Words sonically communicate felt need and exert pressure on the receiver to potentiate meaning and to respond empathically. Symbiotic communications remain the reassuring foundation on which the more sophisticated commensal communications develop. And symbiotic communications continue to function as an important source of data collection and responsive interaction in all human relations.

Parasitic relations

In parasitic relations, "one depends on another to produce a third, which is destructive of all three." Containing or being contained is experienced as threatening and untrustworthy, and must be deflected or subverted. The goal of communication is to evade, even to destroy, meaning and meaningful emotional exchanges. The very act of thinking may be hated as a process that confuses and leads to pain; therefore, commensal dialogue is dangerous, since it stimulates thought and leads to meaning. Symbiotic relatedness may be experienced as inauthentic and entrapping, and the individual experiences a good deal of anxiety and little reliable pleasure in empathic contact with self or other. Parasitic communications may be provocatively direct, as well as subtle and not immediately identifiable.

In the case example, formal, semantic, and paraverbal aspects of the patient's communications illustrate parasitic attacks on commensal and symbiotic links. Mary's use of telephone answering machine and physical absence from the group removes communication from its appropriate time and place, obstructing opportunity for commensal dialogue. Her abandonment threats and withdrawal of positive emotion disturb trust and security, the symbiotic basis of relationships.

Parallel parasitic relational processes occurred in the supervision. Both patient and supervisee were pissed. "What should I do?" Dr. A. implored of me. Like the patient's, her words, on this relational level, were delivered not primarily to communicate and mutually develop feeling, but to relieve feeling by provoking potentially destructive interaction.

I felt an unpleasant something come my way, which, initially, I did not understand. For a moment, I did not like Dr. A. I report my emotional situation not to record negative countertransference but to suggest its relevance in the development of my thinking. In allowing this vague, bad feeling to cohere, I trusted its value in developing my thoughts. And indeed, I soon realized that the badness I felt was a pressure to do something that I could not or did not want to do.

This realization brought personal relevance to my situation with Dr. A and to hers with Mary and group. I did not like what the analyst-supervisee was doing. The analyst did not like what the patient was doing. The patient did not like what the analyst (and her group) was doing. Each of us felt bad and felt the other as bad and not in control. Each of us felt violated and untrusting, and pressured to take non-analytic action.

Like the analyst with her patient, I first had to admit and not freeze my emotional thoughts and fantasies, trusting that they could be relevant and valuable in advancing intersubjective awareness. To think self-consciously about Dr. A's difficulty in thinking and maintain a sense of contact to her, I had to achieve a "decrease of inhibition but also a decrease of the impulse to inhibit" (Bion, 1970, p. 129). That is, I had to feel her attacks on the thinking process and on me, and feel and think about my emotional reactions to these attacks, without mindlessly complying, withdrawing, or retaliating. Indeed, I wanted to comply with the supervisee's demand for me to tell her what to do. I wanted to resist and become sarcastic, or quiet and passive-aggressive. I wanted to blind her with brilliant insights regarding her behavior towards me.[1]

I had felt not nice emotions, thoughts, and fantasies, which I applied to understand and not participate in the parasitic process. Now I could participate with the inner security and relaxed attention appropriate to empathic analytic work. Containing on this level involves preserving and communicating an emotionally balanced state of mind, one that invites the patient or supervisee to participate within it. I wondered whether the patient and the group might accept this invitation from Dr. A.

In the face of parasitic attacks, the analyst needs a container for his or her own stimulated affects. The therapeutic frame of regulated availability, one's knowledge and training, the clinician's legitimate entitlement to assert limits, all may provide this essential function. Particularly important is the analyst's capacity to tolerate hating and being hated, while sustaining benevolence towards the patient and curiosity regarding the interaction. By maintaining a non-retaliatory "disrespect" (Caper, 1997) for therapy-destructive behavior, as well as a caring understanding, in time the therapist may disarm parasitic communication and cultivate longed for but distrusted symbiotic and commensal relatedness.

Further, individuals who communicate parasitically may retain a capacity to reflect on such behavior and may respond positively to feedback from the therapist (and other members of a group). As Steiner (1994) emphasized, even a patient who hates "the whole idea of being understood....needs the analyst to register what is happening and to have his situation and his predicament recognized" (p. 132). An individual communicating parasitically may decide (unconsciously as much as consciously) to be contained within therapeutic parameters or may continue to attempt to challenge or destroy parameters. At times, the individual may decide to do both, and it is left to the therapist to describe how and why the conflict between containing and anti-containing is being played out.

New problems presented in the next supervisory session

A week had passed, and new problems regarding the group had emerged in the mind of the supervisee. A woman opened the session by reporting that she might take a series of sailing lessons on group night. She would be missed, other members responded. An idea from previous sessions recirculated: the group could get together at a singles' bar. But what of Dr. A's reaction? She once had been quite firm about the rule of no after-group fraternizing. Now she claimed to be willing to discuss anything. The members were not convinced. A debate ensued over the merits of what the group assumed to be the therapist's position and why she seemed to be changing it. The discussion then turned to other topics. But Dr. A dreaded what she had heard, and to some extent "froze" for the rest of the session. "The group was lively," she reported, "but I wasn't."

I wondered if some carryover existed from the incident with Mary and the male member. "Oh that resolved itself, Mary is back and in fact she defended me!" Another woman and not Mary threatened to disturb commensal and symbiotic relating. This member expressed the universal and omnipresent conflict over thinking versus nonthinking, the latter thematically developed in the group's tacit blessing of a member's "sailing away," and in the wish for a boundary-violating meeting in a single's bar.

The nestings of clinical problems represented by the container-contained had reemerged, although some of the emotional particulars had reconfigured with different participants. In the therapist's mind, somebody was being bad and out of control, and the therapist feared rejection and group dissolution. There were not nice feelings, and doings, calls to action, asserting mental pressure on Dr. A's relationship to individual patients and group, herself, and me.

The psychoanalytic problem: loosening the "bonds of inarticulation"

The terms "objects" and "object relations" signify thoughts at various levels of abstraction, and the container-contained specifies not a static relationship between thoughts but "a pattern of relationships in the way that mathematicians speak of mathematics as expressing relationships" (Bion, 1970, p. 95). From concrete mental representations of aspects of relationships— of mouth, vagina (the container), breast, and penis (the contained)—the pattern becomes progressively more complex and recurs constantly throughout mental development. "From such relatively simple beginnings the...[container-contained] abstracts successively more complex hypotheses and finally whole systems of hypotheses which are known as scientific deductive systems" (1962, p. 94).

The concept of container-contained describes, then, modes of relating that are dynamic and fluctuating, cognitively multilevel, and interpersonally multidimensional. We come to learn about and represent intersubjective experience at various developmental levels of thought. The pattern of relationships is modeled on vague interoceptive memories of mouth–breast relations, as well on dyadic, triadic, and group relationships. The pattern exists in the commitment to abstract religious, aesthetic, and scientific principles, which still represent object relations pertaining to one's place in the family, society, and universe.

A nesting process is involved, for the container at one level of symbolic transformation serves as the contained at another. For example, the individual serves as container for one's thought (itself a container), but is contained in the larger social network. The nesting process must remain emotionally flexible, mobile, and reversible. Like the empathic [m]other on whom the experience of being contained is based, the container must retain the capacity to remain integrated, while penetrable with fresh emotion. "On the replacement of one emotion...by another emotion...does the capacity for re-formation, and therefore, receptivity, [of the container] depend" (Bion, 1962, p. 93).

To learn from experience, one must link up emerging emotions and emotional thoughts by interacting with the containing minds of other human beings. Interaction is not limited to actual interpersonal contact; it includes thinking as involved in mathematics, listening to music, reading Shakespeare or Freud, etc. The social container of the other, including the parental pair, family, and cultural groups, actively participates in making experience meaningful. In extreme adversarial interpersonal situations, which may include clinical impasse or intense negative transference-countertransference, the social network of the dyad or group is experienced as failing in the containing function. The participants must rely on the internally generated container-contained to maintain self-conscious links to reality, meaning-construction, and the possibility for constructive interpersonal interaction.

Conclusion: the analyst's problems remain

The uses to which a communication is put are critical to understanding meaning, and meaning is often offered ambiguously and ambivalently. The communicative intent and effect of any exchange remains subjective, influenced by the intersubjective context, and malleable upon further reflection. In any therapeutic interaction, it is likely that there are the three relational variations: commensal, symbiotic, and parasitic. While striving to function commensally, the clinician must respond with patience and creativity to the reality that the other may wish to communicate predominantly on another relational level. Also, we must accept that as analysts, we share the human limitation in containing emotional experience and must rely on our patients (as well as on others) to further that which we cannot or do not want to feel and understand alone.

All of us need and fear containing, and scrutinize our environment for suitable objects, human and nonhuman (Mirtani, 1996). In interpersonal situations, we register how and if our emotions and thoughts are being contained, and our success at containing others'. Such mental activity most often takes place without conscious awareness and is communicated by subtle changes in our own relatedness. And thus, the intersubjective process evolves, as ongoing and shifting self-other evaluations mutually influence decisions to participate *commensally*, *symbiotically*, and *parasitically*.

Note

1 In Bion's typology of "minus emotions," my initial reactions fell into the categories of −L (compliance), −H (aggressive acting out), and −K (knowledge used to obstruct meaning making. See also Chapter 5).

Section III

Group process
Moving towards K

Editor's note

Successful group meetings, according to Billow, are ones where leader and members engage in the pursuit of significant psychological truths. These can be historical reconstructions, here-and-now interpersonal realizations, or even common existential anxieties. No matter. To an extent, it is less about the garden than it is about the gardening, more about the open-ended pursuit of knowledge (K) than its attainment. But how do groups come to possess the necessary blend of patience, creativity, and rigor that allow growth to occur? And how can deep convictions be challenged and modified without reflexive dismissal of the other, or masochistic submission? The four chapters in this section deal with group processes and leader interventions that address these questions and facilitate behaviors and felt experiences likely to increase co-operation, creative problem-solving, and psychological-mindedness.

Chapter 8 focuses on *bonding*, the feeling of connectedness necessary for any meaningful learning to occur. For group members to be moved by fellow members or by the leader, they need to be sufficiently confident of their benevolent intentions, integrity, and trustworthiness; they need to feel like the other is doing something *with* them rather than *to* them (Benjamin, 1990). In discussing—and illustrating—his technical approach to bonding, Billow provides an alternative to the contemporary relational focus on recognition, rupture, and repair (e.g., Benjamin, 1990) or the self-psychological/Winnicottian emphasis on accommodation and holding (e.g., Bach, 2016). Instead, he suggests using one's subjectivity creatively and benevolently, while accessing a range of communicative tools. These include, but are not limited to, the use of humor, explicitly supportive comments, and blunt challenges. The chapter also highlights two common obstacles to bonding: misdiagnosing (and pathologizing) patients' legitimate bonding needs and overlooking our own need to feel bonded with our patients or supervisees. Once these pitfalls are identified, bonding needs are met, and anxieties worked through, members and leaders feel safer to explore new ways of being and thinking.

One of the harder things to do in a group therapy session is to identify, and expand upon, the most significant common threads. Such threads are relevant to many if not all of the participants, link members to each other, and deepen the group's discourse. Expanding on Bion's (1963) notion of a "psychoanalytic object," Billow defines a new term the "nuclear idea"[1]—an event, a theme, or a metaphor with the potential to address two questions: (1) What is at the center or heart of current group process? and (2) What has the potential to generate or release the most psychic energy? The nuclear idea may be explicitly acknowledged by the group or its leader (as in the 'checkpoints' example) or implicitly discussed (as in the 'two groups' example); it can alleviate tensions, acknowledge them, or generate new ones. Ideally, it is down-to-earth and experience near. To aid therapists (and groups) in identifying nuclear ideas, Billow suggests tuning in to what is fresh, affectively charged, and unexpected. In line with Pines's (1985) important distinction, it promotes coherence rather than merely cohesiveness.

Stated simply, group cohesiveness implies a degree of closeness between members and a general positive attitude towards the group-as-a-whole. However, groups can unite around a mutual enemy, or admiration for a sports team, and this does not necessarily provide therapeutic benefits. Coherence implies a unity that is based on a shared logic or higher order organization. In the therapy group, this is achieved despite (or perhaps owing to) the other's separateness, and through an agreement to keep learning about, and from, each other. This brings us to the next chapter, which describes the tension between two types of learning: about one's internal world and its correspondence with the external world as seen by others (reality testing), and about the creative/experimental options one has of who to become (testing reality).

Reality testing, which Freud (1917b, p. 233) classified as "one of the major institutions of the ego," continues to be an essential aspect of group work, regardless of stage. In relaying the importance of reality testing to me, Billow contended that a large reason why patients stay in treatment is that they trust the accuracy—and clinical relevance—of their therapists' reality-oriented interventions. Like any good explanatory system, reality testing reduces the level of unexpectedness of events: it helps us better understand ourselves (our psychic reality) as well as others (our external reality). Within the group context, therapists promote reality testing by encouraging honest feedback, providing it themselves, and titrating the amount of "reality" different members are given based on (the therapist's assessment of) their ability to tolerate others' perspectives.

In contrast, testing reality is geared towards trying out new ways of being: a conflict-averse member may try to express dissatisfaction, an overly critical member—express empathy, and a member used to being at the center of the action—be silent. Therapists too can test reality, and their groups benefit from their willingness to improvise and take emotional risks. Of note, testing reality does not have to be behavioral and can also include new ways of being internally. By definition, it is experimental and novel, likely to move into uncharted territory. It reduces our ability to predict how others will respond to us or how we will feel at any given junction. As the chapter illustrates, the leader's role in advancing testing reality is to encourage members to go "as deep as they feel comfortable" and protect them from some of the dangers they may encounter on their psychological and interpersonal voyages.

Concluding this section is a chapter that returns to the central role of the leader in **moving the group towards K**. The four modes of relational engagement—diplomacy, integrity, sincerity, and authenticity—inform interventions as well as an overall leadership stance that both directs and models truth-seeking. *Diplomacy* is defined in the *Oxford Dictionary* (2018) as "the art of dealing with people in a sensitive and tactful way." In Billow's use of it, diplomacy does not necessitate being gentle or conflict-avoidant. Rather, it entails titrating the amount of truth that the leader believes the group can tolerate by leaning on status and authority. Examples include protecting a new or vulnerable member from scapegoating, averting the discussion away from a sensitive topic when the session is about to end, or disturbing stale alliances.

To act with *integrity* (etymologically meaning "whole"), the leader must reject sainthood and asceticism as ideals, and sometimes be willing to "sin" (Orwell, 1946/1981). As the case vignettes show, the leader is neither devoid of self-interest nor attempts to hide it. This can be freeing for members since, as many of us know, being in the presence of saints can be quite oppressive.

Sincerity and authenticity, as modes of engagement, are both used colloquially, often interchangeably, to describe a congruence between what's inside of us and what we present to the world. Here, Billow links sincerity to the either/or, idealization/demonizing stance of the Kleinian paranoid-schizoid position, and authenticity to the more mature, able-to-tolerate-ambivalence stance of the depressive position. Therapeutically, we can appreciate sincerity's importance via its less charitable opposites, hypocrisy, and dishonesty. To feel cared for, members need to trust the leader's communications despite his or her financial (and narcissistic) self-interest. Beyond words, sincerity is conveyed in tone, facial gestures, and actions over time.

I end this note with a few words on Billow's Kleinian slant on authenticity, which has yet to be sufficiently incorporated into our clinical theorizing. The distinction between our "true selves" and the "masks" we wear is, he avers, a false dichotomy. Our feelings, intense, and real as they may seem are not facts, and we are not just pretending when we occupy social roles. To use a rather trivial example from my personal life, when my four-year-old son refuses to do anything I say and gleefully splashes bath water on my dry clothes, I get thoroughly frustrated and count the minutes until he goes to bed. But being authentic means not reducing myself to this narrow version of an impatient father by holding in mind my love for him, the pride I have in myself as a caring father, and the sadness about the fleetingness of his adorable/infuriating four-year-oldness. To live authentically, we need to struggle with the tension between who we are and who we want to be, with being less dissociated, owning our projections, and being less reactive to others'. Though it is always a work in progress, our groups generally reward us for our efforts.

Note

1 An expanded exploration of the nuclear idea can be found in Billow (2015).

Chapter 8

Bonding
The group therapist's contribution

I conceive of bonding as a basic feeling of connectedness, which the individual needs to establish and maintain. Bonding is thus an ongoing aspect of intersubjective experience, a type of mental relationship to oneself and others. Behavioral, verbal, and nonverbal communications serve to establish a feeling of connection between individuals, leading them to feel satisfactorily recognized, cared for, and understood, and thus safe.

The various meanings and import of bonding easily get muddled with related concepts such as identification, group cohesion, and therapeutic and group alliance. Bonding interactions can be progressive or regressive. In this chapter I will focus particularly on the positive aspects.

As Freud (1921) suggested, bonding is based on an inborn need to love and to be in harmony with others: "a group is clearly held together by a power of some kind: and to what power could this feat be better ascribed than to Eros, which holds together everything in the world" (p. 92). Scheidlinger (1964) described a "universal need to belong, to establish a state of psychological unity with others, [which] represents a covert wish for restoring an earliest state of unconflicted well-being inherent in the exclusive union with mother" (p. 218).

Bonding and identification

Bonding is related conceptually to identification, the psychological mechanism that has been hypothesized both as a fundamental process, basic to the organization of the personality, and as the unifying principle of groups.

Freud (1921) maintained that identification was the earliest form of affective bond with another person. He understood identification as based on incorporative mechanisms. Individuals introject aspects of those they love into their egos, who now become their ego ideals. In groups, members consequently identify with each other based on their shared love of the (introjected) leader. But the process of identification may be centrifugal, an outgoing process, as well as centripetal, an ingoing process. In this case, loved aspects of oneself are projected into, and admired, in the other (Freud, 1921).

Janis (1963) defined group identification as "a set of preconscious and unconscious attitudes which incline each member to apperceive the group as an extension of himself...and to adhere to the group standards" (p. 227). Identifications may be established to the leader, other members, and the entire group, as well as to their symbolic representations (Scheidlinger, 1964). Identification may be highly regressive and pathological and lead to mob behavior, dictatorship, and psychotic depersonalization; or, it may be progressive and adaptive, fostering empathic receptivity, democracy, and inner solidarity.

However, the sense of identity, individual as well as collective (group identity), is not identical to bonding. In the psychoanalytic literature, identification is conceived primarily and defined as an unconscious mechanism, and not as a category of behavior (Grinberg, 1990). It is also a relatively permanent internalization of an object representation. Once established in the psyche, it becomes an aspect of the superego or ego.

Bonding may be understood as a cognitive-affective state that precedes and prepares the way for the complex process of identification. Like identification, bonding refers to an intrapsychic state, but it may describe a mode of behavioral interaction, and also, bonding may be quite conscious. Whereas true identification denotes a deep and lasting connectedness, bonding expresses and evokes feelings and thoughts that may be momentary or short-lived, and intense or merely marginal. For example, when attending a sporting event or a concert, individuals vary greatly in the intensity and longevity of bonding to each other and to the performers.

Furthermore, an individual may maintain identification without feeling or behaving bonded. One may have established identifications with one's university, religion, and ethnic group, but no longer feel emotionally connected. In a change of circumstance, such as an alumni reunion, religious holiday, or ethnic strife, the bonding feeling may or may not emerge with intensity.

Even after identifications are well established, bonding may remain an ongoing source of comfort and inspiration, countering paranoid and depressive anxieties. On her last day, a 20-year group veteran reported:

> I carry the group around in my head and talk to it. Whenever I'm sad, or scared or unsure, I tell you and think of what you would say to me and I straighten up. I don't think there is even half a day that goes by without me thinking of the group.

Whereas the group had provided significant identifications, it also retained a mental presence to which the individual was productively bonded.

Case example: from bonding to identification

Frank was an argumentative, opinionated, and self-centered individual, charming but also quick to anger and oppressively dominating. He entered individual therapy as a conciliatory gesture to his wife, who had discovered his extramarital affair and threatened divorce. It took my considerable efforts to get across to Frank the idea that he was not an ideal partner, in a marriage, business, or therapeutic relationship. I was not diplomatic, but blunt and challenging, which he respected since we seemed to speak the same language and not be personally offended by each other. But his wife remained offended and notified him that she was contacting a lawyer and he had better make other living arrangements. He cried, begged and pleaded, and promised to try harder in therapy.

I was surprised that when introduced to group, Frank revealed a hesitant and inhibited personality. Equally unexpected, and unknown to other members, was his immediate bond to the group, which became a focal point of his week and a central topic in our individual work. He looked forward to the group meetings, discussed them with his wife, and inspired her to join her own group.

Frank's individual sessions often were marked by his attempts to involve me in discussions of various group interactions, which I resisted to his vigorous protests: "Hey, I'm new to this game and I don't know each of the member's stories. Why can't you fill me in? Come on." He accused me of being narrow-minded and controlling: "Not everything relates to the unconscious, my parents, and what you like to call transference. I want to know because I want to know. You're creating the obstacles."

"Let's discuss the obstacles to learning the game in the game," I suggested. He insisted that I was really being unfair, putting him in the awkward position of slowing down the group process, and he refused to do that. When invited by a group member to participate, he shyly declined.

Frank's passive fascination with group life continued and, at the risk of exposing his ire to other members, I began to make interpretative hypotheses. I suggested that Frank had trouble understanding the group because this involved identifying with democratic individuals. His life had been about competition and domination. In individual sessions, I called notice to his identifications with a dictatorial, narcissistic mother, also a source of his anger and ambivalence towards women.

Uncharacteristically, Frank did not challenge these formulations or spar with me. He took seriously his difficulty in truly understanding other individuals and allowing them to understand him (see Benjamin, 1990, on mutual recognition). He began struggling with the deep maternal identification that interfered with his resolve to become a "good citizen."

The group experience provided a wake-up call for this middle-age man. Frank became more thoughtful and self-reflective in his interpersonal experiences and attributed it, rightfully so, to his connection to the group.

I emphasize that Frank's bonding to the members occurred first and primarily in his own mind, and was not played out interactionally. Only very gradually—after several years—has he built up new identifications such that he can participate in the empathic give-and-take of group life.

Bonding and group cohesion

Group cohesion, which includes the element of a basic bond or uniting force (Piper, Marrache, Lacroix, Richardson, & Jones, 1983), has been used to refer to different aspects of group experience, including mutual goal orientation, acceptance, and affiliation among members; attractiveness of and identification with the group; and cooperative engagement. While group cohesion rests on such local factors, it arises partially as an epiphenomenon of the local factors. The term might usefully be reserved as a macro concept to describe an attribute of a group, and not of individuals. Bonding describes a process that occurs between an individual and another or others.

Group cohesion aggregates from combinations of member-to-member, member-to-subgroup, member-to-entire group, and member-to-therapist bonds. While the dynamics of member-to-therapist bonding may be subtle and unacknowledged, they primarily determine the other bonding matrices and the ongoing group process. The entire group monitors and attends to each member's affective bond with the therapist; severe disruption of a member-to-therapist bond calls attention to itself and necessarily becomes a focal point of the group work.

Clinical example: a failed attempt to repair a member-to-therapist bond in a cohesive group

Marie, a patient in joint individual-group treatment, had become convinced that her therapist, in supervision with me, was cold and uncaring. Against the remonstrations from therapist and group, Marie terminated individual treatment. Now, several months later, the group was hearing similar news from a male patient: Robert reported his decision to terminate individual work, but also indicated the therapist's approval. His announcement met a round of congratulations, which Marie protested vigorously: "You complained about my quitting individual therapy, why not him?" The members tolerantly explained the difference in Robert's and Mary's respective therapeutic alliances. Marie began to cry: "You people really care about me!" Warm and reassuring exchanges followed. However, Marie did not openly acknowledge the therapist, who felt rebuffed and remained silent.

At this juncture in her reportage, the therapist-supervisee exclaimed indignantly: "I'm usually comfortable with anger from my patients. I've encouraged Marie and she expresses lots of anger. Why isn't she over it?"

I felt jarred, and it took a moment for me to turn my attention to the person of the therapist and to her question. I had been engrossed in her evocative description of the session and was still developing my feelings, and also enjoying them. It felt emotionally rewarding to remain mentally in contact with the caring group and unpleasantly disruptive to connect to the therapist's indignation.

In thinking about my negative reaction, I realized that I was experiencing the therapist as invasive and not receptive in her curiosity. Like Marie, I did not want to respond to her. She was not empathically connecting to the very experience she was describing so well, or to me, and I wanted her to connect. From my supervisory point of view, the problem was not in the patient's unintegrated anger but in the therapist's difficulty in understanding and responding to Marie's bonding needs and to mine.

The group had intuited Marie's overt anger as an articulation of hurt and longing, and they responded with reassuring contact. The members called attention to her difficulties in bonding with the therapist and encouraged Marie to deal with the therapist directly. While Marie continued overtly to rebuff the therapist, she did not rebuff the group in which the therapist played a prominent part. It seemed reasonable to suggest that Marie was indirectly communicating her need for the therapist to express caring, despite Marie's overtly hostile presentation.

I realized that the therapist had difficulty hearing the patient on the level of bonding need, and I, identifying with the patient, and perhaps being similarly treated, wished to withdraw. I had to tolerate the disintegration-reintegration of my caring feelings—my bond with the supervisee—before I could adequately think about her difficulties in caring. For an important moment, the supervisee had become "my Marie," a mental image of one who indirectly and angrily expressed her own caring longings and hurts.

Only after my compassion and desire for contact with the therapist returned, could I with confidence offer the complexity of my own emotional response to further the therapist's understanding of hers. Like Marie, the therapist could not process emotionally that which she understood intellectually: when one feels hurt, it is difficult to seek and offer the love that one wants and needs. Even when the individual is dominated by feelings of hatred, "over all is the sense of obstructed love" (Bion, 1967b, p. 83).

In feeling bonded, an individual can more easily work through an otherwise overly intense emotional reaction. Marie's interaction with the group showed that she did not need encouragement to express anger—she did that most efficiently—but to feel love and to communicate in a direct and positive manner her need for love. While she said to group, "You people really care about me," I heard an implied meaning: "I really care about you, and I can now think about it, for I feel your caring for me."

I suggested that she gently encourage Marie to consider that "you people care" could include "me," the therapist. The words could be effective only if put forth as an authentic bonding gesture. With therapeutic communications on the bonding level, the words implicitly carry the promise of positive feelings. *The conveyance of benevolence must be constant and precedent over any other meaning in the communication.* Sometimes, as in this example, the group is able to carry forth this therapeutic imperative when the therapist cannot (Hearst, 1981, p. 31).

In supervision, the therapist attempted to deal with and overcome her difficulties with Marie. She understood how the group maintained a relaxed and spontaneous symbiotic connection to Marie, which the therapist learned from and struggled to achieve. But the intense negative transference-countertransference overwhelmed the therapist's current emotional capabilities. She could not bond in a sufficiently positive manner to the patient, and Marie eventually terminated.

Bonding may exist without a true therapeutic alliance

When an individual patient joins a group, the therapist often serves as the initial and transitional bonding figure. Freud (1921) maintained that libidinal ties to the leader bind individuals. Yalom (1995) emphasized that the therapist functions as the primary unifying force. But this may not always be so. In some circumstances, an individual may bond first or primarily to other group members, while the therapist remains a distant and distrusted figure. Scheidlinger (1974) and others (Durkin, 1964; Foulkes & Anthony, 1964) have referred to the "mother-group," a regressive perception of the group entity, which occurs during the early phase of group formation, to be supplanted by real object ties among the members including the therapist, and transferences to them.

In any group alliance, there is an element of bonding; although if the activity is simple, the bond does not have to be strong and deep. Bonding may exist without a true working alliance, in that an individual may feel connected to the therapist and be a member of a cohesive group, while going through a lengthy period of challenging the task, frame, or rules, even when evading treatment.

Clinical example: bonding with a treatment-resistant group member

Sheila regularly entered 10 or 15 minutes after the group commenced, with an apologetic flourish and the same unassailable alibi: the boss made her stay late. The boss was an accommodating man, but business was business, and there was nothing he, she, or anybody could do about it. Sheila also telephoned the therapist frequently, alerting her to work emergencies that entailed a still later arrival.

Attempts to enlist the group in dealing with Sheila's resistances fell into a mindless vacuum: What did they think/feel about Sheila's tardiness? Her excuses? Similarly unsuccessful were the therapist's efforts at group-as-a-whole interpretations: Sheila was expressing unacknowledged group dynamics of refusal (Chapter 12), anger, entitlement, and attention seeking. Such clinical interventions backfired, for the members responded with a superior tone that made the therapist feel she was losing control of her group. "You don't get it," the group informed their therapist. "Sheila has a difficult work situation, and not everyone can rearrange their lives to meet your group schedule." "Sure, we don't like being interrupted, and we miss Sheila when she can't be on time. But we can accept it." "It's always nice to see Sheila when she arrives."

But the group leader did not feel nice. She remained anxious and expectant, greeting Sheila's tardy arrival with a sarcastic comment or a nonverbal expression of pique. The therapist feared that unless Sheila changed her behavior, her own anger would chase the patient away or, worst, alienate the entire group. There were, then, two clinical problems: one involved the patient and her difficulties in establishing a working or therapeutic alliance and the other involved the therapist's reaction, which interfered with her bonding to the patient.

I asked the therapist why she could not tolerate Sheila's behavior, since the rest of the group could. The therapist sardonically replied that the group members had not read the psychotherapy texts that we faculty had assigned in her training. She could not simply ignore a member's persistent acting out, she reminded me. I agreed and shared my conviction that no one, not even Sheila, was ignoring her actions, but that different meanings to them were being assigned.

Clearly, the therapist valued the meanings promulgated by the texts, supervisors, and institutions of our profession, which would indicate that Sheila's actions disrespected the time boundaries of group, semantic communication, and verbal insight. But the therapist was disrespecting the meanings important to Sheila and broadcast by her behavior. Sheila meant to have her words and behavior accepted at face value and not have them interpreted. In essence, she valued words for their capacity to evoke interaction: to garner attention and reassurance that she was different from the other individuals and special.

Whether the patient could be on time or at least tolerate verbal exploration of her behavior, and therefore accommodate to a working alliance as defined by the therapist and our profession was one pressing issue. But another was whether the therapist could in good conscience accommodate to the needs that Sheila felt were pressing and quite meaningful. An accommodation had to be reached, for the risk was a loss of the remaining positive connection between them.

"Say more. If you could show me how to do it, I would do it." The therapist's enthusiastic and immediate acceptance of an as yet untendered treatment plan suggested that I had become one of the texts that, not surprisingly, a novice group therapist may rely upon. I accepted without comment or criticism the presenter's response, which I understood as an expression of her own bonding needs. In serving as a different kind of text to which she could bond, perhaps I could aid her bonding to the patient.

I advised that, rather than ignore or criticize Sheila's behavior, the therapist should call positive attention to it. At the beginning of the next group, even before Sheila's arrival, the therapist was to announce that she had retired from the job as group truant officer. She was off Sheila's case! When Sheila arrived, the therapist was to replace her usual disappointed silence or questioning glance with a welcoming greeting. Someone most likely would explain to Sheila the therapist's change in attitude, at which time the therapist could connect directly to Sheila, and convey relief in revising the relationship. Something like: "It's great not to have to bug you. I feel better already."

As I did in the previous clinical example, I stressed to this supervisee that these interventions be applied only if offered authentically. The therapist had to recover and communicate a caring for the patient and an inner freedom (Symington, 1983) to be with her and to enjoy her, uncontaminated by judgmental anger or a need to do the "right" thing. There would be time to help Sheila and the group understand Sheila's experience of being in the world: the thoughts, feelings, fantasies, and behaviors she was expressing and evoking—positively and negatively—in others.

I hypothesized that the members valued the cohesiveness of their group, which was threatened by the growing rift between patient and therapist. Like in the clinical situation involving Marie, the group attended to the bonding needs of a seemingly intransigent member in an effort to cement a therapeutic alliance. It seemed likely that once patient and therapist were confidently bonded, other members would be released from carrying forth this aspect of the therapy. Eventually, another member and not the therapist would apply a questioning attitude or become perturbed by Sheila's behavior and its effect on the group.

Bonding as therapeutic technique

I have emphasized throughout how the therapist often must take an active role in establishing and maintaining member-to-therapist bonding. The concept of bonding also refers, then, to a therapeutic posture or technique, utilized to establish a positive transference and therapeutic alliance. In the context of individual therapy, Mitchell (1993) wrote that most clinicians

> try at times to bend the treatment to the person… I believe it most commonly entails a responsible and realistic effort to find a way to engage the patient, to reach him, to make him feel connected enough, secure

enough, to participate in an analytic inquiry into his experience and difficulties in living.

(p. 177)

In the group context, Foulkes and Anthony (1964) termed the "supportive" factor, and Scheidlinger (1964) the "experiential," both referring to the therapist's fostering a climate of permissiveness, acceptance, and belonging. Yalom (1995) stressed that "underlying all consideration of technique must be a consistent, positive relationship between therapist and patient. The basic posture of the therapist to a patient must be one of concern, acceptance, genuineness, empathy" (p. 106). But this therapeutic posture, Yalom clarified, does not preclude confronting the patient, showing irritation and frustration, even suggesting that a highly resistant individual consider leaving the group.

The therapist's bonding involves not only affection, concern, and affect attunement but evidence of the capacity to interpret the emotional state of the other. Freud (1913) suggested that "everyone possesses in his unconscious mental activity an apparatus which enables him to interpret other people's reactions, that is, to undo the distortion which other people have imposed on the expression of their feelings" (p. 15). Modell (1984) suggested that empathy also involves theory that allows us to have knowledge of our patients' minds and their feelings that they may not.

To empathically accept the group's bonding wishes and needs, and to understand them and not be provoked into premature action, requires a capacity for what Balint (1965) called "primary love", Searles (1979) referred to as "therapeutic symbiosis," and Sandler (1976) as "role responsive." To establish and maintain a culture of bonding, the therapist must accommodate to the individual member's contact needs, longings, and fears, without mindlessly submitting to or prematurely interpreting them.

Accommodations may be subtle, communicated by bodily and tonal responses as much as by overt action or actual dialogue, and may be directed towards unexpressed rather than expressed wishes. The group therapist must differentiate between expressions of genuine needs for contact and regressive exaggerations or defensive minimization of needs, and between fantasies involved in bonding wishes and pathologically entitled actions employed to gratify such wishes. In many instances, the dynamics and behavior of entitlement may be fruitfully—if not always immediately—interpreted.

Clinical example: acknowledging and enjoying bonding

The following was presented at a case conference seminar. Rachel, an analysand, had willingly accepted her analyst's invitation to a newly formed group. But now, several months later, she declared to him in an individual session her intention to give the group three more sessions before terminating. Patient and analyst agreed that the group had quickly and positively come together, and there was meaningful interaction among members. All seemed to be benefiting from the treatment. Did Rachel not feel this to be so? he inquired. Rachel replied that indeed, she already had learned from and enjoyed the experience, but "I just like individual much better; I get your full attention."

I asked the analyst-novice group therapist if he gave Rachel his full attention in group. He reported that he had purposefully minimized his involvement with her. She was a very attractive young woman, and he feared attending to her would betray his other female patients, as well as unfairly dominate the males. Everyone would be upset by his behavior and would want to leave group.

It became apparent that the therapist was anxious not only about giving Rachel special attention but also about receiving special attention from any of the members, particularly from Rachel. He had encouraged and responded well to the intense interactions among the members, concentrating on intrapsychic, interpersonal, and group dynamics, but not on himself. The therapist's relationship with each individual patient—the essential factor for sustaining and advancing therapeutic work—had not been sufficiently acknowledged and addressed.

Showing interest in Rachel would call attention to the therapist. Other members would monitor and react in unpredictable ways to his bonding and move him into unchartered territory. Certainly, a new dimension would be added to his group, and the challenge interested him.

I believe the class noticed, as I did, his unverbalized appreciation for my offering a stimulus for his professional and personal growth. In parallel process to what was imagined for the therapist's group, a display of intimacy between group member and leader took emotional center stage. I enjoyed the bond with the presenter, while appreciating that inevitably, conflicting emotions were being stirred up in his classmates that would become an aspect of the group dynamics of our seminar. I also was comfortable with the likelihood that, in his mind, I was going to remain part of the action in both the current class session and his forthcoming group, most likely, a center of his attention.

The presenter reported in a subsequent class meeting that he was finding it much easier to look at, talk to, and respond to Rachel. He was no longer pretending, to himself as much as to the others, that he was not involved in an intimate, therapeutic relationship with Rachel, one that was special to both of them. He became acutely aware that other patients and not only Rachel were vying for his attention (disapprobation as well as approbation). Rachel was just one of many who wished to be acknowledged and to have the therapist enjoy the bonding relationship. With the realization that he was and would remain a center of attention, the crisis with Rachel resolved itself. He found that in relating to Rachel easily and naturally, she did not demand, or require, special consideration, and she became a secure and active participant in the group.

Notice that it would have been hurtful and inaccurate to interpret Rachel's determination to leave group as a pathologically entitled need for attention. Indeed, on considering the total situation of the transference-countertransference, we could say that Rachel's dissatisfaction was a sensitive response to the therapist's withdrawal of bonding. Her resistance to group signaled a legitimate need for the analyst to make an authentic relational gesture.

Further discussion of cases: bonding is ubiquitous in transference-countertransference

> Bonding, attachment, affect attunement, and mind reflectivity are but a few of the innumerable, valuable contributions that have begun to change the way we feel about the relationship of the infantile aspect of the analysand and his or her relationship to the analyst.
>
> (Grotstein, 1999, p. 191)

As each case example illustrates, therapists (and supervisors) also have a complex of bonding needs and anxieties that are brought to the work. Like other group members, the therapist longs to contain and to be contained, to be connected and in relationship. Indeed, to the extent to which the therapist does not feel and understand one's own basic relational needs, but defends against or acts them out, he or she is handicapped in establishing and maintaining bonding or allowing the patient or group to shift from a preoccupation with bonding to other types of interactions.

Each of the cases required the therapist to understand and respond enactively to group members' bonding needs and fantasies that were expressed, but not necessarily semantically represented, and which might have been vigorously denied if verbally articulated. In the first case example, Frank protested when I encouraged him to talk about his growing bond to the group, as if his verbal acknowledgment of caring would shame him.

In the second example, the bitterly resentful Marie longed to bond with a therapist who could contain and detoxify her anger, but she resisted admitting her longings. The therapist needed to follow the group's lead in pursuing Marie; the members' words were concrete reassurances of caring. In the third case, the late-arriving Sheila could not challenge her boss or process challenge from her group therapist. Her need for support and attention took precedence over negotiating boundary relations (and violations) on the job or in the group, or even talking about such negotiations. And finally, in the fourth example, Rachel's inclination to withdraw from group was a meaningful response to her therapist's emotional withdrawal. The therapist's behavioral correction was essential—his words alone, not sufficiently meaningful. In each case, I monitored parallel process and attempted to maintain a mutually constructive bonding experience with the patient or supervisee, one that I did not necessarily call attention to or verbally articulate.

Concluding remarks

Bonding wishes and anxieties, as well as their fluctuations, remain a part of all human relations. We monitor how connected we feel towards other people and their connectedness to us. Such mental activity takes place with and without conscious awareness, and subtle changes in bondedness are communicated in behaviors, words, and silences.

The group therapist's words (and silences) are particularly powerful. They often define the emotional atmosphere of the room and allow for bonding wishes and anxieties to be expressed, bonding needs to be secured, and bonding resistances and fixations to be worked through. As the members bond and the group coheres, multiple peer and therapist-based identifications solidify, and, at the same time, members begin to differentiate from each other and define themselves. Nonetheless, the dynamics of bonding are continuous and inevitable; they are a source of anxiety and comfort, resistance and growth, despair and inspiration.

Chapter 9

Developing nuclear ideas

In the course of leading a group, ideas flow in and out of my consciousness. Some seem to originate from within me, although many emerge from the verbalizations and behaviors of others. Even if the group appears to move on, an idea may linger and begin to impinge. Since it is now asserting influence on me, unavoidably it affects group process. So I tend to think about why the idea has captured my attention: what it has to do with the clinical situation—present and past—and to my psychology, to the extent to which I understand it. Emotional and symbolic reverberations energize my thoughts, and realizations sometimes occur that surprise me. I consider how the idea relates to what others are saying and doing—linking together, if I am able, unfolding intrapsychic, interpersonal, and whole-group processes. If I wish to communicate, I must test whether the idea is comprehensible to other group members.

The nuclear idea

The nuclear idea expands on Bion's (1963) "psychoanalytic object," which he conceptualized as emerging from the patient's discourse and behavior and brought to meaning by the analyst, who uses observation, theory, his or her own emotional experience, and intuition. Both aim to establish a shared focus and invite symbolic thinking, though the nuclear idea places greater emphasis on the therapist's subjective experience and extends to group rather than solely to dyadic psychotherapy.

I conceive of nuclear ideas as emerging from the nucleus of the group process: from intersubjective forces and locations that cannot be fully specified, yet may be possible to observe, name, and utilize clinically. They arise from the indeterminacy of the network of communications and interactions, that is, from within the "dynamic matrix" (Foulkes & Anthony, 1964) or "culture" (Whitaker & Lieberman, 1964) of the group, co-created by the therapist's participation and influence, and expressed in the group's "idiom" (Bollas, 1989), its particular language, symbolization, and enaction.

A nuclear idea may evolve from any mental phenomenon that captures attention, and thus may be felt, fantasized and thought about, on conscious and nonconscious levels. It may focus initially on an observation, a feeling, belief, or memory that takes place in group, and which may be about group, or a personality, such as a group member or leader. An idea materializes: something has transpired—an existential and intersubjective moment or sequence of moments has been partially articulated in words or behavior. The therapist may take the opportunity to conceptualize further and negotiate meaning with the co-participation of other group members.

A nuclear idea entails a process of thinking and developing thoughts. This process may begin and be abandoned early on, or more fully evolve by some or all members of the group. When well developed, a nuclear idea possesses *experiential*, *symbolic*, *affective*, and *metapsychological* resonance.

The *experiential* dimension provides empirical and communicable reference. The leader needs to determine if, and to what extent, the members are hearing, seeing, and talking about a similar or different experience. The *symbolic* dimension refers to levels of embedded meaning, conveyed in speech (metaphor, verbal imagery, etc.), enactions, and group and personal narratives. The nuclear idea represents and stirs strong feelings: the *affective* dimension ensures that the idea carries here-and-now emotionally significant weight. Last, *metapsychological* significance emerges when thoughts extend to general principles of self, group, and societal organizations. People come to think about how they think (and do not think) and when and why.

Developing the nuclear idea provides a framework for how the therapist—and the group itself—goes about the task of containing (see also Chapter 7). My contention here is that groups organize themselves—with the therapist's participation and influence—by developing nuclear ideas. They are vehicles through which members individually and collectively come to self- and group-reflect. Nuclear ideas energize and may determine the direction of group process. As concept, technique, and process, the nuclear idea supplements the lenses through which the therapist comes to understand group experience and base his or her interventions on.

Four clinical vignettes

"Two groups"

A veterans hospital outpatient psychotherapy group changed leaders, as one psychologist, Lewis, replaced another, Rebecca, who left the area. The members missed Rebecca, of whom they spoke reverently, yet took to Lewis immediately.

Lewis supported the members reviewing Rebecca's person and leadership. This continued long after the group evolved with newcomers. Even after several years, the old-timers would reminisce about "Rebecca's group"

and how it differed from "Lewis's group." Recounting the dangerous behaviors they had eliminated or modified, this subgroup of self-described
"rough guys" (including several females) declared that Rebecca had "saved
our lives." Rebecca had put up with "no crap." "We had to clean up our act,
watch what we said, and how we said it." "She was very strict about rules
and following them."

Lewis also queried the group about his leadership, which the senior members described as "more hang-back," "relaxed," "not such a rule stickler."
"Rebecca locked the door, while you [Lewis] allow us to come in late." Still,
"you can be a ball buster." "If you think someone has an issue that they
don't want to talk about, you make us come back to it." "Rebecca did a lot
of digging, now we do your fucking work."

One outcome of these discussions surprised the members: they had become and remained "well behaved," even though the style and gender of
leadership had changed.

Discussion

The core members of Rebecca's group had been through and shared a violent period of adjustment—they were old hands at dealing with their own
chaos and that of the new members. Perhaps because of Lewis's inviting
and non-authoritarian style, it became easier for the members to become
his investigative allies. And perhaps, they did not also need "tough love"—a
phrase used repeatedly in describing Rebecca—not because what Rebecca
did was unnecessary, but because the old members were more mature and
modeled (and perhaps enforced) maturity for the new ones.

In terms of enaction and *symbolic* influence, the two leaders—most likely
unintentionally—took on parental roles related to earlier and later developmental phases of socialization. Rebecca was a "toilet training" parent.
A clear set of behavioral rules and expectations—a reinforced "yes" and a
firm "no"—provided a basis for what the members had called "cleaning up
our act," a process that was apparently absent or traumatically damaged in
these veterans.

Lewis established or reinforced latency ideals of mutuality and cooperation. In doing "his fucking work," the seniors verbally and enactively transmitted behavioral norms and expectations— now internalized—to the new
members. While not abrogating authority and enforcing it when necessary,
Lewis democratically shared investigative leadership, and it was the group
members themselves who initiated the nuclear idea of the "two groups." Most
likely, Lewis encouraged its clarification and elaboration without forethought
or conscious awareness. He was both leader and led, augmenting and creatively surrendering (Ghent, 1990) to the force of the idea of the "two groups."

To emphasize this point, Lewis did not make the leader of the old group,
the ongoing group, or the comparisons between them an explicit nuclear

idea. Here the leader's role was to recognize and enjoy—allowing the members to think for themselves: to introduce and revisit without ever naming the idea of "two groups" and the effects on their thinking and behavior. The members' pungent language captured key qualities of the respective leaders and their impact on their groups—how they operated *experientially*, as well as the *affective* impact of their personalities and decision-making.

The nuclear idea of the "two groups" functioned as an unnamed metaphor, linked experientially to the sensory-affective features of the therapists but stimulated by and based on their leadership behaviors, both imagined and real. It operated as a material entity and as a complex "relational image" (Migliorati, 1989, p. 198), utilized in affectively intense exchanges that referenced the group and also extended to extra-group psychological functioning. "Two groups" thus possessed the essential features of a *nuclear idea*: *experiential, symbolic, affective,* and *metapsychological*, bearing on and energizing the here-and-now therapeutic process.

The "uncomfortable role" of being in group

I had the opportunity to lead a demonstration group via Skype. The group conference took place in a city outside the United States. In an introductory exchange, the attendees expressed interest in hearing about "truth," "love and hate," "rebellion," and "connection," and I said I would try to address these concepts in either the small group or debriefing.

The room had been set up in preparation for the telecast: I faced a row of participants, with their backs to the large audience of observers. I suggested rearranging the chairs so that the group of eight was rearranged in a semicircle. While this improved the observers' sightlines, my view of several of the members became eclipsed. Further, while I could be clearly seen in close-up, the group members, at some distance from the camera, were blurry on my computer screen. Since nothing else could be done with the technical arrangements, we began, with 50 minutes allotted.

Not obscured by the electronic compress of our several-thousand-mile distance was a familiar jolt of start-up apprehension, which I took as my own magnified by the group's. A woman's first remarks perhaps spoke for all: "I feel uncomfortable, I can't explain why." Not waiting too long, I asked her if she could try. She repeated herself, and then asked if others could talk. I encouraged her once again to continue. She again appealed to the group, saying indistinctly: "I'm finding it hard to stay in role." Some mumbling among the group members followed, which I could not understand. Then, a man (his back to me) confessed: "We were assigned roles." Another member: "It's difficult not to be yourself."

I responded: "Me too. I was assigned a role and I want to be myself, and I'm uncomfortable too." The room resounded with laughter. "We're all in the same boat," I emphasized. The man tentatively suggested dropping role assignments, which met with exclamations of relief and no dissenters. I referred to the process as a constructive *rebellion* (Chapter 12): modifying the rules of engagement seemed appropriate for the brief time we had together and could make it more likely that we could reach some emotional truths.

A woman addressed the group: "I don't like the new arrangement." "But you went along," another woman responded. "Yes, that's what I do, I go along, then withdraw and sulk until I can't stand it, then protest." The group seemed to enjoy her honesty and began to inquire further about this aspect of her psychology, about which she claimed to know nothing further.

The protesting woman was in my full view, and I said that she seemed angry and asked with whom? "I don't know … I guess you." Although we were talking about anger, our exchange was amiable, and she seemed pleased to be addressed directly. Another woman turned to her: "You could be scary, but I'm glad you spoke up." A third woman said: "Yes, you made it easier for me."

The man who had revealed the role-playing spoke up. "Maybe I shouldn't have said anything." I said, "Are you apologizing?" "I started it," he reminded us. "You seemed to be intimidated." "No, yes, you're right." He turned enough for me to see the indistinct image of his profile: "I'm the youngest person here." "And the first man to speak," I emphasized, and then I asked him his age: "Twenty-nine," he said, and I told him he was old enough to be a full member with equal rights. His thank-you seemed emotional, and I felt that our exchange had been intimate, with some special significance for him, possibly related to the theme of being oneself.

And then from the remaining woman who, until then, had been silent: "I'm bored." I said that might be because she had not taken a chance to "connect" (I was referring to the term introduced by an audience member). Another woman interrupted: "I want to connect, but I am distracted by the audience. Several of them are raising their hands [also indicating boredom]." I told her that they were envious and she could tell them to fuck themselves. My remarks drew another round of laughter from the room, and apparently the hands went down. "That feels better," she said. The woman professing boredom then engaged with several others; she said she no longer felt that way.

I asked if anyone else was bored. An older man said he wasn't bored but rather confused: "Is this supposed to be psychotherapy? Should I talk about my problems?" I said that given our time frame, we wouldn't have time for "problems" and that he should just connect to feelings and to others. The woman who had first spoken in our group addressed him: "You were one of the reasons I was uncomfortable. We know each other from other places and haven't always gotten along. I like that I am in this with you and getting to know you differently." With encouragement, she elaborated on what she had discovered about him.

Everyone in the group had taken the opportunity to talk and address others, and after inviting them to do so once again, I closed the session.

Discussion

I heard the opening remarks as speaking for all: "I feel uncomfortable, I can't explain why." This shared and expectable discomfort gave birth to the germ of a nuclear idea. When a participant revealed that the group volunteers had been given roles to play as patients, but instead wanted to be themselves, I heard an opportunity to include myself and to refine the *nuclear idea* by treating the disclosure metaphorically, metapsychologically, and self-referentially: "Me too. I was assigned a role and I want to be myself, and I'm uncomfortable too."

I had floated a nuclear idea: we were discomforted not only by being put into these roles of demonstration leader and members but also by being in any group and needing to be ourselves, to think for ourselves, and to make meaning. The use of the nuclear idea put us on task to reach multiple learning goals: it called attention to the painful quandary of any therapeutic or quasi-therapeutic situation addressing the need and discomfort of being and learning about oneself; it invited the members to share in the discovery process; it lessened the asymmetry between leader and members; it provided an example of the therapist's use of self; it opened the door to metacommunication: symbolic language and thinking; and finally, it modeled risk taking, constructive *rebellion*, and the open expression of intense feelings.

When I suggested that the bored audience members could be told to fuck themselves, I was merely extending the nuclear idea in the form of a whole group interpretation. By implication, I was calling attention to a typical and unsurprising dynamic between two types of "uncomfortable roles" in a large group that may impede thinking: envious spectators who cannot actively participate and the demonstration group members, with specific responsibilities and expectations, assigned or not.

"Checkpoints"

We were several hours into a two-day Institute held in Jerusalem on the topic of "reconciliation." The members had expressed interest in my writing on "passion," yet I found myself unable to reveal, stimulate, or feel any. In response to increasing conversational lulls, I suggested that people might be anxious. A woman immediately responded that she was "perfectly relaxed" and suggested that it was I who must be feeling anxiety. My acknowledgment brought no interest or curiosity. Someone suggested that it might be a good idea to return to the theme of the conference. "Everyone here wants peace, yet the process seemed so sad and difficult," another woman lamented. The Gaza residents talked about their difficulty getting past Israeli checkpoints, even to attend a meeting on reconciliation; the Israelis countered with justifications for the barriers. Each side related stories of hardship, loss, and terror.

When attendees from other countries attempted to moderate the rising antagonism, the Arabs and Israelis concurred that these suggestions were unfeasible, given the political climate in the Middle East and the influence of the "military-industrial complex." Intellectualization replaced anger—but no passion.

After a while, I said that despite obvious ethnic and political tensions, the main barrier in the room appeared to be between everyone else and me. I could not locate, much less get through, a checkpoint and become part of this group. After some denials, reassurances, and hesitations, several members came forth with their doubts: I was an American, a visitor, and an outsider; how could I understand their anguish and loss? I acknowledged that I probably understood less than anyone else and would learn and gain more than anyone else during our two days together. I invited the group to deal with me directly when I went "off base."

The nuclear idea, which attended to the group's *refusal* (Chapter 12), located the impasse in an inhibited need to "check out" the leader; it became my point of entry. Now the group could attend to other barriers. The members checked out sources of difference and conflict related to ethnicity, citizenry, age, gender, political leanings, and personality. The women came forth to complain that the men—Israeli and Arab—had been doing all the talking. Two young Arab students confessed to being intimidated by their professor, sitting across the room. An Israeli housewife–community organizer confronted what she assumed were bellicose attitudes of the two high-ranking male soldier-psychologists from her country.

Was reconciliation possible? remained a question throughout the two days, but now we were checking each other out openly and mutually, painfully learning about the glaring and consequential personal as well as sociopolitical forces and affiliations that are ineliminable aspects of our identities.

Discussion

Supplementing the typical paranoid/depressive dreads and excitements accompanying formation, our group was subject to specific determining influences: fear of and anger towards ethnic and religious difference, and a collective, traumatic disillusionment with leaders, local, national, and international. I had been serving as the personification of the distrusted leader, and a "foreigner" too. Calling attention to the "checkpoint" located the predicament a leader must face with an untrusting and angry group.

The nuclear idea provided a point of entry for the messenger and the message. I shifted from being a shared threat and common target to being a sufficiently safe physical and mental reference who could be confronted and verbally "checked out." The salutary effect was to destabilize the preexisting ethnic subgroups and prejudices so that members could relate to me, and then to each other, as individuals.

"Not being missed"

From a long-standing group: "I'm just letting everyone know that I'm going to miss the next couple of weeks," said one of our members of four years. He was surprised when people inquired as to his plans. I was surprised by his surprise and asked him: "Why are you surprised?" A female member of many more years piped in: "I can understand that, I don't expect people to be interested in me when I'm not here. But I'm interested in you." "I'm not surprised, I feel the same way, I will miss you, but I know I'm not missed," echoed several others.

I found this curious, given that people regularly began with "Where's so and so?" "How's so and so?" Absences were noted and talked about. In individual sessions, group mates recurrently referred to and inquired and worried about other members. "Everyone seems to miss everyone else, but nobody feels they're missed," I summarized. Several members initially dissented, but they reexamined their feelings in the interlude that followed: "My father practiced 'children should be seen and not heard.'" "I don't know why my parents had children, we seemed to be ignored." "My sister was the pretty one; I was supposed to be smart, and if I wasn't, forget about it, I mean, forget me." "It was about my mother, never about us."

When I asked one of the speakers how her feelings affected her group participation, others joined in, so that our discussion extended to how members conceived of and thought about our group's culture and process. Members had registered but had not previously talked about the group's greeting and departing rituals: how and if they were addressed in the waiting room and who said good-bye and to whom. Only some members anticipated a friendly reception at the start of the session. Group etiquette included "taking turns," monitoring frequency and duration of "talking about oneself," and "attempting to interest others, but never being sure." Post-session introspective preoccupations more than occasionally involved review of possible injury of others and fear of guilt-inducing retribution.

No matter the mutual reassurances and disconfirmation, members echoed lingering doubts concerning their clarity, perceptiveness, and value to others. One individual's ironic evaluation of our discourse brought appreciative laughter: "What an 'up.' No wonder I love this group!"

Discussion

"Why are you surprised?" I asked the member who was the subject of inquiry, not expecting resonance from so many. I had stumbled upon a group mythos—a belief shared by the majority of members, which was captured by the nuclear idea: "Everyone seems to miss everyone else, but nobody feels they're missed." My intention was not to interpret, direct group process, teach, or confront the members with reality, but to rather provide an opportunity to assess and publicize the depth of the commitment to an emotional belief that I had been ignorant of and had surprised me. My words were spontaneous and ironic, perhaps obvious, yet they captured an important and unexamined emotional truth located in the member-to-member relationships. Here was a group where each member testified to the value of the others. Reiterating the sense of not feeling missed in the face of contrary data made vivid the power of trauma and the difficulty of modifying or eradicating its effects on how we think and what we think about.

As therapists, we often do not know where an inquiry will take us. With little therapeutic effort, the nuclear idea segued to throw light on group cultural interactions, which unbeknownst had reinforced preexisting self-stereotypes and strategies of group participation.

Not mentioned in our discussion, but perhaps universal, is the harsh reality of not being missed. Not only Oedipus or those traumatically neglected or abused but the child in all of us deals with the ungraspable fact of not being wanted for oneself or missed. As parents once claimed their sexual relationship, our loved ones claim their private spaces. And too, a future looms wherein we—like our long-departed group members—will not be remembered.

Our group left the nuclear idea before such metapsychological and existential elaborations were consciously thought about and explored. A nuclear idea may stimulate an infinite network of associations; we had articulated and interpreted some but not all of its emotional elements. While an exploration of a nuclear idea may be carried out adequately, it cannot be done all at once, and never completely.

Groups organize themselves around nuclear ideas

Let us review the four case vignettes.

1   "Two Groups." The nuclear idea, arising casually and remaining unnamed, assumed essential holding and transformational containing functions. The pungent discussions of "Rebecca's group" and "Lewis's group" functioned as an ongoing and fertile source of formulating and clarifying individual and collective meaning. The culturally transmitted, enduring mental relationship between the members and the nuclear idea of the two groups (associated with core ideas relating to the respective leaders) stabilized the transition and the relatively smooth initiation of new cohorts, spurring cohesion and coherence (Ezquerro, 2010).
2   "Uncomfortable Roles." The nuclear idea revealed and made manageable a locus of anxiety that could have otherwise blocked learning during a short-duration demonstration group. I was an electronic figure, burnished by the aura of the "invited presenter" (Billow, 2013c). Acknowledging my own discomfort reduced our emotional distance and fostered

empathic bonding. We were "in the same boat," I had declared, a containing reference to our shared discomfort, which we then addressed realistically as well as psychologically (and metapsychologically).

The justifiable rebellion against the sponsoring organization's role-playing stricture, the benevolent intragroup confrontations, and my playful "tell them to fuck themselves"—these were enactions directed to reduce discomfort that made sense because of the clarity and safety provided by the nuclear idea.

3   "Checkpoints." Until the introduction of the nuclear idea, group process was marked by the *parasitic* variation of the container/contained. The unproductive intellectualizations, denials of anxiety, and emotional flatness suggested that the participants found our new group untrustworthy, antagonistic, and unsafe. Thinking and thinkers were avoided or attacked, as in the silent hostility directed towards me. The "checkpoint" idea encapsulated important sociopolitical aspects of the attendees' experience that were both metaphoric and real, perhaps too real and too dangerous to contain in language without the group leader's active interventions and benevolent presence. I tolerated the participants' projections without retaliating by withdrawing my subjectivity, such as by falling silent, claiming not to be affected by anxiety, or offering lofty interpretations. As a metaphoric extension of a political reality, the nuclear idea invited the attendees to carry out a "checkpoint" in words, rather than to surreptitiously halt the process and sabotage the group.

4   "Not Being Missed." A nuclear idea has the potential to serve as a *selected fact* (Bion, 1963, p. 11), to the extent that it clarifies, reorganizes, and brings illuminating depth to prior and ongoing events in the group. The experiential data, fantasy-based and emotional, had been submerged in the minds of the various members. Each member's characteristic defense patterns and anticipatory fantasies contributed to the inhibited participation that characterized a dimension of our group. The nuclear idea brought to light but did not resolve a "common tension" (Ezriel, 1950). Nor could it, for "not being missed" remains an everlasting source of existential anxiety, common to us all.

Still, in being broadcasted, the nuclear idea unified the membership, and group process moved in an unexpected direction. Members linked the nuclear idea to unresolved historical relationships, revisiting trauma, expressing anger, and mourning.

The nuclear idea extends discourse to the metapsychological

A nuclear idea may involve a premise, a working hypothesis, a strategy, a nonconscious working through, or an exploration and interpretation of group, subgroup, or individual traits, fantasies, and dynamics. But it is more than a conflict, tension, "theme" (Whitaker, 1989) or an interesting process that gets addressed by naming and connecting to individuals, subgroups, and the whole group. Developing a nuclear idea becomes a living event of self/other awareness that changes the psychologies in the room.

The nuclear idea vitalizes thinking and being, particularizing the vague or theoretical, and making abstract and universal the concrete. A "common tension"—such as being a part of "two groups," "uncomfortable in role," in need of "checkpoint," or feeling "not missed"—clarifies group process. But presented and treated as a nuclear idea, the formulation extends the scope of thinking. The nuclear idea of "two groups" is far-reaching, condensing the past and providing a forward-directed model of "good behavior." "I feel uncomfortable in taking a role" broadens to the metapsychological (and sociological) question, "What is the nature of being in a group?" Derivatives of "checkpoint" reflect intense internal, interpersonal, and sociopolitical realities, fantasies, and cultural myths that are both ancient and as current as today's newspaper. "I feel I'm not missed" relates not only to group realizations and negotiations but also to spiritual dimensions that are timeless and irresolvable.

A relational stance, which makes the therapist's subjectivity available for inspection, provides a model of an emotionally reflective self. When incorporated in a nuclear idea, the therapist's subjective experience offers metapsychological reference. For instance, my report of feeling unable to get through a group "checkpoint" also implied that I would not stop thinking for myself, even if my thoughts were unwelcome. Treating the "checkpoint" references metaphorically and metapyschologically involved accessing and publicizing some of my fantasies, anxieties, affects, and thoughts in relationship to the group participants' barriers to me and to their own thinking. Perhaps, in revealing a metapsychological dimension of my subjectivity, including allusions to my own helplessness, the nuclear idea put the group in a less dependent (and frightened) position. The members became willing, and able, to observe their own (non) thinking and, in so doing, to think for themselves.

The "uncomfortable role" vignette provides another example of the nuclear idea's extension into the metapsychological. My self-report of how I felt also conveyed a sense of how I thought, and that I would share rather than withhold my thoughts about my thinking. My therapeutic action encouraged other members, who came to report on their thoughts about thinking. One woman spoke of her "going along" with the thinking and action of others; another spoke of her anxiety about broadcasting thoughts in the presence of the first ("you can be scary"). A man spoke of his uneasiness of being the youngest and presenting his ideas. Others acknowledged impaired thinking processes: boredom, distraction, and confusion ("Is this psychotherapy?").

A nuclear idea provokes the curiosity drive and extends its reach from the personal, interpersonal, and social to the metapsychological. Without assuming formal leader status, all group members may participate as drivers of this function. They are not leaders of the group, but they may initiate and even lead this discourse (as in the "two groups" and "not being missed" vignettes). Each group member is capable of being a thinking, interpreting subject, capable of doing conscious as well as nonconscious psychological work.

The nuclear idea is the type of intervention that expands the category of what is thinkable (Ogden, 2011)—"a point of departure for new meanings and places not yet known" (Levine, 2012, p. 27), for generating new thoughts and new ways of thinking. And, since its goals are transformational, and not merely informational, the nuclear idea often stimulates, rather than resolves tensions and conflict.

Summing up

The lexical representation of the nuclear idea is often simple in grammatical structure and straightforward in experiential group reference, but generalizable and complex in symbolic and affective resonance. Something has transpired—an existential and intersubjective moment or sequence of moments—that subsequently becomes named and (partially) articulated. It is built on, refined by the group interaction, and linked to a shared database of here-and-now verbalizations, nonverbal behavior, and enactments. As a thought or a series of emotional thoughts that are thought about, nuclear ideas are self and group reflective. They offer opportunity for the leader or therapist to focus, refocus, or challenge the group, orienting the members towards the search for meaning, on personal, interactional, group, and metapsychological levels. As we have seen, the nuclear idea can be the organizing principle directing the inquiry, the focus of the inquiry, or the result of the discovery process.

A nuclear idea has to catch on, to function in dynamic relationship with thinking, in order to involve the group or some members in an emotional experience associated with learning. It cannot be rushed or imposed; it emerges from the intensity of the clinical experience. It is provisional, tested in terms of its affective saliency and capacity to generate interest and thought. It can go flat, be ignored, or applauded, and is not an oracular pronouncement.

That which may potentially be developed as a nuclear idea may not seem to interest particular members, or involve all members equally, or be optimally significant to the group and its process. Nuclear ideas differ, then, in depth, breadth, creativity, and relevance to group and the particular needs and wants of the individual members.

The nuclear idea (1) gives opportunity for new meaning and depth to any experience that has occurred before or is ongoing in intrapsychic and group relations; (2) focuses participants' attention and provides a mode of entry; (3) establishes a shared activity and common goal of understanding; (4) privileges group members as potential sources of transformation;

(5) conveys a sense of order to and mutual appreciation of the group; and (6) creates interest in and valorizes attending to other nuclear ideas, such that metapsychologizing becomes part of group culture and process.

Developing nuclear ideas circumvents (and may even anticipate) the type of meaning deprivation that leads to a profusion of exaggerated *basic assumptions*, *common tensions*, and *focal conflicts* and which encourages unproductive *rebellions* and *refusals*, and static *resistances*.

All group members of a psychodynamically oriented group share in the invitation to attend to, develop, and harvest nuclear ideas, and to their quality. Nonetheless, the therapist's influence remains primary. In offering him- or herself as a metapsychologizing subject and relating likewise to other members, the therapist sets up a culture and process in which the group comes to listen for and develop *nuclear ideas*.

Chapter 10

Reality testing and testing reality

We are trained as psychotherapists to examine reality: to become expert observers who help our patients become "in charge," addressing and overcoming defensive distortions and unrealistic strategies. Whether vocalizing or not, we listen to our own inner voice of reality, ever alert to the often-deleterious effects of a mind or a group preoccupied with infantile wishes and fantasies.

However, therapy needs to veer away from *reality testing* and to protect clinical process from overly energetic problem-solving. Striving to be "realistic" and solve problems may foreclose an experimental attitude—one that that embraces *testing reality*. Whether merely in thought and feeling, or in actual behavior, *testing reality* brings a broadened view of what may be available to live a vital, creative life. It entails discovery and construction, actual or purely conjectural. It is open, spontaneous, and unbounded; it tests limits.

When applied to inner life, *reality testing* seeks to reach understanding, clarify distortions and the influence of past traumas, and prepare for appropriate behavior. *Testing reality* proceeds with the faith that anything that draws attention—feelings/thoughts/fantasies that we judge unrealistic, immature, immoral, or primitive—potentially has emotional truth value (Billow, 2015).

It would be difficult to imagine a situation where both processes are not going on. Still, their disjunctions and conjunctions influence the clinical situation and therapist-patient tensions and dynamics. Each approach brings opportunities for—and limitations in—fostering constructive process and meaning-making.

Testing reality may predominate over reality testing: two clinical examples

Protecting testing reality in a long-term group of high-functioning adults

"Therapy or divorce! I can't live like this anymore," Ben's wife threatened, more than once. He entered group volunteering little other than that his children were very difficult and he needed our help. He missed many sessions, due to traffic problems, business meetings, even Mets and Yankees games. When arriving late, he annoyed members by offering opinions without fully absorbing what had been taking place. The women particularly, who I assumed spoke also for his wife, declared themselves to be "bored" and "turned off" whenever he spoke. While acknowledging the group's legitimate complaints, I supported Ben by emphasizing the value of his insights and encouraged him to defend himself or fight back.

At the beginning of one session without Ben, several members questioned why Ben came at all, and Marvin insisted that I not allow him to continue. Joan said Ben was "vacant" whether he was there or not and he did not matter, like her father, who had been passive and emotionally absent. She asked why it bothered Marvin so much.

Ben arrived in the midst of this exchange.

MARVIN (*TO BEN*): We were talking about you too, and why you stay in group since you miss so much.

JOAN: And come so late when you do.

BEN: I'm glad to be here, when I am.

MARVIN: Yeah, but it isn't fair to the rest of us.

LIZA: You never tell us when you're going to miss. I always call [therapist] if I have to. Do you? I don't think so.

MARVIN: You never tell us much, what are your problems that you are working on? I'd really like to know.

BEN (BECOMING EMOTIONAL, RATHER THAN APOLOGIZE, SAY HE WOULD TRY TO DO BETTER, AND WITHDRAW, WHICH HAD BEEN HIS MONOTONOUS PATTERN): Look, I appreciate your wanting me to be here, but I'm not going to do it. I'm not going to do what you want because you want it. I had to suck it up with my father, stay out of sight. He'd be drunk, smoking up the house, and ready to beat the shit out of me. I come when I come, and when I want to—I want to when it isn't an incredible hassle. You don't know my day. I drove 400 miles seeing clients. No matter what you may think, my way, not yours. Don't try to control me. It pisses me off.

Tom said, "It's like 'fuck you.' Like you're still a member of a street gang."

Ben, now a successful financial advisor, took some pride in correcting Tom's version of his teenage years: "I was my own independent agent, stealing and torching cars, I didn't need a gang." Ben offered no appeasements and no empty promises to do better. Not everyone was happy with Ben's assertion of independence, but we agreed that a new voice had spoken.

For the months that followed, Ben continued to "torch" us with his unaccounted absences, but when present, a different Ben emerged: more confident, verbal, and, for the first time, consistently helpful in addressing the conflicts of others.

MARVIN: You know, I'm starting to miss you when you're not here, and before you just pissed me off.

JOAN: I don't tune out when you speak.

Discussion: enactments test a multiplicity of realities

Ben did not care about our "reality," he had declared, which had been obvious, but until now, not acknowledged. He was not ready to address the problems that brought him to group, and not interested in verification or being monitored. But he had stayed—and likely not only because of fear of his wife's leaving him. Ben was enacting, playing with and putting into action emerging subjective data not otherwise available for discourse, neither in his mind nor in the group setting.

Enactments refer to that dimension of experience that is lived out without necessarily being understood. In my opinion, they represent a fundamental element of all behavior. Enactments reveal "multiplicities" (Hoffman, 1991) or "visions" (Schafer, 1970) of realities existing among members (including the therapist) and expressed in all aspects of clinical life: its structure, culture, and process. They provide sources of data that inform about how reality is perceived and being tested. While enactments are never fully understood, we may usefully identify and think about them.

Ben's lengthy enactment revealed repressed and dissociated dimensions of his inner reality, which he (unknowingly) rebelled against in the safety of the group. He had expressed defiant behaviors for much of his life, but never before revealed the emotions that had driven—and for a while would continue to drive—such behavior.

Members, individually such as Ben, and those who collectively banded against his behavior, tested whether and how their communications were received, understood, and reflected upon. We may appreciate from this clinical example how enactments may signify the emergence of new forms of engagement and experience, if and when they are tolerated and eventually brought to understanding (Davies, 1999).

An adolescent group tests forbidden realties

Two young adolescents introduced me to the practice of adolescent group treatment. Robert was an impulse-disordered 13-year-old with enuresis. Lucy, of similar age, was socially inappropriate, with a mild thought disorder possibly due to organicity. These two immature teenagers found each other in my waiting room during the intermission between their respective appointments. They huddled around the boy's portable video game which, glued to his hand, had been an impediment to our making contact. They asked if they could take a portion of their individual sessions and share them; I assented.

Several months were spent focused on the game, without much talk or wish for my inclusion. They wanted to know if I treated other kids and wanted them to join us for longer sessions. Again I agreed, adding over time Steve, an inhibited and semi-mute schizoid boy with an uncertain sexual orientation, Tonya, a 14-year-old girl adopting crass behaviors, and Sam, 14, with a history of stealing from his adoptive parents.

Now three years later, I describe a beginning of a session that was not unusual.

TONYA: What are you looking at, you dumb, four-eyed bastard? [*I wear eyeglasses*]

STEVE: I was thinking this week, Billow deserves to be cut up in little pieces and thrown down the toilet.

BILLOW: What did I do this week?

(Silence)

BILLOW: I guess you missed me, and you're giving me the same treatment I gave you all week: silence. I don't make it easy for you and you're not going to make it easy for me.

TONYA: *I'm* easy! [*The boys laugh awkwardly.*]

STEVE: What did he do this week? He was born.

ROBERT: No hatched, in a test-tube.

TONYA: He's one of 'them'.

LUCY: He probably beat his kids.

TONYA: No sex with his wife.

SAM: He gets drunk as soon as he leaves here—probably, stoned.

ROBERT: He's stoned already.

SAM: So am I.

STEVE: What a pervert.

TANYA: You're the pervert, Steve.

STEVE: And proud of it.

TONYA: I know he's [*therapist*] a pervert.

ROBERT: We ought to cut off his nuts.

TONYA: What nuts? He's a dickless wonder.

ROBERT: Get the magnifying glass and the tweezers.

Discussion: testing reality through play

Winnicott (1971, p. 46) defined the task: "Where playing is not possible then the work of the therapist is directed towards bringing the patient from a state of not being able to play into a state of being able to play." The video device, a form of isolating play in individual treatment, had been replaced with a group-created display: "dis the therapist."

Hamlet, proclaims: "The play's the thing/Wherein I'll catch the conscience of the King" (Shakespeare, 1961, II, ii, 905). As central figure, I served as outcast, eunuch, pervert, stupid, clumsy, clown, untouchable, villain, evil monster, and so forth.

I had to be alert to, tolerate, and also confront the convergence and amplification of primitive emotionality, fantasy, and behavioral potential, represented by the group's split transference, in which I was both the defiled and longed for object. Could an adult be discovered who was not inhuman, unbalanced, or "small"—one equipped to cope with their manifest hostility and not retaliate? I interpreted their loud chorus of obscenity, but, most importantly, showed them that I was not drowned or drowned out by it. At some point, I might verbalize with sarcasm my appreciation for the group's interest, professing to be complimented by its preoccupation with my sexual life, such that it was.

I good-naturedly accepted their testing me, but I concentrated on advancing reality testing too. I talked over them and interrupted, linking their profane verbal play to the realities of their inner and outer worlds. I stood for every hated and feared adult—their parents, teachers, cops—I insisted, and for themselves as well. "Shut up, Billow," they replied, with true affection.

In relatively harmonious group phases, the members satisfied that I remained "complimented," that is, unrattled by their introductory volleys, shifted towards reality testing. The teenagers shared and adjusted perceptions about favorite movies, music, parents, and the "straight" kids from school. They gave constructive advice to each other.

I could be praised for interventions and interpretations that were most often simple, addressed to one individual but really applying to all of them. For instance, "Steve is the angriest person in group, that's why he's the most quiet. He is scared of himself and what he might do to others." Steve: "Yeah, I'd like to kill my father, and one day I will." Or, "Tonya puts up a good tough front, but she's a mush [softie] inside. She just wants to be loved, let's face it. She's a big phony." Tonya (*smiling*): "That's why he gets my parents' big bucks."

A well-working group tends to monitor and challenge members who represent the extreme ends of testing reality and reality testing. So, while the adolescent group freely expressed fantasies of rape, pillage, and murder, even those teenagers who engaged in delinquent behavior would caution against it. They celebrated each other's social successes: Robert passing 11th grade and free from court supervision; Steve coming out to his parents and withstanding his father's gay-bashing; Tanya hooking up with a steady boyfriend and renouncing, in her word, "sluthood."

In using the group to engage in both testing reality and reality testing, members connected to stable, trustworthy, and knowable external and internal worlds. They discovered that even their most antagonistic words and antisocial behavior could make sense. I believe the group was instrumental for some in surviving their difficult high school years.

Further discussion of the two cases: the influence of the group and its leader

In their protest against reality testing, both Ben and the adolescents tested realities that seemed to take us far from conventional therapeutic goals. Ben's "my way not yours" and the adolescents' insulting rebelliousness had become destructive routines, left unaddressed by a "facilitating environ-ment" (Winnicott, 1965). In the new context of group, they gained or re-gained their potential as testing strategies. Ben's disappearances and the adolescents' profane language and behavior were witnessed (Chapter 17), eventually understood, and applied to relevant social contexts outside the group. Given fortuitous therapeutic group circumstances, then, testing re-ality may come to make sense and be subject to reality testing.

The members in Ben's group carried out reality-testing functions. They confronted him with his behavior and its effects on others, and pushed him to self-disclose. After years of refusing, he did reveal himself, although his behavior did not change immediately. I tended in the other direction, pa-tient with his testing reality and nonplussed by his willful obliviousness. I welcomed Ben whenever he appeared, openly encouraged and appreci-ated his participation, remained reflective but noncommittal when members asked about "rules" regarding attendance and absences, and unfazed by the ensuing controversies over my leadership.

At various times, it fell to me to protect the adolescents from themselves. This meant understanding the realistic sources of their anger, while also de-fusing its reckless intensity. The group was not in danger, but various mem-bers were, and in a non-accusatory and direct manner I regularly challenged their behaviors with humor, irony, and interpretation. To my initial and con-tinued surprise, the group supported my confrontations.

Testing reality may challenge actualities

Individuals often come to therapy for difficulties in reality testing, for situ-ations involving perception, judgment, and decision-making. They want to solve problems; testing reality sometimes causes them. Opening up unsus-pected potentials, testing reality invites entry into unknown circumstance with unpredictable outcomes. While reality testing offers clarity and relief, testing reality may present existential risk, for an individual, and for the stability of the group as well.

Testing reality threatens a member's sense of self

Lois took some pride and much dissatisfaction in being the mature part-ner in a discordant marriage of different religious and social class back-grounds. A former public-school teacher and officer of her church, Lois was responsible, practical, and reality-oriented, while Stuart ineptly tested reality's limits. He was "wild and out of control," Lois scolded, sobbed, or screamed in the marital sessions, but several times, it was Lois who punched her mate before I could intervene. Exacerbating the contentious relationship was the prospect of more home-alone time together, for Stuart's displays of poor judgment and childish behaviors led to an early retirement from his wealthy family's business.

I arranged for the couple to join separate groups. While Stuart needed to tune in to reality to understand the effects of his impulsive behaviors on himself and others, Lois, isolated and lonely, had to find a way to embrace Stuart's positives, and also to expand her narrow sphere of interests and activities.

Welcomed by her curious group, Lois omitted the unpleasant details of Stuart's behavior and her own. The insightful members could decode her underlying frailty and despair, and Lois seemed to receive an infusion of poise and confidence from their gentle pursuit. Not lost on her or me, but left unspoken, these intriguing members were similar in attitude and lifestyle to those in her suburban community who, Lois felt, had shunned her.

For several years, Lois participated without much self-revelation and retreated to the background during heated group interactions. In our concurrent individual treatment, however, she was quite different. With embarrassment and anxiety, she revealed an inner world of erotic feelings and fantasies, many now directed towards me. When sexual dreams involving other men in group emerged, Lois worried that I might be hurt and would lose interest in her. We made considerable analytic progress with these anticipatory fears, and Lois overcame her reluctance to sharing with the group.

Relaxing a tightly held, defensive grip on external reality, Lois opened up a channel of thinking and being, for herself, and for the group as well. Her "x- rated" dreams (her term) stimulated productive group interchanges involving romantic feeling and fantasy, and fostered frank discussions of the members' sexual functioning and practices.

Lois ventured into a weight-reducing program, braved her suburban culture to join a tennis league, and, when she became an officer of the parent–teachers association, developed enjoyable, mildly flirtatious relationships with several male administrators. However, school commitments lessened as her children moved on, and she began to search for other workable goals. She decided she could accomplish them without further therapy and, with regret, left treatment. I saw Lois intermittently afterward, mostly to temporarily resolve flare-ups with her husband.

Lois gradually withdrew from her suburban community, depressed, and sequestered within church, extended family, and the television. She regained her weight and became hobbled with diabetes. With continued attendance, encouragement, and support from his group, Stuart managed to establish and enjoy some degree of independence. He developed a tolerant coterie of older, sports-loving retirees, which Lois blessed and denounced.

Discussion

Internally and interactively, the formerly obese Lois had "shaped up," becoming more her own self and more like other individuals in her group and community. She had tried *on* and tried *out* a notion of self in a social context (Nitsun, 2015) and liked it. So how to explain her regressive decision to leave her group?

Within the confines of her combined therapies, Lois had become realer and livelier than in "real life." She knew that there was no realistic risk to her familial and religious commitments. But like a fashionable new outfit that she dared not wear outside the showroom, she had judged her emerging self as a "not me." Without relational roots and images to support independence (and a sufficiently friendly superego), Lois could not sustain the psychological tensions that Erikson (1962) described in reaching a new stage of *developmental actuality*. This involved breaking bonds of hostile codependency and actualizing a normalized, mature self. To maintain an internal "sense of reality"—the narrative of obedient daughter, long-suffering wife, and dutiful mother—she sacrificed her potential to carry forward developmentally.

Directing two approaches to learning

I describe three sequences of a day-long experiential group in a European city. In the first sequence, I offered reality testing for group negotiation; in the second, I encouraged testing reality; and in the third, I intervened to address a member's testing reality that I assessed as a threat to both approaches to learning for the entire group.

Sequence I: negotiating reality

I took the remaining empty seat and found myself next to Peter, who had arranged the visit and secured participants and site. He asked all of us about the timing of coffee breaks and ordering the lunch. Given the morning's time limitations and the group's goals for the day, I suggested that we forego the short morning break, which always extends into a long one, and that people could pee, get coffee, and check in with their cell phones, as they felt necessary. People voiced relief that I had avoided a lengthy debate and that we could move on to the program: a short lecture and the process group, which I now describe.

Peter broke our brief silence by saying that he would like to change seats. "I was disappointed that we ended up next to each other. I don't want to feel that we are co-leading or that other people link us together as a pair. I want freedom to participate."

I said that I felt the same way and for the same reasons, but here we were. Could we try to work this out in words, since this is what we want from our group members? "Sure, let's give it a try," he responded. He gratefully assented to my suggestion that someone else take care of coffee and lunch arrangements, and two colleagues volunteered. Peter responded emotionally to this resolution, declaring tearfully that he was relieved not to always be "in charge." He did not follow further, and I did not push.

Other participants picked up the theme of being "too much in charge," but it veered to the circumstantial, as sets of members revealed their respective roles working together as co-therapists, taking minimal risks. To get things moving, I asked facetiously whether we were going to work in pairs, or could each person be "just enough in charge?"

Discussion

The exchanges with Peter and the group established a *consensual* basis of reality testing: the focus was on negotiating group procedures and boundaries of behavior. I stated a preference for goal-directed work over coffee breaks, words over motor action, and independence over pairing. My view of reality—and how I supported it behaviorally—was affirmed by the group. Sufficiently trusted to be the conservator in charge, I could shift to being a challenger as well.

Sequence 2: expanding reality

"I want to go deeper," Jon declared and, referring to the man on his right as his co-therapist, continued: "Axel has a phrase when a group stays on the surface that seems to help...." He faltered nervously, and Axel completed the anecdote.

Turning to me with tremulous voice and imploring look: "I wish I didn't depend on him so much."

"Now is a chance to depend on yourself, to go as 'deep' as you feel comfortable with."

"I don't feel comfortable at all. [sympathetic laughter] Everyone's looking at me, not wanting me to talk. That's what I felt from my mother. But I said I would today, to break out of the mold and become a better group leader. I'm having some trouble now."

"Is there somebody here who's reminding you of your mother? It could be a man, too, even Axel or me."

"No, the whole group. Not true. It is you and you, [addressing two of the women] I feel you think I've talked too much already and am taking too much time."

The elder of the two women professed bewilderment, while the other, a same-age peer, partially confirmed the reality of his fantasy: "Well, yes you are right. One part of me wants you to continue and another part says shut up, you *are* taking too much time." [laughter]

"So I should stop now. Besides, my mother isn't a bad woman, she also loves me."

I interceded:

> Yes, we know she isn't an axe murderer [laughter], but she doesn't sound entirely loving, and [referring to the woman who had spoken] neither is she, but it took courage for her to share her mixed feelings. [to Jon:] Are you going to stop talking?

Jon took my encouragement and described his maternal relationship with a painful realism. Others continued in resonance, developing further a theme from *Sequence 1*: "My parents never should have stayed together...I have to be 'in charge,' take care of them both. I hate it." "I care for my [elderly] mother more than she cared for my five siblings or me." "I'm always holding things together, afraid my groups are going to fall apart. I'm like my uptight parents. Why were they so worried about us [siblings]? It keeps me from being creative, like you, Jon, even here."

Near the end of the morning's session, Maggie confronted a man who had been too much "in charge," analyzing others and remaining non-disclosing. Maggie had been an insightful and challenging participant, and I expressed some disappointment in saying to her that the interaction would remain a "cliffhanger" [laughter], to which we could return to after our short lunch break.

Discussion

A personal anecdote mirrors *Sequence 2*. Our twin grandsons (identical), 13 months old, were busy exploring the new spring season in their backyard with their nanny; I seemed not to be noticed. One ran confidently to the bushes and shook and pulled. But the other approached and stared longingly, his little body trembling with fear and desire. He grabbed my hand and directed it to touch the green needles. He then let go to happily explore the bush on his own; later, we repeated the same sequence in another part of the yard.

Group leaders provide an available hand to support members as they explore and follow their inclinations. While often stimulated by the here-and-now external reality of the group "yard," subjective realties also are tested. Not everything or everyone we touch in fantasy or actuality is soft and welcoming. We map out actions accordingly.

Sequence 3: reality asserted

"Seventeen people are too much. I'm going to sit quietly in the back of the room and observe," Maggie announced when we convened. Moving from her seat, she placed herself at considerable distance behind the group circle.

"Nothing to do with this morning," she maintained, as bewildered members questioned, interpreted, and implored. "Ignore me and move on," Maggie insisted. Given that we had begun the day with the controversy concerning changing seating versus verbal discourse, and that Maggie had shown herself to be a sophisticated and constructive participant, I was surprised by her behavior, and then alarmed. What could come next if she continued to follow her inclinations? I wondered to myself.

Interrupting and speaking over the members' entreaties, and cupping my mouth as if speaking through a megaphone, I called out: "Hi Maggie, how are you out there!" I shouted loudly: "The group really misses you. As you see, they won't go on without you. [pause] You are calling more attention to yourself, even if you don't want to." I was willing to continue until she budged.

"Okay, I will return to my seat," Maggie acceded to my verbal barrage. She registered the members' relief and approval, and we seemed to move on; of course, derivatives followed, including an uncomfortable pause.

Another woman finally spoke up. She was the elder of the two women who had been Jon's transference target. Referring to the morning's session, she addressed Jon:

> Your mixed feelings about your mother made me nervous, particularly when you singled me out. [cries] My son hardly speaks to me. I've tried to deal with what happened, but he won't. I'm grateful he lets me see my grandchildren. I was too much "in charge." I didn't want you [the group] to think that of me today.

The group became reality focused, offering sympathy, resonant experiences, and suggestions. We were approaching the end of the day and finding a symbolic reference, I linked together many of our varied interactions: "Being 'in charge' has to do with today, and how you relate to others and yourself. Your options are limited with your son, much less with us." I referred to Bion's (1962) distinction between solutions to problems and solutions to problems of development. "As adults, we all have problems, without immediate or fully satisfying solutions. We've been working on them together. Your son is an adult but he is not acting as an adult; he has problems in development."

Discussion

Working with an individual to solve problems, or a group to reach "enabling solutions" (Whitaker & Lieberman, 1964)—may be a first step (resolving housekeeping issues of coffee and bathroom breaks), an emergent necessity (confronting Maggie's behavior), or remedial, (clarifying the elder woman's relationship with her son), while also solidifying therapeutic relationships.

We meet the individual and the group on whatever levels are possible. However, to function with integrity, the therapist must attempt to extend reach from merely addressing conflict to a wider and deeper focus on the growth of the mind and relatedness.

In the debriefing, members expressed surprise that I could be laissez-faire and casual—such as by allowing people to go to the bathroom, get coffee, or check their phones—and forceful, even directive at other times—as in asking Peter not to change seats, encouraging Jon, and challenging Maggie.

I shrugged. "If you have to pee, you have to… I guess these days that goes for the cell phone too. [laughter] The serious question concerns what is worthy of our attention as members and leaders to further the goals of the group and the individual members?"

I said that in the interactions with Peter, I had put forth my preference for talking, but that there was a realistic basis for action, such as changing seats. I was "in charge" of my beliefs about optimal individual and group functioning—and let them be known. But it was important to establish that also the leader could defer and could wait to see what developed. As a group, we could deal realistically and perhaps symbolically with Peter's decision regarding his seating and my response to it. Working with Jon allowed me to extend the group's boundaries into the symbolic and transferential, and disturb valences towards pairing and regressed dependency.

Regarding the situation with Maggie, I felt impelled to take charge and assert power and control (a not always pleasant dimension of leadership *diplomacy*). Maggie's behaviors had an experimental purpose, unknown to me and perhaps to her as well. If there were no time limits, it might have been appropriate to let them unfold. But in a time-limited group, I assessed her tactics as a type of rebellion that stimulates group processes of reality-defying *anarchy* (Billow, 2003). Her attention-getting maneuvers would make it difficult to think or talk about anything else, sabotaging the goals of our group, which were to address problems in development, both professional and personal.[1] The intensity of her emotions and self-presentation blocked her own self-exploration and inhibited the creative work of others.

Conclusion: embracing both approaches to emotional learning

Of course, clinical experience should engage both approaches to emotional learning, and the best of our interventions do just that. A definitive answer clears up unnecessary confusions and provides mental space to explore; still, any communication from the therapist—even when to pee—should attempt to stir curiosity, generate new possibilities, and increase the likelihood of group discourse.

In reality testing, group process appears well-structured, coherent, and linear in that meaning gradually develops and is clarified. In *testing reality*, the group may appear to be thematically and even behaviorally disorganized. The meanings that emerge may seem to arise spontaneously and unpredictably, and may coexist without a drive for consensus or urgent validation. While *testing reality* can be rebellious and loosen social constraints, it can provide new possibilities in engaging with reality and enhancing interpersonal skills.

Again, the two types of emotional learning are rarely discrete, particularly in the group setting wherein all communications are experimental and risk public scrutiny. Just by showing up in a group, each member exhibits some willingness to test reality. Some individuals dip their toes, some go ankle deep, and some immerse themselves in the flow. It is the therapist's job to make sure no one drowns.

Contributing their knowledge, intuition, and empathy, group members inform and challenge my reality testing and aid me in testing reality too. I witness and learn from their inspired actions and interactions. They stimulate my experimenting with my thoughts, feelings, stance, attitudes, words, and silence. I enter each individual or group session with some excitement and some anxiety, with the confidence that I will be tested, and also that I will test out something unknown about myself—in thought, word, or deed. And through this process, I will become more effective in addressing the challenging realities of our work.

Note

1 Looking at this interaction theoretically, my verbal barrage served as a group-as-a-whole intervention. Communicating with Maggie on her wavelength, I could jam her "noise" with my own, and the group communicative *node* (Chapter 12) could resume operation.

Chapter 11

Four modes of therapeutic engagement
Diplomacy, integrity, sincerity, and authenticity

"Tell all the truth, but tell it slant," wrote Emily Dickinson (1960, pp. 506–507). "The truth must dazzle gradually, or every man be blind." By this, she meant that we have a limited capacity to tolerate truth. Individuals and groups need truth for security and growth. However, truth may be premature, be incomplete, or not relevant to the immediate situation; truth may hurt, mislead, or obstruct. The leader has the special role of managing truth: evaluating and responding to the truth needs of the individual and the group.

I put forward four modes of engagement available for the leader: *diplomacy*, *integrity*, *sincerity*, and *authenticity*. They inform the struggle to seek, confront, or modify ("slant") truth. These strategies of discourse (Austin, 1962) or modes of speaking and listening are influenced, of course, by the intersubjective processes of the group. The leader monitors discourse for truth through the lens of subjectivity and responds to various aspects of interaction that often are subtle and out of awareness. Consensus among the participants concerning what is said or what is meant may be absent, and the significance debatable. Finally, the effects of the modes of engagement—how truth is reached, delayed, modified, forestalled, or even avoided—are not always immediate or readily visible.

I propose that all interventions are captured under one of these overlapping rubrics; the four modes are exhaustive but nonexclusive. They supply conceptual references for the interactional stance one has adopted, allowing the leader to be more aware of what he or she is doing and why.

Diplomacy

Diplomacy is concerned with establishing and maintaining relationships and alliances. Interpersonal relations entail negotiating the not always resolvable divergences of interests and goals, and between what can be known and what is safe to communicate. Diplomacy respects the motivations, affiliations, and beliefs of different people and subgroups and the roles they occupy. While ideally, empathic and truth-seeking needs of different constituencies will come to support one another, versions of truth, and even the need for truth, may continue to vary or even clash. Issues of power now come to the fore, as do the leader's authority and status in the group culture. Still, to some extent, power is shared, albeit unequally. In being diplomatic, leadership is strategic: influencing the group not to express its power in forms of retaliation.

In the diplomatic mode, a leader situates certain truths and not others as primary or ideal. Certain truths may be emphasized and explored, while others are minimized, shaded, or withheld. Diplomatic interventions are not always popular or balanced evenly among all participants. In the following example, I was experienced as turning against my own constituents and favoring a new member.

Case example: responding to different truth needs

Claire, in her early thirties and engaged to be married, recently joined our group but now had second thoughts. "Everyone here has children or is planning to. I don't want any; you're going to think something is wrong with me." Her declaration stirred interest and an incipient interrogation. "This is what I feared, that I would have to explain myself."

I too was interested in exploring the meanings behind Claire's decision, but there was truth in her apprehension, and I felt it important to call attention to it. "Yes, no one would question why one of us would want to have a child. 'Childless' seems to define something negative." Claire felt the support of my intervention, but several of the women took issue with me. "I feel you are suppressing me. I just want to learn about Claire." "Should I feel uncomfortable if I talk about being a mother and how wonderful it feels?"

Claire reassured the second speaker that she loved children and enjoyed hearing about them. But she was stung by the accusation of suppression, which she felt was directed to her: "I don't want to suppress you..." and she broke off, near tears but also frozen with anger.

Again, I heard truth in Claire's ostensible misidentification. The first speaker was angry with Claire for her position: announcing yet refusing to explore her decision. There also was justification in the first speaker's anger towards me for defending Claire, in effect, redirecting the conversation. I matter-of-factly acknowledged both standpoints, neither of which seemed untenable. Claire was not willing to have a child or to talk about it at this time. She had declared her turf, and I secured her right to it. I suggested that perhaps more than one person was angry, with me particularly. My summary statement served its purpose of cooling the situation sufficiently, and the session proceeded with relatively peaceful coexistence.

Discussion

The strategy behind my assertion of power and authority was to forestall an open confrontation between a prematurely interpreting group and a member who would *secede* rather than abdicate a position of *refusal* (see Chapter 12) so as to prevent a fissure in developing group cohesiveness. At this stage of the initiation of the new member, it was important to identify the mutual hostility but not encourage its exploration. In taking an active stance and a clear position *vis-à-vis* differing truth needs, I could deflect some of the anger to a safer target: me.

The dimension of self-interest in diplomacy

The interests and goals of the leader may not be entirely congruent with those of some or even all of the constituencies, and they may be partially or entirely self-serving (as in issues of fee, vacation schedule, etc.), without necessarily being false or against the group's welfare.

Case example: disentangling leader-member entitlements

"How are you contributing to the group?" I asked Randy, cutting short his recount of an ongoing struggle with his wife involving his noncooperation with household tasks. "Maybe they [other members] can relate to their issues," Randy offered unconvincingly. Another man rejoined sarcastically: "It doesn't relate to me, I take out the garbage and don't have to be asked." Ignoring the group's resonance, Randy continued. I interrupted again: "Randy, you're making yourself the butt of the group, it's not good for you and it's not good for the group. Isn't this what you do in your marriage?"

He launched once more into his story, and I said he had to stop and respect my leadership. "But no one else is complaining, Rich. You're making me angry." I responded: "I understand that, but you'll have to control yourself and give other people a chance to talk." Randy: "You don't talk this way to other people." "I don't have to," I countered. Randy: "All you care about is your group, the big bucks." "Not 'all', but some," I acknowledged, "I care about the group and I care about supporting myself, now let's move on."

DISCUSSION

"Diplomatic" is not synonymous with "nice," supportive, or nonconfrontational. In the psychotherapy situation, the leader safeguards the group's emotional and interpretative impetus. Whereas I was willing once again to address Randy's entitlements and also acknowledge the truth in his identifying mine, my primary motivation was to "govern" the group system. My principles and practices served strategic purposes: in the service of the group, but also were self-serving, expressing my values, and to some extent satisfying my own aesthetic, emotional, intellectual, and fiscal needs.

The role of falsity

We make distinctions between factual truth and emotional truth. At times, one may be valued over the other. For example, in most exchanges between people, emotional truth and understanding between them is more important than exact attention to facts. But if a point of fact is crucial to understanding, then the factual truth comes first. Emotional truth implies a degree of tactfulness: factual truth does not.

Perhaps alluding to diplomatic communications, Samuel Butler (1912/1951) penned, "Truth does not consist in never lying but in knowing when to lie and when not to do so." We may be honest but merciless, and one must be careful how to ask for or volunteer truth when it can be hurtful. Questions, however, do not always seek truthful answers. Even when they do, minimization and shadings of feeling and meaning, even white lies, lubricate and may make possible beneficial social relations. Straying from what is exactly true and completely honest is not necessarily malicious, self-serving, or harmful to others. In the following example, I sorrowfully came to understand the depth of Butler's pithy statement.

Case example: diplomatic falsity

"Rich, I better see you. I've been too embarrassed to come to group or make an individual appointment. I've been going for tests. I'm sorry to have to say this—they put me on Aricept and Namenda."

It was terrible news, although I was not surprised. At age 57, my father was a practicing physician who could no longer tell time. I was intimately familiar with the trajectory of Alzheimer's. Dorothy had been complaining of memory problems for over a year. Her individual sessions were marred by references to group members with "what's her name? I can't remember." I had ceased attributing dynamic significance to her lapses. And now the medical data were emerging. "What should I do," she asked. "I guess I better go back and say good bye."

"Do you want to leave?" I asked.

"No, not at all. I just feel I can't participate like the others."

"So what else is new?" This had been a typical complaint of Dorothy, who was a Midwesterner in a group with many members who were, in her words, "sophisticated New Yorkers." But my communication was not honest, since I believed that there was something "new" in her difficulty, which I ignored, and chose to mislead her.

DOROTHY: That's true.

BILLOW: Why don't you take your time and decide what feels comfortable for you? Would you like to stay?

DOROTHY: Of course.

BILLOW: So stay.

DOROTHY: I don't want to appear "out of it."

> "Me either!" I interjected playfully. But, fearing what I believed to be the inevitable sequelae, I added seriously: "If you lose interest in the group, or feel that you're not connecting and we can't do anything about it, I'll help you leave."

DOROTHY: I'd hate that to happen.

BILLOW: Me too.

DISCUSSION

I misled, evaded, and encouraged and participated in collusion against factual truth. My pragmatic goal is to respond to what I felt was Dorothy's need (and perhaps my own), to feel comforted and cared for. I could tolerate the truth, but I felt it was in her best interest to forestall pointless pain, so that she could continue to benefit from group membership and the stimulation and support it provided. Dorothy had the freedom to make her own choice: when to embrace factual truth which she did a few sad months later.

Integrity

In engaging from a mode of *integrity*, salience resides in the leader's moral and ethical principles, in reference to his or her professional, political, ethnic, and religious affiliations. *Integrity* would seem to present little ambiguity concerning truth and falsity, since the leader may refer to and rely on a clear set of conventions. But as I will emphasize, integrity involves strength and consistency, but also flexibility; it emerges not only from principles but from how they are applied.

Integrity without judgment, self-examination, and relatedness is not sufficient and can be, in fact, inappropriate and even damaging. Integrity may manifest as rigidity and blindness to personal contingencies, and even be of questionable moral value. While integrity denotes being true to one's principles, such principles may be false, that is, ill-chosen, ill-applied, or wrong. As the "Mayfair Madam," Sydney Biddle Barrows (1986) acknowledged: "I ran the wrong kind of business [prostitution], but I did it with integrity."

Integrity and self-knowledge

Samuel Johnson (1759/1985) clarified that "integrity without knowledge is weak and useless, and knowledge without integrity is dangerous and dreadful." For any leader, *self*-knowledge is important; for the clinician, it is the lens through which one evaluates emotional truth and falsity and responds to the contributions of others.

In the following example, the group therapist, Jerome Gans (2006) carried out a painful introspection so that he could function with thoughtful integrity rather than moralistically. Gans first came to understand the truth that he, too, had an unethical part of his personality.

Case example: Understanding one's own conflicts
regarding integrity

A group member:

> My wife's insurance is paying for my therapy but it doesn't take effect until April. Could you bill the insurance company for eight sessions in April rather than the four we met in March and the four we met in April?

At one time Gans (2006) would have quickly responded, "No," motivated by unspoken moral outrage: "Who does he think he's dealing with, asking an ethical guy like me to participate in such underhanded shenanigans" (p. 22)?

Gans concurrently worked at a facility where many of the medical staff were double-billing their patients and finding other ways to inflate income. He found himself tempted, "frightened by the intensity of my own greed and the seeming ease with which I could rationalize it away" (p. 21). Getting in touch with his own fraudulent impulses provided crucial self-knowledge and stimulated curiosity about the member, rather than an internal rush to judgment.

Gans linked the request with traumatic incidents of corruption in the patient's family history. When the patient brought up his request again, Gans responded: "How could you ever win with a request like that?...If I do not comply with your request you will probably be annoyed with me and, if I do, you will have a corrupt therapist" (p. 22).

DISCUSSION

Had Gans not understood his urge to react moralistically, his engaging from a position of integrity would have been premature and defensive. Hiding behind a screen of integrity is hypocritical, whereas engaging with integrity may include temporarily laying aside certain ethical or moral truths, in the service of developing meaning. A harder-won emotional honesty may emerge for all participants, the "sinners" and the "sinned against."

Integrity applied systematically

Embedded in the complexities of every psychological situation are ethical dilemmas: dimensions of truth and falsity, both bold and shaded, exist in leader and the constituency. In the following example, a leader found herself caught between conflicting systems of ethics, her loyalty to the group member and respect for his confidentiality, and what she interpreted as state-mandated legal procedures. In retrospect, neither system captured the nuance of the psychological situation in which the therapist as well as the group and the member and his wife were embedded.

Case anecdote: a leader's problematic "will to a system of integrity"

Scott occupied many group sessions vilifying his wife, who had been, and possibly continued to be, unfaithful. Now he reported an incident in which his wife, tussling with their adolescent daughter over control of the television remote control, left a bite mark on her arm. The next day, the therapist telephoned and requested that Scott appear immediately in her office. She explained: "I was troubled all night by what I heard, and I think I might be required to call Child Protective Service to report abuse."

Scott became enraged and could hardly respond. "My wife and daughter have a great relationship! You know that! She's not an abusive mother. You must hate her as much as I do!" He stormed out of the office: "I don't think I can come back to the group."

Although often reticent and even secretive about group, Scott shared this incident with his wife, who responded sympathetically. At the same time, she empathized with the therapist: "I'm sure I don't have the best reputation with her" and encouraged him to return to group and attempt to work it out. This did not entirely please the husband, who, while mollified towards the therapist, now had to present a different view of his wife to his group. For, even when hearing falsities about herself as an unfit mother, she had remained steadfast, empathic to her accuser, and loyal to her husband and his need for therapy. To reconciliate with the wife—and with the group and its therapist—all would have to inspect Scott's mantle of moral outrage—his "truth" and how he misused it.

DISCUSSION

Cohen and Schermer (2002) described the "moral order" of a group, referring to its norms, values, beliefs, and ambience, and which supplies a context for each member's group self and the group's collective conscience and ego ideal. In my view, the leader most often personifies this ideal and, due to tendencies in one's personality as well as to projective pressure, may reflexively take on a moral mantle. Rulebooks are ever-present, symbolic, but also real. They guide but also may mislead. We are all susceptible to a "law and order" mentality and must assess our urges for fairness and "equal treatment for all," and wishes to advise and protect.

Sincerity

Sincerity is the mode that conveys the leader's positive or negative emotionality. "One cannot both be sincere and seem so," Andre Gide (1902/1996) averred. He meant that *sincerity* is categorical—either you are or you are not. In my conceptualization (based on Melanie Klein's metapsychology), sincerity derives from the idealization and devaluation characteristic of the paranoid-schizoid position, preceding the full-fledged depressive position. In the former, others are recognized and preserved mentally as loved objects, or omnipotently denied, while splitting rather than mature thinking remains prominent as a mode of organizing experience ("either/or," "good/bad," etc.).

I contrast the mode of sincerity with that of authenticity, described later in this chapter, which represents achievement of the depressive position. The hallmark of the depressive position is the capacity not only to love or hate but also to experience ambivalent feelings while maintaining a balanced and humane outlook. Authenticity involves mental integration of conflicting feelings, thoughts, wishes, and motives, directed to loved objects, competitors, and even enemies.

Sincerity is communicated by, between, and under the leader's words. It may be felt and conveyed immediately, activated by the leader's interest and compassion. It may be ongoing and constant, amplify over time, or be withdrawn. However, we may think we are being sincere without being so, for changes in feelings often precede awareness, yet are obvious to others. A leader's sincerity may be perceived as lacking or insufficient to meet the immediate relational needs of the group or member.

Sincerity may represent a leadership achievement

According to Yalom (1995), above and beyond all other technical considerations, the therapist must maintain a benevolent attitude towards his or her patient. Here I stress that any leader may adopt this attitude without sincerely loving in a manner required by the relational context. In the following case example, I cared; I offered good enough interpretations, and the patient reported "getting better." All was true, but none of this satisfied her particular developmental need to be idealized: considered as special, attractive, and delightful.

Case example: insufficient sincerity

June (age 61) lamented to her group: "I don't feel you are excited to see me. People are delighted to see each other, but no one is delighted to see me." June was the respected "senior member," a slight limp from childhood polio added to her gravitas.

"You are 'soo' reserved," a group member responded truthfully, while a chorus of others added, ineffectively, "We care for you."

The theme emerged in her individual psychotherapy:

> I'm feeling blank, nothing. Weekend was pretty good, the kids brought the grandchildren, but not that exciting. I never have enough time. Always a stack of work on my desk, this committee and that. I can't enjoy myself because I think about all I have to do.

I reminded her of her feeling that I, and her group too, did not enjoy her. "Yes, it is not that you don't like seeing me. But I guess I feel most people could take me or leave me." I asked whether she *believed* that I did not enjoy her, as well as *felt* it. She considered the question and decided that she really believed it:

> It's a matter of caring, you don't care that much. My parents took care of me, maybe overprotected me when I got polio, but never made me feel pretty and that I could have that kind of effect on them.

"So that's what you want!" I replied, and then brought us into a truth of our heterosexual adult life: "You want me to find you sexually attractive." June did not directly respond, but I believe she had allowed me to offer and herself to receive a sexual thought. She ended the session without her usual tense facial expression and its trace of bitterness. I sensed that we both felt more relaxed and connected to each other.

DISCUSSION

Beauty and its appreciation exist in every person, no matter how stifled by social forces or physical limitation. In Stephen Sondheim's musical play, *Passion*, a handsome visitor, Giorgio, arouses in the ailing and homely Fosca a love that proves irresistible to him, and he ultimately yields without regret. We cannot love, or love sufficiently, or effectively, without reciprocity of feeling, real or imagined. I, or our group alone, could not reignite June's libido from its embers. She too had to supply energy. Like Fosca, June took the chance to reconnect to her desire, which included her desire to be desired. She became more appealing when I could feel her as emotional and interested in being experienced as sexual. Derivatives of erotic feelings are natural and expectable, an enjoyable aspect of bonding with others, and at times a dimension of sincerity.

Ruptures in sincerity

We cannot will our feelings and are rarely pure of heart and mind. Feelings spring from sources other than Eros or Thanatos and may conflict with leadership ideals and sincere intentions. The leader's love—openness to others, interest, concern, and enjoyment—is revealed in the subtleties of timing, tone, and cadence, which amplify, modify, or even contradict what is verbally spoken (Chused, 1992; McLaughlin, 1991). The sincere leader learns by ruptures and, when opportune, attempts to repair them.

Case example: competency disguises a rupture in sincerity

After five years of intensive combined psychotherapy, the thrice-married Ralph began to grasp what I dubbed a "Fox News" dimension in his personality, a reference to the politically conservative American television network and their bullying commentators. But here he was again bellowing and fiercely finger-pointing at Julie, a group member and wife-substitute, such that I had to intervene. In an attempt to exculpate himself, he reminded the group that he had not behaved this way in quite a while and that even his wife said he was better. That satisfied the members sufficiently to move on to other interactions.

Several weeks later Ralph asked me in an individual session whether something had changed between us. "You seem a little different, not distant or uninvolved, but maybe more work-focused or business like."

Associating to the incident in group and realizing the truth of his observation, I said: "I don't think I've recovered from the last 'Fox-News broadcast'." My acknowledgment sounded to me defensively light-hearted, so that I added a corrective: "You're right. I don't feel the same way about you. I think you are going to have to repair our relationship."

"I apologized, what do you want! Now you're being hard-assed like Fox-News," he retorted.

I wondered whether I was abiding by the talion principle, paying back for what I had experienced as his hardness. I asked: "Did you apologize? It doesn't feel like one to me."

Ralph continued: "I checked it out with Julie after group, and we're okay."

"We're not okay, at least not yet," I acknowledged.

Ralph teased: "Oh, you're pouting. Just like my wife."

I did not try to hide my amusement and smiled. I offered him what I understood to be the current state of my feelings: "Your bringing this up might help. I don't know yet."

DISCUSSION

It took me a while to realize that something had come alive again in our relationship: my *sincerity*, and I liked the feeling. I even liked saying: "I don't feel the same way about you," which I recognized was true in my consciousness, but no longer true in my unconsciousness. I had become one of Ralph's walking wounded, hurting from his ruthless treatment of Julie (and me, via my identification with her). Ralph felt my lack of involvement, and he pursued me, becoming playfully seductive, which apparently I needed in order to be able to love him again.

The limitations of sincerity

Wilde wrote, "All bad poetry springs from genuine feeling" (Trilling, 1972, p. 119). Sincerity is always simple, and sometimes simplistic. Consciousnesses of positive or negative feelings and their public expression do not necessarily advance relationships. The target of our love or hate may be unready, or undeserving, and in not moderating or holding our emotional response in thoughtful abeyance, we may distract or obscure that which is cogent. Sincerity has its risks. One can be self-deceptive and sincere, ineffective, inappropriately seductive, willful, or misleading.

Case example: sincerity has unpredictable effects

A senior therapist had established a warm working relationship with Helene, a patient in combined treatment. Helene had endured several miscarriages and, nearing 40 years old, she feared becoming infertile. Being the trusted witness to Helene's travails, the therapist felt increasingly uncomfortable withholding her own parallel experience. At a moment she felt it particularly beneficial, she disclosed that she also had married in her late thirties and described similar difficulties in childbearing. Helene seemed reassured when the therapist revealed that she was the mother of two thriving teenagers.

Now, pregnant again and half way to full term, Helene came into a group session announcing that the fetus had died, and she would have to have an abortion. The therapist cried along with the patient, which touched the members, who concurred that the therapist "really cared."

Was she crying for Helene or for her earlier self? the therapist wondered. She felt herself to be false, undeserving of the credit for "caring," since the group did not know of her own reproductive struggles and identification with Helene. And, in her atypical display of emotion, the therapist was concerned that she drew attention to herself, depriving the anguished Helene.

The patient had a different take; much later, Helene revealed apologetically that, if she could not deliver a healthy child, she would be a disappointment to the therapist.

DISCUSSION

No matter how sincere our feelings and intentions, and how directly we express them, we cannot be fully aware or certain of our motivations, meanings, or interpersonal consequences. In expressing certain truths, we may omit others and falsify ourselves.

Authenticity

Whereas *sincerity* is categorical and simple, *authenticity* is dynamic and complex: tension exists between self-awareness and expression. Authenticity bears upon how the leader approaches and avoids truth, in the context of frame, technique, and propriety. Communications are mediated by appreciation of the dimensionality of emotion, the influence of the irrational and unconscious, and the inescapability of social role.

In his monograph, *Sincerity and Authenticity*, Trilling (1972) analyzed the differences between these terms. *Authenticity* suggests

> a more strenuous moral experience than "sincerity" does, a more exigent conception of the self and of what being true to it consists of, a wider reference to the universe and man's place in it, and a less acceptant and genial view of the social circumstances of life.
>
> (p. 11)

Trilling's conceptualization implies that authenticity is difficult and remains ambiguous. It requires "strenuous" mental activity, an "exigent" (i.e., demanding) standard of being true and of representing truth. A "less acceptant" view of human interaction is requisite for authenticity: the recognition that neither leader nor constituent can simply love or hate and remain sincere. Uncongenial circumstances of social life inevitably get stimulated by group and must become part of authentic experience.

Remorse and reparation: the pathway from sincerity to authenticity

Interpersonal relations stimulate covetous, angry, and censorious feelings, thoughts, and behaviors, even towards those we love; so we feel guilt and sorrow (Klein, 1975). Authenticity requires mental and sometimes behavioral efforts to repair the harm we have caused, both imagined and real. In tolerating the depressive position, the leader operates from a mode of authenticity, rather than mere sincerity. Informed by what Bion (1961) referred to as the "painful bringing together of the primitive and the sophisticated that is the essence of developmental conflict." (p. 159), the leader strives to synthesize the irrational and rational, narcissistic and socialistic, and blunt and cultivated aspects of one's personality.

Case anecdote: the member's passion and the
leader's reparation

Seth summoned courage to report that he had felt "ambushed" when I began the New Year with the announcement of a raise in group fee. "I had no choice," Seth protested. "It would be fairer if you had discussed it first in group." Other members disagreed: "This is what other doctors do." "It wouldn't make a difference. It is Richard's right to set the fee." "We don't have to stay."

I was surprised and became interested in Seth; he spoke up forcibly rather than play out his usual agreeable self. He had made a fair point and, despite my support from other group members, I felt embarrassed and remorse for hurting him. But I was also annoyed, as if he was being ungrateful for making so much of the issue. After all, my rates were not exorbitant and he was benefiting from my efforts. I knew that aspects of my conflictual response were "primitive" and irrational and that I needed to remain "sophisticated" as well. My act of reparation involved tolerating the mix of pleasant and unpleasant feelings towards Seth and supporting his efforts at being authentic (as well as my own). I responded by saying that I had not realized that he had felt ambushed, and that I would do as he suggested next time, even if no one else seemed to care. Seth was delighted: "I didn't expect to be heard."

DISCUSSION

In struggling towards a mutually authentic relationship, Seth had become less acceptant and genial. He now required others (myself particularly) to be more acutely reparative: anticipating and recognizing our effects on him, and thereby modifying our behavior, no matter how we might feel or wish to behave in the interactive moment. Seth had become a person capable of expressing and integrating a range of emotional thoughts and in so doing contributed to the authenticity in our relationship and within the group.

In striving for authenticity, the leader endures and encourages others to tolerate and suffer through the breakdown of pre-established attitudes and behaviors. Supporting the secure connections and bonding relationships characteristic of sincerity, the authentic leader also disturbs them, to drive change and stimulate creative growth.

Sincerity is spontaneous yet deliberate. Authenticity is mediated, but paradoxically happens without full awareness or certainty. Words and actions are partially derivatives of an unfolding (and evolving) unconscious. Authentic communications represent the leader's most profound insights and powerful intentions. Yet, they remain only best guesses of what the leader feels, thinks, and decides is appropriate to express, to be reevaluated and revised over time and further experienced within the life of the group.

"Every profound spirit needs a mask," Nietzsche asserted (Trilling, 1972, p. 119). Leaders and constituents wear masks, that is, roles that are social and mutually contracted, and which allow individuals to relate to each other in ways not otherwise possible. Within their respective roles, they participate in and bear witness to the struggle to develop and communicate truth.

Conclusion

Leadership involves holding the tension of truth as one understands it and deciding at what level—how, when, and how much—to convey truth and to whom. We navigate the four modes to cement bonding, build trust, allow relationships to evolve thoughtfully, and strengthen abilities to think creatively and relate constructively to the ongoing challenges of relational life. They represent the leader in interaction: how he or she approaches and avoids truth. Inevitably, significant truth about the leader also is revealed.

Section IV

Impasses and opportunities

Editor's note

The spirit of therapy, as advocated by Billow, is dialogic and mutual: through close encounters with trusted, informed others, we revisit and revise narratives, amend cherished ideas about self and other, and expand interpersonal and intrapsychic freedom. However, the process of change never happens smoothly, and therapeutic impasses are inevitable. By impasses I am referring to situations where the flow of feelings and ideas (LHK) among participants, or within an individual, is stymied. And since Billow's approach to the growth of the mind is an intersubjective one, these are precisely the situations that warrant close examination and creative solutions.

Therapeutic errors, shortcomings, and misattunements, real or perceived, if not equated with moral sins or dismissed as resistance, can provide useful links to transferences and unresolved traumas. To harness these opportunities, Billow focuses on the therapist's role in nondefensively recognizing and acknowledging his contributions: In one of the case illustrations, he accepts a group member's unflattering admonishment ("I'm afraid I've heard that comment more than once regarding my technical finesse"), and in another he concedes his reluctance to forfeit analytic, or status, entitlements. These interventions serve multiple purposes. First, they model an attitude of "I can be wrong, and you can be right," and a preference for cooperation and compromise. Second, they help ease patients' minds sufficiently so that they too will be more likely to take in the therapeutic testimonies of others. And third, through example, they broaden what can be incorporated into one's view of personhood. If successful, such efforts result in a greater integration of impasses, resentments, and entitlements, placing them in a larger context, without the anxious grasp for resolutions.

Chapter 12 begins with a proposal to revise the saturated term resistance. While Freud considered resistance "anything in the words and actions of the analysand that obstructs his gaining access to his unconscious" (Laplanche & Pontalis, 1973, p. 394), Billow suggests that it is useful to distinguish among clinical phenomena that are subsumed under the umbrella term "resistance." He describes three constellations that more closely describe clinical phenomena: *resistance* (in a narrower sense), *rebellion*, and *refusal*

(Billow, 2010b). Each describes a discontinuation of the intersubjective give-and-take, though they vary in intentionality, combativeness, and openness to dialogue.

Resistance, in the narrow sense, titrates the amount of emotional awareness one is able to tolerate. The reasons for resisting awareness are often quite compelling and may have to do with maturational and situational limitations. For example, as a young man—really just a boy of 20—I partook in military operations in Southern Lebanon as part of the Israeli army. I was only minimally aware of being frightened, or of my beliefs regarding the legitimacy of these actions. I was not prepared to face my insecurities, my fear of disappointing authority figures, and disapproval of the political process. Greater access to these thoughts and feelings came much later. At that stage of my development, and without the participation of mindful others, I could not find a way to think about my resistances and was unprepared to rebel or refuse[1] without being self-destructive.

Of the three Rs, rebellion (Billow, 2003a) is most closely associated with the possibility of therapy being more democratic and egalitarian. Billow views rebellion as an attempt to challenge the leader, group, or social network's authority and counsels to consider what may be usefully addressed, no matter the nature of delivery. Complaints, censures, and other forms of criticisms, friendly or hostile are not reduced to enjoyable acts of discharge or tension relief (Bernstein, 2007). Instead, rebellion offers opportunities to clarify differences and negotiate disagreements. In one example (Chapter 15), when a patient complained: "Why do we always have to analyze?" Billow inquired what she would rather do and was thoroughly surprised by her answer.

Unlike the rebellion in the previous example, where the patient had a different idea about how to spend her time in therapy, refusal (Billow, 2007) is best captured by the obstinate phrase "I don't want to!" though it needn't be that explicit, or juvenile. In chapters 12 and 13, Billow examines refusal and related phenomena that block the passage of ideas among people and/or restrict the introduction of new psychological ideas about oneself. For the refuser, the threat of intrusion is felt more poignantly than the interest in innovation. Consequently, the refusers and refused become less available for mutual influence, narrowing the space for meaningful analytic work. A change of mind is still possible when refusal is brought into the open: recognized, normalized, negotiated, or, at times, simply accepted.

Chapter 13 introduces the term "nodule," which Billow defines as the psychological clogging of communicative channels or nodes. Unexpectedly, individuals become preoccupied with powerful thoughts and feelings or go blank. Such dissociative states, lacking self-awareness, constrict thinking about—or engaging with—others' perspectives. Like the experience of being in a crowded subway, though surrounded by others, one's attention is hyper-focused inward. Also, if abruptly prodded, scary irruptions of negative affect may ensue, often evoking in others alarm, disbelief, or panic. As with refusal, recognizing and tolerating nodules and shifting discourse to verbal exploration may protect the dyad or group from the nodule's potential destructive impact. If the therapist does not over-rely on the patient or the group to do the work (a common thread throughout the book), he or she will, over time, be rewarded with collaborative efforts to revitalize emotional communication.

Fond of snow metaphors, Billow has cautioned me on several occasions that if, as a leader, I want the road cleared, I ought to be willing to pick up a shovel. A willingness to lead and take creative risks does not, however, guarantee cooperation. Following the treatment narrative of an intransigent adolescent, Chapter 14 explores the issue of falsification. Though perfectly willing to come to intensive treatment, very little seemed to bother, excite, or interest Simone. Her seeming indifference posed a somber therapeutic challenge since, as Billow concedes, it is not easy for therapists to tolerate being "whatevered." Simone's purposeful renunciation of creative thinking, manifested in stock phrases, conventional language, and clichés, and unresponsiveness to empathic or confrontational interventions, required the therapist to stretch his view of what constitutes effective, or even professional clinical behavior. Citing Bion (1970), Billow highlights the tension that arises between two equally problematic pitfalls: Colluding with the patient's pernicious view that nothing matters (especially not words), or becoming a moralistic, super-egoish, or nagging authority figure.

To conclude this section, we selected one of Billow's earliest papers on entitlement, which remains a relatively underexplored facet in treatment impasses. Commonly referred to in a pejorative sense, like a child who believes the world revolves around them, Billow explores the different, not necessarily pathological, aspects of entitled attitudes, in both patient and analyst. Impasses may ensue when either party feels wrongly deprived of their rights: analysts usually feel entitled to analyze and have their interventions considered, while patients feel entitled to warmth and acceptance. Presumably, underlying these entitlements is a universal wish to love and be loved. Faced with the threat of succumbing to the other's demands, coupled with the loss of positive bonding, either party is liable to (re)experience feeling overpowered or deserted. The goal is, of course, to move beyond manipulative power plays and moralistic accusations, towards a healthier, less desperate and demanding, even enjoyable, sense of entitlement.

Note

1   A few years later, I joined "Courage to Refuse," an organization of conscientious objectors, and refused to serve in the occupied territories of the West Bank. The act of political refusal (which in this chapter's terms is actually a rebellion) was more available to me, partly because I had the support of like-minded individuals in my academic setting.

Chapter 12

The three Rs of group

Resistance, rebellion, and refusal

Resistance (Billow, 2010a), *rebellion* (Billow, 2003a), and *refusal* (Billow, 2007) are familiar yet ambiguous words, often referred to without theoretical or clinical precision. I have adapted these terms to separate and identify psychological dynamics—demeanors, tensions, strategies, and therapeutic processes that have traditionally been huddled under the umbrella term "resistance." Individuals and groups resist, rebel, or refuse with varying motives, including those that are quite reasonable. The patterns and processes that emerge may serve as an impetus rather than an impediment to discovery, debate, independent thinking, and new modes of relating. Also, I do not necessarily associate any of the three Rs with positive or negative qualities. For instance, a resistant patient or group member may drop out prematurely, minimally participate, or put a pall on therapeutic interactions, while rebellious or even refusing individuals may commit energetically to the therapeutic process.

The following reports on an afternoon's workshop I led at a regional group therapy conference. I describe a painful emotional juncture, not unique to me, I am sure. The situation is this: the therapist or leader has gone too far, feels he or she has gone too far, or has been accused of going too far. The offended group member generates a network of sympathy and support, and attention turns antagonistically to the leader. Questions are raised regarding the leader's professional and emotional balance, principles and practices, personality, unconscious dynamics, and motivation.

A workshop on "formulating the unformulated"

Entering my assigned room, I felt heartened by a full roster of attendees, a few recognizable from previous presentations. Our topic was "Formulating the unformulated," and I invited people to determine how we should proceed. After a spirited debate and a sharing of interests, the group decided on the afternoon's format, a combination of experiential and didactic learning, with emphasis on the former. I agreed, and added that, most likely, I would be more active than in leading an ongoing psychotherapy group, both because of the large number (22) of participants and in order to call attention to the role of the leader.

The early give-and-take revealed many sophisticated participants, well versed in psychoanalytic theory. For example, several volunteered that they wanted to alter their "paranoid" and "schizoid" outlooks that they habitually brought to group experience. The room seemed to relax and affably settle in when I encouraged people to stick to their feelings and, for now, leave me to bandy about the Kleinian and Bionian formulations.

But one woman, Myra, regularly interjected herself and insisted on framing process in these terms and asked me to comment and clarify. As to be expected, members wanted to know more about Myra, why she wanted to know, and why now. Ignoring the curiosity about her, she simply reminded the group that I had written a book on relational group psychotherapy, and therefore I was an expert. She spoke with an accent, which added to an impression that she was different, perhaps foreign to an experiential workshop. However, her questions were easy to field, and for a while I succeeded in relating them, and her, to ongoing group process. Her interruptions continued and members turned to her with alternatingly caring and hostile attention.

For whatever reasons, Myra was not translating the feedback in a useful way. She seemed not to understand and frayed members' patience. I nipped a spirited, but indirect, attack led by Peter, a man sitting to my right, with a sardonic aside to the group at large: "If we were concerned with scapegoating, rather than unformulated experience, I could not have written a script for a better foil." I told Myra I would try to answer her interesting questions later and turned to engage a segment of the room which had not yet spoken.

But Peter protested angrily at my cutting him off. What was I saying to him? I replied that I was aware of interrupting him, and that I had assumed he would understand that it was not about him, but an effort to protect Myra, and keep the group from being mired in the easily "formulated." He said he did understand, but did not like the way I had done it. I sympathized and said I was sure that I could have done it better and apologized for offending him. Sitting next to each other, we literally were face-to-face, and thus, our moment of intense intimacy was observable to all.

Michael, sitting across the room, broke our brief silence by checking in with Peter, how did he feel about my response? Peter replied that he was satisfied by my explanation and our exchange. Michael then complimented me for handling the matter straightforwardly. Peter clarified that he realized that I had been trying to move the group into a more feeling level, and that he had a tendency to intellectualize. Still, he did not like being interrupted and, while he agreed with Michael that he liked my directness, he was holding his judgment about me in abeyance.

Jane, a woman flanking my left, seemed to have little doubt about me. She said she was shaken by the interaction and felt I had lost control of the group. She declined to comment further. Karen introduced herself, saying that it was too bad Jane felt that way. She liked Peter's directness, both that he could confront me so early in the group and that he could be reasonable and self-reflective. Michael concurred and reiterated his positive feelings about the group. "I'd like to continue," Karen interceded. Michael said, "go ahead." She said she was not comfortable speaking in groups and wanted to speak up and say that, before she lost courage and retreated. Now she felt uncomfortable!

Karen's acknowledgment brought out several who said that it was difficult to break the ice and speak up. Karen said that they would get much more out of the experience if they did, "see, I'm already saying more than I usually do!" Her warmth seemed to encourage others to introduce themselves, describe some of their life issues, and enter into affecting dialogue with the group at large.

As if to cool the developing emotional intensity, a person cheerfully told about herself, a hiker in the Sierras. She connected to another person with extensive camping and wilderness experience. A third spoke of fly-fishing, a fourth, a photography expedition to Africa. Conveying a sense of making an intervention almost too obvious, I suggested that the group get back to our indoor adventure. As if I had said the opposite, Jane launched into her own lengthy travelogue, which seemed not only to disappoint but also to stun the group. Despite several polite attempts to redirect her conversation, she found a cohort to continue an exchange. At some point, I interceded and asked them if they could relate more directly to what they were feeling in the group.

While her partner voiced appreciation for my stepping in, Jane became irate and attempted to draft Peter by referring to our early interaction. Peter supported my leadership, however, and, along with others, attempted to work with Jane, explaining what she was doing, asking her to be more direct. She seemed dejected and confused, and still not a bit happy with me. In order to move things along and avoid another scapegoating, I complimented Jane for letting us know how she felt about me.

Several of the less secure participants took a chance, speaking briefly about the group experience or their personal lives, while conveying a touching vulnerability that stimulated the group's cautious curiosity. Tom, who had described himself as "schizoid," reported a life crisis. He married late, and now he and his wife had their last chance to conceive. He had lived a life without having to care for another, and could he do it? Eric shared that he had just become a father, and he began to cry when he considered how it felt. He knew he was different than his own father, who cared, but could not show it. Perhaps Tom needed to think about his relationship to his own father. Karen commented that although Tom did not say much, he conveyed a great deal of caring, and that she thought he would be a great parent. As if to prove her point, Tom thanked Eric for his insight regarding fathers and gently attended to Eric's sadness.

Michael joined in the midst of the exchange between the two men, informing the group that although he was even older than Tom, he remained ambivalent about settling down and having a child. Several women were interested, he informed us, maybe he was in love with at least one of them, but he was not sure if he was ready, or that he ever would be ready. Eric thought that would be too bad. Yes, it would be, Michael rejoined poignantly, but took the conversation no further.

Ben turned to Karen and commented how much he enjoyed her participation. Even when she was not saying anything, she had lively eyes. Karen, taken aback and quizzical, smiled in return. Michael volunteered that he too noticed Karen and agreed that she was contributing a lot to "process." His reference redirected attention to an abstraction, the group entity, and away from the couple. Addressing Michael, I said that I believed he could take something from the afternoon's workshop that eventually might help him in making a decision about his life. I commented that he tended to get in the middle of exchanges between other members. And then, as an afterthought, I added that he was functioning as the group's "Oedipal child."

Michael at first seemed interested in my insight, but shortly became enraged. "You have some nerve to call me 'Oedipal,' you don't know my situation. I have been in analysis for fifteen years, with several highly qualified and well-known people. You know me for a couple of hours, where do you get off analyzing me."

Concerned by the intensity of Michael's response, several members tried without success to soothe and reason with him, to bring out what upset him so. Peter turned attention to my leadership. "We didn't contract for psychotherapy," he reprimanded.

Gail, a woman who had spoken only briefly, explained that I was interpreting an "enactment," something that occurred in group and in all human relationships, whether or not involving psychotherapy. She went on, "that's the beauty of group, the deepest issues may come out after a few moments. Michael calls attention to himself whenever two people start to connect."

"I feel like getting up and leaving, but I won't," Michael continued.

Ben attempted to mediate the situation. He said he hoped Michael would stay and try to work this out. He understood how Michael felt, but he believed that I made the comment in the spirit of trying to connect and be helpful. Ben suggested that Michael might be reacting to how, as much as what, I said. Ben had been in another of my workshops. He observed that mostly I put my comments as mere ideas to be considered, or not considered. But I had spoken differently to Michael, with an air of certainty.

My use of "Oedipal" bothered several people who spoke up. It sounded "clinical." Why did I use the term? How was it helpful?

Gail said that I was a psychoanalyst and the term did not necessarily mean the same to me as it might to others. "What is so bad about the term, anyway?" Karen declared, and some others silently concurred.

I too was perplexed, for the group had begun with many members speaking in psychoanalytic shorthand, and I assumed liberty to use the vocabulary.

"It sounds like name calling," someone replied.

Ben said that he believed I meant "Oedipal" metaphorically, and not literally, but psychoanalytic terms should be avoided, because they carry with them a lot of baggage. Particularly when the leader says them, they mean more. How was Michael doing?

"Not very well. I don't need this. [To me] You don't know anything about me. I am a widower….my wife died many years ago and I still carry around unfinished business. Maybe I'm still in mourning. I haven't been able to really commit since then. I don't know if I want to build my own family." Michael continued to talk earnestly to the group. While feeling supportive and encouraging of him, I also felt clumsy for my intervention and guilty for having opened his wound.

Peter turned attention back to me; he wondered if I was angry with Michael, and that is why I spoke to him that way. I said that as far as I was aware, I might have had too much "desire" to connect with Michael and be helpful. Perhaps my desire is what Ben heard as certainty.

Peter remained unconvinced, as if I did not know my own feelings, which was, of course, a distinct possibility. I asked Michael if he felt I was angry with him.

"No, I think you like me and are interested in me. I liked you, until now, I still do. I think you were genuinely trying to be helpful. But it felt like a kick in the butt."

"I'm afraid I've heard that comment more than once regarding my technical finesse."

Michael replied: "In all fairness, I've heard more than once that I need a kick in the butt."

"Well, we both got our butt kicked this afternoon," I said, as we exchanged warm smiles.

Ben commented that he was glad that Michael stayed. Had he left, it would have been bad for him, and for the group. He was grateful that we had a chance to work on what happened. I asked him why this was personally important to him. He said it meant a lot that an authority figure could be flexible and listen, and even acknowledge mistakes and shortcomings. His own father was quite the opposite: rigid and self-righteous.

Ben responded positively when I suggested that although he knew something about his relationship to his father, he had used the group experience to formulate unformulated feelings and thoughts. While it seemed evident that, like Michael's (perhaps Jane's and Peter's as well), Ben's reaction to me had an "Oedipal" cast, I chose not to share my opinion. I turned to the group, saying that I was aware of time constraints, and that the participants also might want to formulate their experience. Some members did so, while others opted to comment on the most recent interaction, pick up and continue earlier links, or merely say good-bye.

Myra did not ask any more questions; rather, she reported having been intensely involved during the session, although she was not ready to put her feelings into words. Jane said that she could: she had remained angry and disappointed in me. She turned to several of the younger participants, letting them know that their struggles reminded her of her earlier self, and of some of the choices she made and had not made. Members reflected that she was communicating differently, and touchingly, and they raised the possibility that her "formulating" had to do with the leader's influence on group process. Jane stiffened and did not address me directly.

Peter remained somber, and he was one of the few who did not participate in the remaining half hour. However, as people were exiting, he revealed himself to be an editor of a forthcoming book on group therapy. To my surprise, he asked whether I would contribute a chapter.

Still, I left the workshop not convinced about the durability of the repair between Michael and myself and the meaning of the group experience for all the members. And, although the participants rated the workshop highly on their review forms, I remained vaguely rattled and in doubt regarding what people thought of it and of me. Perhaps uncertainty is a valuable, even necessary dimension of the pursuit of truth, an aspect of formulating—and reformulating—the unformulated.

Discussion

There are, of course, many different ways of thinking about, organizing, and analyzing group process retrospectively. In concentrating on the influence of the leader and dynamics of resistance, rebellion, and refusal, I necessarily neglect or minimize other important group, subgroup, and intrapersonal factors.

Resistance

Psychoanalytically, "resistance" refers to words and actions that obstruct access to unconscious sources of truth. While Freud first considered resistance as an obstacle to be overcome, he came to realize that resistance could be used as a vehicle to reach these repressed truths. The transference, in part a resistance, could be analyzed, and like dreams and free association may be traversed as another "royal road" to the unconscious.

While an individual may halt associations, not remember dreams, and suppress or otherwise withhold attitudes towards the leader and others, group members intuit resisted truth. "Everyone possesses in his unconscious mental activity an apparatus which enables him to interpret other people's reactions" (Freud, 1915, p. 15).

Bion's extension of Klein's seminal idea of projective identification has provided a conceptual vehicle for understanding resistance (inter) subjectively. Truth may be inferred from gathering in, or "containing," another's projections. Bion posited projective identification as a fundamental mode of communication: how we understand and convey emotional truth unconsciously, pre-consciously, and pre- or nonverbally.

All group members emit and receive projective identifications, hidden under, among, and within our words, silences, gestures, and actions. Their evocative effects on group process and culture are palpable, immediate, and cumulative, yet also, subtle, ambiguous, and delayed. Projective identifications provoke potent counter-reactions, and interacting networks of emotional communication and miscommunication are to be expected and not immediately understood.

In the workshop's brief time span, basic unconscious themes regarding genesis, growth, parenting, family, sexuality, and competition were expressed and partially developed. Birth themes even were presaged by the workshop's title: "Formulating the unformulated." However, to some extent, the group idea is pre-formulated, rather than un-formulated. In anticipating a workshop, each participant mentally affixes to a vague entity, a group-as-fetus. And, upon entering the workshop space, the fetus almost immediately becomes the baby born—the roomful of people becomes a "group."

Perhaps the most difficult, and saddest, aspect of the leader's job is to separate sufficiently from this neonatal group to become its leader. While the group struggles with babyhood, to maintain connection and to feel secure, the leader struggles with parenthood, to separate and to feel adequate. Certainly, the leader has birthing anxieties, fantasies, and wishes in proposing, preparing, and entering a workshop: Will I deliver a healthy, truth-seeking group? Can I adequately nurture such a group and challenge the group's inherent antagonism to what they need? Will the group love me?

In the workshop, I quickly came to feel as if I were a good parent to some members and a bad parent to others. My sense of "playing a part, …in somebody else's phantasy" matched Bion's (1961, p. 149) description of the experience of being the object of projective identification. Bion counseled the therapist to mentally "shake" out the accompanying numbness, to think objectively. When Peter chastised me for interrupting, I felt numbed by many sets of accusatory eyes, including my own. It was quite possible that, despite my conscious intention to be objective and not to retaliate, I divided the room into good and bad children in terms of how members treated me as good/bad parent. Eric's message to Tom, to think about the father–son relationship, applied to me as well.

I had to accept that my words and actions were partially derivatives of my unconscious, and only retrospectively could I begin to become aware of the enactments that I contributed to (Chused, 1992; Renik, 1993). In our controversial interaction, Michael and I met at an emotional crossroad, an intersection of our father–son psychologies. In retrospect, we came to understand that we had engaged in mutual "butt kicking"—certainly a less lethal enactment than played out between Oedipus and his father.

In his landmark book, *Transference and Countertransference*, Racker (1968) suggested that a neglected aspect of the Oedipus complex was the analyst's wish to be king, not only of other people but also of one's own unconscious. So, the best I could do as leader was eradicate, as much as I could, not my own Oedipal complex, but my resistance to increasing self-awareness of it.

Bion (1965, p. 168) coined the phrase "proto-resistance" to describe a crucial feature of the analyst's subjective experience, an anticipatory anxiety regarding the antagonism of a patient to an interpretation not yet made. The question remains then, whether I was anxious enough in relating to Michael and other group members. Perhaps Ben was right, in that I was too certain, or Peter was right, that I was frustrated with Michael and angry. In the workshop, I raised the possibility that I had too much Oedipal "desire" to connect with him and be helpful. Only a certain amount of truth may be introduced into experience. It is among the leader's primary tasks to offer protection from too much truth, or too little. Like other group members, I remained in conflict regarding pursuing truth, and also reacted characteristically when meeting resistance to my own truth-seeking needs. I take consolation from the thought that, while my unconscious conflicts, character structure, misunderstandings, and empathic failures contributed to the multileveled resistances in the group, they also provided vehicles for working them through.

Another thought also consoles me, which is that my intervention with Michael was accurate, appropriate psychoanalytically, and suitable for a workshop with sophisticated professionals. Bion (1965) put it thus: "Freud stated as one of the criteria by which a psycho-analyst was to be judged was the degree of understanding allegiance he paid to the theory of the Oedipus complex.... [T]ime has done nothing to suggest that he erred by over-estimation; evidence of the Oedipus complex is never absent though it can be unobserved" (pp. 49–50).

No one said the truth was easy. Interventions often are as difficult for the leader to offer as for groups to receive, and sometimes we feel and are made to feel bad for making them. Confronting resistance, counter-resistance, and "proto-resistance" remains an uncertain, confusing procedure, and often a mark of the success is ongoing discomfort and self-doubt. The journey from unformulated to formulated is fretful and incomplete.

Rebellion

Group members feel intersubjective tensions that arise from differences in beliefs about how their group should function, and at times they rebel against the group process. There are different pathways of rebellion, differentiated by their processes and outcomes: defiance, secession/exile, anarchy, or revolution (Billow, 2003a). Rebellion denotes a strategy of social action, adopted by a faction, when other avenues of influence seem futile or unattractive, a judgment that depends on the group's genuine receptivity to discussion and change, and equally on the state of mind of the rebelling faction. While rebellion represents a mental attitude, it is useful to think of group process, and rebellion, as an attempt to move the group in a different direction.

In rebellion, unlike resistance, the ideas and feelings that are expressed, and the behaviors that are planned or enacted, are not to be considered primarily as psychological phenomena, with unconscious levels of meaning, to be brought into conscious awareness and appreciated for their symbolism. Rebellion focuses attention on the idea of the group: what kind of group is this and is it acceptable? The basic premises and values of the group are at the center of the controversy, to be acknowledged, and addressed on that level.

Since I consider rebellion as representing a possibly valid challenge, and not necessarily a resistance or a stage of group life, my conceptualization is at some variance with the idea of rebellion as it has figured in the major theories of group formation and process (e.g., Agazarian, 2012; Bennis & Shepard, 1956). To give a most prominent example, Freud (1921) postulated that rebellion against the leader is necessary for group formation and process; members must work through unconscious resistance to feel and verbalize their wishes to overthrow the leader and indulge their sexual and aggressive fantasies.

Resisting awareness, expressing a vexing self, or even deviating from the existing group culture does not necessarily constitute rebellion. As we know, persistently resistant or difficult individuals may spend years challenging the opinions of the group therapist or other members, while regularly attending and finding benefit in the treatment. Others may feel bonded, yet disobey the task, frame, or rules, and even may dodge treatment. Neither situation necessarily represents a true rebellion, since the members are not motivated to address or influence the group's principles or mode of operation. Quite the contrary, they may enjoy the group as constituted and have no wish for change, despite their protests and difficulties in living within it.

Thus, I emphasize that the conflict of therapeutic assumptions and values leading to rebellion may exist quite apart from resistance, dynamic and character issues, or transference-countertransference per se. The conflict may represent reasonable differences in beliefs in what constitutes an effective group experience. Exposing and discussing the differences in perspectives, and what are believed to be incongruities in underlying or basic values, becomes an essential aspect of the group process. Psychodynamic issues underlying the clash also may be analyzed in due course.

However, in human relations serious misalliances may be unavoidable. The various pathways of rebellion are not always subject to modification via negotiation, compromise, and analysis. For example, our group worked around Jane's stubborn defiance, which remained unresolved. Michael threatened secession, and if the group truly was unsafe, secession was the choice pathway. Similarly, if an individual or faction had used the group for harm of self or other, I would have exiled the offending membership. In revolution, the premises of the rebelling faction come to overpower and dominate the group, which goes on to a new phase. However, revolution may rise organically as part of the group's development, and hence, the group's transformation may not always be immediate or obvious, or result from a single or dramatic event.

The conflict leading to the action pathways of rebellion may not involve antagonism to all forms of truth and manners of pursuing it, but to the particular group approach or to the type of truth pursued. In our group, Myra wanted didactic truth, and initially she defied adhering to the agreed upon experiential format. Peter initiated rebellion against me. "What was I 'saying' to him by interrupting?" he asked defiantly. It was not clear whether he objected in principle to a leader's interrupting, anyone interrupting, or my oblique mode of interrupting. Still, I found his reasons for defying me—as far as I understood them—sensible and possibly valid, and I apologized, and directly explained my behavior.

"How did Peter feel about my response?" Michael asked. While I suspected Michael of kindling lingering embers of discontent, I accepted the legitimacy of his inquiry. Peter supported me, and the fan of rebellion passed to Jane. I had "lost control" of the group. I heard in her declaration a revolutionary clarion for new leadership, which brought out the loyalists. As spokesperson, Karen promoted my principles: speak up, share feelings, self-reflect, and others followed. But Jane broke the intimacy with her insistent travelogue and would not adhere to my injunction to relate her feelings to the group. She clung to her view of group process, and once again mounted an unsuccessful challenge to my leadership. I felt I had to protect her from the group's counter-insurgency.

Then, another challenge occurred, this time instigated by my "Oedipal child" remark. I could not be sure whether Michael's outrage was a rebellious ploy to oust my leadership. Peter's chilly assertion that I was practicing uncontracted psychotherapy amplified my threat of exile. Ben served ostensibly as the great compromiser: I could continue to lead, but avoid all psychoanalytic terms. My theory and technique of group leadership was up for debate. A revolutionary troika of men—Michael, Peter, and Ben—set about to decide the fate of our group.

Was the rebellion phase specific, an occurrence that would be directed against any leader? Were the three men jockeying for status, power, and influence? Or, was the rebellion against me specifically?

Of course, I was a rebel too. While, on the one hand, the group leader is a primary agent in fostering a sense of continuity, cohesion, and regularity, he or she is also a powerful agent of change. The group leader symbolically, linguistically, and behaviorally may traverse the various pathways of rebellion, taking multiple roles of defiant instigator, anarchist, exiled outcast, and revolutionary.

The putting-into-words process is a most important act of rebellion. To avoid sounding omniscient or oracular and to encourage feedback, the leader needs to interact spontaneously and maintain a vernacular, down-to-earth, even playful manner. Still, "clinical touch" cannot be defined, and two group leaders may think alike and make similar interventions at similar moments with quite different results. It was possible, as Ben suggested, that it was not my words, but how I used them, that needed challenge and investigation.

Group leaders have destructive as well as constructive rebellious tendencies, independent of group phase or similar behaviors from other members. Certainly, my version and approach to truth might have contributed to the group's rebellion, and to my response to rebellion. I had formulated an idea that the group could not yet tolerate, and to insist upon my idea would have been unnecessarily provocative and without political purpose. However personally unnerving, I thought it important to encourage and participate in the group's discussion of my normative assumptions, leadership principles, personality, and human limitations. The group faced and lived with conflict between the leader and certain members, and their clashing versions of truth. Rebellion, not quashed or resolved, to some extent enhanced the group experience.

Refusal

Certain truths, and certain modes of truth seeking, may be experienced as destructive. Refusal establishes a mental boundary between what is considered appropriate and inappropriate for intrapsychic or interpersonal dialogue. Unconscious as well as conscious processes of feeling, thinking, and meaning-making are refused entry, left undeveloped, or obstructed. Working with refusal requires appreciating how and why truth-seeking interactions are being rejected.

The refusal to feel, to think, and to make meaning—to confront and search for psychic truth—is more pervasive than we recognize. Refusal may be conscious and overt, or it may be disguised via confusion, indecision, ambivalence, intellectualization, distraction, emotional withdrawal, compliance, and cliché. Refusal is a strategy of the three basic assumptions, as members refuse the instruments psychoanalytic theory uses to uncover resistances and cope with rebellions: thought, language, and those who use and respect thought and language. While refusal is a common, obvious, and even pervasive aspect of individual and group psychology, refusal is infrequently considered as a primary relational mode. And, perhaps because group members may refuse outright, forcefully, and persistently, the group leader may refuse to think about refusal and make it a sustained focus of inquiry.

We may contrast refusal with both resistance and rebellion. Resistance involves symbol and symptom formation, transference-countertransference, and other derivatives of unconscious activity. Rebellion eventuates in challenge, debate, and the possibility of sociopolitical action. Refusal thus differs from resistance, which forestalls conscious but invites unconscious thinking, and from rebellion, which invites conscious but not unconscious thinking. Refusal remains antagonistic to unconscious and conscious versions of truth. Whereas in resistance and rebellion, the group leader becomes immersed in conflict and process, refusal engenders intellectual void. However, sudden flare-ups and impulsive threats and behaviors may be expected.

In the workshop, a number of individuals exhibited the refusal mode. Myra was the first to go against the group will, and she refused to examine her behavior or to link it to ongoing group process. Her communications remained concrete and circumstantial. For example, when questioned helpfully by other members, she responded by referring to my so-called expertise, as if that would explain her insistent intellectualizations.

Like Myra, Jane rebuffed dialogue and concluded as self-evident that I had lost control of the group. Later, I made a procedural suggestion, to return from the outdoor to the indoor adventure, that is, the here-and-now. Jane stunned the group by doing the opposite, inducing another member to join her in travelogue. I directly interceded and requested that the pair relate to their feelings, which relieved Jane's cohort, but Jane became irate and refused, and attempted to induct Peter. He refused to partner her, but he did not function in a refusal mode, since he utilized thought and language to link to her and seek meaning.

My fateful words, "Oedipal child," ignited Michael and released a dark cloud of censure that spread over my intervention and me. "Psychotherapy!" Peter decried. "Clinical!" echoed a chorus of the self-righteous, and they could not—or would not—think about how my use of the term possibly could be helpful and not destructive.

Gail brought up the concept of enactment, referring to Michael's repeatedly inserting himself in the middle of two-person relationships. She spoke of the "beauty" of group process, and others agreed that something important had been revealed. But for a subgroup, beauty was not truth, and truth not beauty, and they remained a congregation of the unconverted. They thought I was thoughtless and, for a while, refused to think further about the possible constructive purposes of my interventions. I thought them thoughtless. To repair the breach, I could not refuse to think about refusal and convey respect for the reasons behind it. With the group's help, I found words, an attitude, and a mode of connection that encouraged a return to formulating thought.

Concluding remarks: antagonism to truth and antagonism to falsity

As group leaders, we feel intersubjective tensions activated by social participation, representing the currency and history of our own intrapsychic and interpersonal struggles to seek and avoid truth. Like other members, the leader is capable of understanding a great deal about another, oneself, and the group at large, without pursuing that which is painfully immediate and most meaningful.

Even when factually true, our communications may serve falsity by being misleading, inauthentic, irrelevant, or cliché, so providing a buffer against genuine mental interaction. Recognizing our own limitations in—and repudiation of—thinking is not easy, for we hide ourselves from ourselves, as well as from our groups. We may contain our anxiety and be quiet, or answer conventionally, with the best of conscious rationales: to maintain therapeutic space, provide a (relatively) blank screen, preserve the therapeutic alliance, let group process emerge, and so forth. And, should we boldly utilize our subjective experience in making interpretations, or otherwise self-disclose, we may be consciously as well as unconsciously avoiding, and yet also inadvertently conveying other aspects of personal experience (Frank, 1997; Greenberg, 1995). Neither action nor inaction relieves the therapist of the ambiguous relationship to truth and its absence.

Truth emerges from how and why the leader pursues (and avoids) truth, and which truth, and the leader's success in engaging other members in the truth-seeking process. In being professional, significant truth about the leader also is revealed: how the leader understands and responds to challenge and defiance, his or her investigative and interpretative pacing, tact, empathic gestures, and bonding efforts. Issues of the leader's authenticity, his or her sincerity and insincerity, and truth and falsity, are open to public scrutiny and affect group process. Ambivalence to truth is a prominent element in intersubjectivity, functioning at varying levels of awareness and in different relational modes such as resistance, rebellion, and refusal, awaiting mutual discovery.

Chapter 13

Psychic nodules and therapeutic impasses

I introduce the term "nodule" to call attention to a particular type of irruption into the individual or collective's psychology while it is engaged in other psychic and interpersonal activities. Something happens that punctures the ongoing flow of experience, hijacking the individual and group focus. This interruption may occur with vivid sensory and emotional immediacy, disrupting the individual or group.

The nodule takes hold of a segment of an individual or group's mental life, preventing associations from usefully integrating and furthering self-reflection. Rather, associations crystallize as preoccupying affects and feelings, bodily states, actions, and action tendencies. Whether accompanied with pain or pleasure, anxiety or relief, the subjective experience can be activating and engrossing, while simultaneously numbing.

Psychic nodules may develop as a unique response to a new and difficult situation, or something that reappears at specific moments and relates to past or ongoing trauma. They may be intense but brief, repetitive, or ongoing, lasting over lengthy personal or historical time periods. While this chapter will concentrate on the individual and group experience, a political society also may be "taken over" by a nodule, engulfing its citizens. A contagious spread effect or "force field" suppresses and blunts contradictory states of feeling and thinking, such that the social entity functions in heedless unison.

Psychic nodules have been implicated, although not identified as such, as a dimension of trauma and dissociation (Dell & O'Neil, 2009), impairing group functioning (Bion, 1961), and contributing to leader-group enactments (Billow, 2012; Grossmark, 2007).

Nodules disrupt nodes

A *node* is a convergence of pathways—a focal point—of a network through which communication flows. When analogized to an electronic device, such as a router, a node is active and capable of sending, receiving, or "rerouting" information. In contemporary psychoanalytic theory, the mind is often conceived of as a node, an organizing configuration of shifting or oscillating nonlinear states of consciousness-nonconsciousness (see, for example, Bromberg, 2009).

The influential English group theorist, S. H. Foulkes (1964; Foulkes & Anthony, 1965), conceptualized the group similarly, as a "matrix," an informational network of individuals linked together by their interactions and communications. The matrix may also be considered as the superordinate node, a dynamic complexity of interacting communicating subnodes, to varying degrees impinged upon by disruptive nodules. As with other types of dissociative phenomena, nodules are pathological to the degree that they persist in limiting or foreclosing the capacity to hold and reflect upon different states of mind (Bromberg, 2009; Stern, 2009). At times, they create therapeutic impasses and may lead to confusion, disorganization, and anarchy in the group. In this chapter, I report on the combined individual-group treatment of three individuals struggling with intense and repetitive irruptions, and their impact on their respective groups.

Three case studies

Erik: trapped within a seductive and troubled mother's orbit

Erik was a proverbial jack of all trades who found himself, in his late twenties, ambivalently attached to a family business, a pregnant wife, a therapist, and a group. While at times focused and intensely tuned in to other group members, Erik could drift off in somnolence or communicate elusively. With some alarm, the group discovered that one personal topic—his relationship to his mother—could not withstand exploration. When pressed by another member, Erik could curse a "fuck you" or, more threateningly, lurch forward, as if to get up and leave, or hit the offending questioner.

Erik frequently signaled his need for attention and appreciated being pursued. However, connecting or reconnecting to him could be problematic. He could halt mid-sentence and follow with a lengthy wordless pause that bewildered and embarrassed him, which he could rarely recover from or receive help for.

Such episodes of mental "jamming" illustrate the nodule's propensity to "clog" the mind's information and communicative apparatus (the node) with inadequately processed data. Erik's suspension of language—the verbal freeze-ups—suggested to me a fierce internal struggle that he could feel but dare not form into communicable language. The cumulative residue of an over-stimulating and engulfing mother confined Erik and shut off his access to an independent mind that could think about the mother–son relationship. A nodule "took over," leaving him troubled and restless, easily depleted, exhausted in mind, word, and body.

Erik's dramatization of the nodule affected the whole group, damaging its nodal functioning. In the words of one member, Erik was too scary to reason with at these moments, or afterward. The members felt helpless and silenced in response to his bewildering gaps and the sudden standstills. Devolving into a refusal mode (see Chapter 12), the group became nonverbal and felt unsafe.

Technical approach

Erik required time, patience, and a buildup of trust before we were allowed entry into the guarded walls of his mental life. Additionally, he required active monitoring and intervention. His provocative and frightening shifts in mood—the drifts of alertness, muteness in the midst of intelligible discourse, sudden flashes of anger—could be misinterpreted as primarily histrionic bids for attention. Both he and the group needed protection from premature confrontation or exploration regarding his behavior and its underlying meaning.

We made therapeutic progress when he allowed nonspecific statements about his defenses and dynamics: how he was apt to keep us—and "life" itself—away, and how he must have done likewise in his childhood to escape "family pressures," perhaps stimulated by his parents' problematic marriage and wrenching divorce. Cautioned by the fierce displays of protectiveness toward his troubled mother, I was careful not to name names or suggest blame or responsibility. Other group members followed suit.

Intervals of noninterpretative accommodation seemed unavoidable, and so I yielded to his agitated demands for the group floor, greeted late entrances, and accepted his refusals, as in supporting his wish to "rest" or even nap during group sessions. When Erik froze in mid-sentence, I relieved his humiliation and the group's distress by reassuring Erik that he could think about what was on his mind, and we could return to the topic later or at another time, and alerted the group to move on.

The group provided here-and-now access to Erik's vulnerability and to his underlying anger and its primary target. We witnessed his impatience and irritation when certain female members tearfully sought out sympathy and rejected his laborious attempts at advice and rescue. I sometimes intervened with playful irony: "Mmm, you get caught in a well of sympathy for damsels in distress. You need some help to pull you out." Or, "You've been in the theater [as an actor], you're really drawn to melodrama." Such interpretative comments did not necessarily please Erik or his female foils, but they relieved tension and began to explain Erik to himself and the group; they also normalized and linked Erik to other members. Certainly, Erik was not the only group member weighted by residues of a symbiotic–parasitic relationship with a narcissistic and compelling parent.

Erik's increasing participation in the communicative node, the group "matrix," supported his capacity to think, even while in the nodule's grip. He began to feel and untangle its psychic qualities and describe them verbally. However, after years of intensive psychotherapeutic work, Erik remains vulnerable to regressive moments and a resurgence of the symptomatic moods and erratic behavior that signify the lingering presence of the nodule and the cumulative trauma that it recapitulates. Still, he listens better and tolerates rather than disrupts and jams the mental activity of the working group. In these instances, communicative channels, although reduced by one member, remain undamaged; other group members are free to resonate, to stay on topic or move on. Psychological thinking is directed to those who are ready to receive it.

Marcia: fighting the "waves" and bracing against the nodule's force

"You don't understand; let me explain what I mean." "You don't understand, and I don't think I'm making myself clear." "Sorry to cut you off. I didn't realize." "Let me talk…Let me finish…I don't talk much about myself, I need to do it today."

The group came to accept these remonstrations with humorous resignation. Calling her "a siren," one group member would hold his ears as an insistent Marcia stated and restated her opinions, talking over speakers. Others (including me) were equally direct: "Stop, you're ranting"; "It is like you are spinning out of control and can't stop"; "We got it!"; or even, "Shut up already." Marcia rebutted us all: "I don't want to do group your way."

Even when yielding to interruptions (to her interruptions!), Marcia negotiated the terms: "I'll try to hear you, but don't tell me I'm 'spinning.' Think of another word. Not 'ranting,' that's worse. I know I do this sometimes; that's why my [ex-]husband hated me, but he criticized me no matter what."

Marcia rested comfortably with the knowledge that she was not hated, but rather enjoyed and valued for her good-hearted empathy and insight, and she affably ignored the group's confrontations. "I just needed to get this out; I don't need feedback." "I'll talk about this with Rich in individual," she said with some resolve, "Thanks, let's go on."

Marcia's static, a wall of disconnected words, alerted me that she was responding to some sort of irruption that she could not tolerate. I then assumed that she was defending against psychic material that she believed would engulf and overwhelm her. However, while personally affected, she did not produce disorganization in the group. When she stopped talking, other members resumed. Static ceased without data loss; other nodal channels resumed functioning, undamaged and operational. Still, nothing useful seemed to accrue from these repeated occurrences, and I attempted to address them when Marcia would allow.

Technical approach

"Is this how you want to spend our time?" I challenged, as Marcia tripped from topic to topic during individual sessions. "I wanted to tell you about my day and my plans for my new kitchen. It's fine. I'm not in any rush to get cured, and nothing needs to be 'accomplished' in a session."

I could feel captured or allow myself to be captivated. "But don't you want me to feel good about myself for doing something?" I teased, but, also, I was speaking from a true feeling. I had come to enjoy Marcia's lively reportage and the byplay between us, without wishing to forfeit all desire to move us from her monologue to our dialogue.

"Get over it; why do you need this for your ego?" she rejoined. I said that I did, and that I was not going to give up trying to convey my sense of what was happening. She did not want to be controlled, and neither did I. "Fair," she smiled, and I echoed her. Even when Marcia appreciated my interposed clarifications, she gave an impression of disagreeing. "I'm not arguing with you," she protested, "I don't know why people say that to me sometimes." She felt criticized if I tried to ask why, and I was reduced to trotting out the same unavoidable question: "Who are you arguing with?" And the answer was always: "My mother. We know this. She told me how to think, how to be. She monitored my friends and criticized everybody. I get it. No need to go over this again," to which I responded, "Apparently, we do."

To get us past the formulations that were too familiar to us, I sometimes concentrated on what I thought was her bodily experience (Billow, 2013b). One illustrative incident:

BILLOW: I don't know if you will appreciate the image—when you were talk-
    ing to me I thought you were feeling that you were standing firm against
    the waves [I gesture by putting up my hands].
MARCIA: You don't have to say more. That was exactly the feeling I
    had with my mother growing up. I can't believe how much she still
    affects me.
BILLOW: You didn't let her swallow you up. I guess that goes for your fear of
    me, even though you tell me you don't have any.
MARCIA: Yes, I see it. I'm talking before you interrupt and tell me I could
    have done it better. That's what she would do.
BILLOW: I think it is more than telling you what to do. You live in terror of
    drowning—losing yourself as a separate person.
MARCIA: My house was suffocating, even though it wasn't that small. I
    couldn't wait to get out and was made to feel guilty when I did.
BILLOW: So you haven't really "gotten out." You don't want me or any-
    one else to take you over, and you live in constant fear that we might
    try.

Marcia remained quiet and reflective.

BILLOW: At one time, if I attempted to link themes, or say anything, you
would have held me off, as if I were the waves coming at you.

MARCIA: I only do that for two reasons: If you don't get it exactly right,
or if you are telling me how I am supposed to do it, disguising it as an
interpretation.

BILLOW: Like if I had said, "I'm not your mother and I'm not fighting what
you're saying."

MARCIA: I would have heard you saying that I shouldn't talk the way I
wanted to, that you were correcting what I was doing in the session.
When we talk about this, I can see her—it's that vivid, right in my face,
I can practically touch her—But I don't want to, I want to get away, and
I feel bad even saying this.

We came to understand that an unrecognized but ever-present sense of feeling pressured—a vague anticipation of being controlled—could launch a
verbal stream. Almost any dialogical engagement still has such moments of
foreboding, for the nodule lurks, hovering.

In truth, it was not my ego, but Marcia's that needed support. To rescue
her from maternal merger, I persisted with the language function (Lacan,
1953/1977). While making efforts not to embarrass her, I called attention to
her verbal behavior—to her interruptions and argumentations—and how it
shuts others out and halts exchanges. "[Marcia:] Okay I get it, let's move on."
I invited her participation post-irruption or carried on despite her negative
input. In forcefully inserting myself as a thinking subject, I enactively and
verbally addressed her developmental deficits, not only in relationship to
her mother, but also to her real and symbolic father, and consequently to her
own capacities to engage in useful discourse.

Marcia has become aware of how, when, and why she utilizes language to
"get away," in her words, and not let "inside" what I—or anyone—may pressure
her "to be or to do." To some extent, then, the group and I have entered her ego,
helping her cope with cumulative trauma and mitigate the nodule's force.

MARCIA: I remember everything, not only what you say, but how you say it
and your look, and think about it, even when I change subjects. You're
right; I need to trust more. I'm more intimate with you than with anyone else, maybe not as much in group, but I think a lot about group
afterwards.

However, even after a decade of combined treatment, discussions may be
undermined by her verbal torrent. Thinking about the psychic issues stimulating the nodule can bring it "too close," in her words, and I become its
representative rather than interpreter.

Ralph: "going dark"—expelling the nodule (a cycle of encasement-projection)

Here was Ralph again, bellowing and fiercely finger-pointing at Julie, a new group member describing her marital turmoil, such that I had to intervene. In an attempt to exculpate himself, Ralph reminded the group that he had not behaved this way in a while. "My wife says it is 'going dark,'" he explained, only partially acknowledging Julie. "It's like I don't exist, and then I explode, and she turns on me if I complain or tell her what she's doing [wrong] with our kids. She blames me, when it's her fault." Finding her husband in Ralph's acrimony, Julie declared that she was "proud for not collapsing" as she does in her marriage. The repair seemed to satisfy the members sufficiently, and we moved on to other interactions.

Ralph continued to "go dark" whenever Julie began to speak and seek help. While he made efforts not to erupt, he could look unhappy, slack, and without energy, with lusterless eyes. Sometimes Ralph roused himself to offer Julie valuable observations and advice, although they were delivered with such harshness that I wondered why nobody but me interceded. Even Julie seemed to have accommodated to Ralph. "I know he just tolerates me, but I haven't given up!" I was on my own to challenge Ralph, for which I received his hostile belittlement, wordlessly witnessed by the group.

Ralph effectively closed off certain channels of communication. Other members acted as though they did not hear or did not see, and rarely commented on his behavior or its effects. The group had crafted "switching devices," redirecting attention and discourse. By changing channels, they preserved the node, but with a reduction in communicative reach. The situation was not optimal; too much information drained off from these repetitive interactions. As unpleasant as Ralph's ill temper could be when directed at me, I owed it to him and the group to make sense of his darkening moods and their intersubjective consequences.

Technical approach

With Erik, the nodule's emergence handicapped functioning, and he strove to control associative gaps and leaps. His sudden verbal explosions or blockages frightened him as well as other people. Ralph had no such motivation to modify his behavior. Unlike Marcia, he could not ward off the dreaded nodule and evade its enveloping grip. The best he could do for self-preservation was to swell up with righteous anger and "blow out" the reincarnated mother and its representative. "She was crazy," he exclaimed, rarely altering or developing a narrative, "never satisfied and edging for more from my father, and from me too. Always more, more money, better houses, better grades from me, an honor student. I don't blame him for wanting to be left alone." Language became a weapon used to eject and attack with painful memories, images, and feelings, now linked with hatred to the other.

Ralph saw nothing wrong in treating such individuals with the verbal abuse and withering disdain he had observed (and often felt) from his father. He became scornful and volatile when I challenged his pat reconstructions and asked him to reconsider his assumptions—"you're never satisfied, you are being like my mother and you deserve it"—and yet I had to find a way to confront his dogmatic subjective truths. They provided the self-justifications for his rages, the cold rejections, and the self-imposed isolations, behaviors that threatened his second marriage and brought him into therapy.

Via identification and psychological transmission, Ralph duplicated his father's irruptions—a varying strategy of verbal attack, interpersonal banishment, or psychic self-retreat (Steiner, 1994). "Get her out of here, shut her down," Ralph railed during individual sessions, "before I kill her." The fantasy persisted that he could expunge the nodule—by my behavior or his—but not merely talk about and gradually relieve its psychic hold. "I am exploding even to think about her, and I blame you for wasting my time, there [in group] and here. You criticize me when I am trying to help Julie—she's too stupid to get it."

"Too new at this stuff, and too afraid," I defended her, at risk of reigniting him, which I did.

"Poor baby...," Ralph mocked me.

She can't hear the truth, and never will. Somebody has to say it. It takes all of me to sit still when she tells us how "proud" she is of herself. For doing nothing. I'm in control, say it, you cheap bastard, say it. Nobody complained. You are the only one who says it [who comments on Ralph's intolerance]. You're too sensitive, I mean it.

"Let's check this out," I suggested. Ralph had provided the opportunity to confront what had been for me a puzzling lapse in group discourse and for him, consensual validation. When I brought this up, members came forth tentatively: "You used to scare me, but we worked it out." "You can be scary, but I know you care." "I see that Julie handles what you say, so I can relax."

No therapeutic mileage here, I concluded, and changed tack: "What about how Ralph treats me when he's mad?"

"I know you two love each other, but I don't like it." "I wait to see if Rich is okay; it makes me anxious." "I freeze up; it is like when my parents fought and I couldn't do anything [begins to cry]." "It is disrespectful and a waste of time, [angry] just stop it, Ralph!"

"You stacked the deck, Rich," Ralph declared with cold contempt. "I'm not bad and if I had been, you [other members] would have complained. So fuck you, Rich, and all of you too!" No one claimed he was bad, members insisted, and I joined them in reassuring Ralph of his genuine value to our group.

But a blocked channel of communication had opened up. I was freer to query the group when Ralph became "dark," turning particular attention to how he related to me, since I had become a primary target of his unhappiness.

Now, members elaborated, associating to their own histories. But Ralph remained unconvinced, combative with anyone who challenged him, and I came to feel guilty for hiding behind other members' subjectivities.

I soon had opportunity to address Ralph directly: I said that he was being violent in how he was talking to me, and that I deserved his respect. We could disagree, but did he also want to hurt me? Ralph said he knew that I did not take it personally. I said that I did: I felt pain and upset, how could I not? My disclosure caused tremors in the group. Some members did not believe me and agreed with Ralph that I was using "technique." Others reported being shaken and worried.

I reiterated: "I can take it, but it hurts and I lose confidence in our relationship. [To Ralph:] It makes me feel that I mean nothing to you—that I am nothing." Ralph and several others found my declaration implausible. "Ralph never misses a session." "He respects you and even quotes what you say." I shrugged ruefully, as if to say this is still how it feels to me, which it was.

The session ended without consensus regarding my believability, and without assurance that Ralph would alter his conduct. But apparently, I had succeeded in engaging him without establishing a retaliatory sequence of mutual guilt-tripping. Something real got through—perhaps me as a caring person and not primarily as a cerebral entity, "the therapist." Likely, our strengthened bond has given Ralph some control over his irruptions directed towards me, as when I rematerialize as the critical mother or aloof, abandoning father (the latter, another nodule, which he is just approaching).

Ralph still exhibits incidents of "darkening," fierce shifts in self-state as the nodule takes hold. But dissociation is not as fixed as it once was. He has achieved some consciousness of the precursors and manifestations of impotent rage—which he understands, at last, as a reactive internal force that neither he nor his father adequately coped with. He more willingly accepts feedback and finds relief when we bring attention to his mounting tension and unhappiness. Observing ego function restores, with some impulse control and occasional gratitude.

Nodules: encased and projected

A nodule materializes each time as if the first, asserting its presence without foreknowledge or self-understanding. It hits with blank sensory force. Like grits of sand that do not form into a pearl, the nodule remains an irritation not affected or transformed by repeated exposure. With therapeutic intervention, its compacted elements may come to be felt, visualized, and conceptualized—linked to the dynamics of the individual and the group, but the nodule does not easily resolve.

While it disrupts concentration, the nodule itself is difficult to concentrate on. A trauma has rematerialized, as has the difficulty in thinking about and working through the constituent elements that have entered the mental register. In terms of group process, cohesion may be maintained, but coherence, the meaning-making process, is negatively affected (Pines, 1985).

Like Erik, one inhabits the nodule and is inhabited by it. Erik demonstrated a history of implosion-explosion when confronted with psychic material that stimulated the nodule, informing us of an underlying mental intolerance of the mother, with whom he was also too closely identified. Marcia projected the nodule outward, resisting social influence. She could feel and "see" the nodule, anxiously and only partially fending it off, as she had done with her actual mother. Ralph exemplified both sequences. He withdrew from or attempted to expunge the nodule, mentally beating it—and whoever represented it in word or presence—into momentary nonexistence. All three attempted to eject and escape from a chaotic state of mind, one which had become a dimension of the nodule itself.

Miscarriage of the language function

The three individuals used words and bodily movements for evacuation—to get rid of the object—"as if nonrepresentation could free oneself of the threat it [their respective mothers] represented" (Williams, 2010, p. 448). Through his erratic "fuck you's," sudden pauses, silences, and threatening behaviors, Erik alerted the group that he had disordered his own body and mind, and might treat others similarly. Marcia's incantations—her stream of words—fended off and screened out valuable input, which she confounded with soul-destroying maternal communications. Ralph's harangues beat down, ejected, and banished what he perceived as an invasive nodule and those who attempted to transform it into useful meaning. Even thinking of Julie—without her actual physical presence—infused Ralph with the psychological reality of a maternal bad object who undermined his sense of existing.

Conclusion: the therapist works to repair the node—the group follows

Given the intensity of group life and the therapeutic process, we expect irruptive experience. The three individuals under review are high-functioning, empathic people and good citizens of their groups and outside communities. They have benefitted from combined individual-group psychotherapy. Yet, for each of them, a well-defined but unconquerable nodule, stimulated by the group experience, could take charge.

The therapeutic situation became an intersubjective enactive "field" (Baranger, Baranger, & Mom, 1983), encompassing all participants and creating impasses. Erik silenced his frightened, bewildered group, which for a lengthy period depended on my interventions to reassure members and resurrect communicative channels. Marcia overpowered her group repeatedly, although only momentarily halting our discourse. Ralph's "going dark" switched off the very channels of group communication that could have lessened the nodule's grip; the members proceeded as if unaffected. Interventions proved unsuccessful until I revealed my painful subjective reactions.

It is a therapeutic advance when a nodule can be sufficiently tolerated by the stricken member to partake in verbal exploration. But when the individual either will not or cannot, the therapist must not wait for the group to do the work. He or she may need to intervene, immediately and persistently, to secure and maintain empathic bonding, monitor and protect all individuals, provide psychic relief, and make anxiety manageable. Impasses often do not resolve quickly or completely. If the therapist succeeds in making sense of what is going on and is able to reduce field effects, that is, collusive denial, evasive action, and other refusals, constructive co-participation of other members will follow. The group itself will then participate in resolving or lessening the effects of nodules on the affected individual and others.

Chapter 14

A falsifying adolescent

"Where are you going?"
"Nowhere."
"Who are you going with?"
"No one."

As parents, we have come to expect this exchange with our adolescent children. Indeed, bald adolescent falsifications are typical, even conventional. The dialogue is not without meaning, however, and serves communicative goals. In the questioning, the adult signals ongoing interest in—and concern for—the youth's life and welfare. In the falsifying responses, the adolescent reasserts motives for separation, privacy, and independence.

Later, I will discuss the treatment of an adolescent patient who, I discovered, had not been asked these questions sufficiently and who wanted to be asked. This left her in charge of how much I was going to hear, which was plenty, and how far we were going to develop meaning from what she had to say, which was often minimal. As I reflected on our early interactions, I found helpful Bion's ideas regarding the *container-contained*, which guided the strategies I adopted to advance the analytic work.

Column 2 of Bion's (1970) grid, designated by the Greek letter psi, refers to statements "known by the initiator to be false, but maintained as a barrier against statements that lead to a psychological upheaval [i.e., growth and change]" (p. 9). The individual may pretend not to understand, when he or she fears thinking about the truth and its consequences. The individual may omit, slant, or exaggerate relevant data, leaving both speaker and listener confused or drawing false inferences.

While in Aristotelian logic, truth and falsity are categorically distinct, not so in human relations. Bion neither emphasized how one's version of truth can be wielded as a hurtful weapon nor noted how falsity may facilitate the building of constructive relationships. "How do I look?" a provocatively clad adolescent girl asks her inwardly wincing father. Questions such as this do not always seek truthful answers, and even when they do, diplomacy, minimization, and shadings of feeling and meaning—even white lies—lubricate and make possible social relations. A marker of mutual growth between parent and adolescent is observed when each can understand and accept the other's fictions and disguises—the respective social selves of everyday life (Goffman, 1972). In the case that follows, I show how both truth and falsity may be used in developing a psychoanalytic relationship.

Truth seeking in development

> The customary answers given the child...damage his genuine instinct of research and as a rule deal the first blow, too, at his confidence in his parents....he usually begins to mistrust grown-up people, and to keep his most intimate interests secret.
>
> (Freud, 1907, pp. 135–136)

The individual's capacity to tolerate truth seeking reflects the history of the caregivers' interest and success in responding to the child's truth needs. Only a certain amount of truth may be introduced into experience, and it is among the parents' first and most important tasks to protect the infant and growing child from too much or too little truth. From the start, parents introduce make-believe into the infant's world, creating (or in today's jargon, co-creating) "his majesty, the baby" and fostering mutually idealizing, bonding scenarios. However, to advance truth seeking, the parents must gradually dethrone the infant. We may hypothesize that certain depriving caregiving behaviors—for instance, those involving physical absence, delay of immediate satisfaction as in partial weaning, and so forth—stimulate thinking and a reality orientation.

In childhood and adolescence—indeed, at all stages of development—to seek truth and to challenge the human tendency towards falsification, the individual requires authentic communicative interaction. In some measure, the Establishment, consisting of parents, school, religious institution, and government, represents and upholds reality, including the values and standards of the status quo. But the established order must also encourage challenge and dissent, and must stimulate and respond to emotional truth and the individual's search for it.

Parents and societal caregivers who unduly rely on *psi* may reward conventionality, to the neglect and discouragement of curiosity. In response to a psychosocial network that is suppressive, manipulative, or merely inadequate in fostering truth, the individual may become evasive and tentative as a form of self-protection. The need for significant truth remains unintegrated and dissociated. To escape from the resulting emotional and mental deadness, the adolescent may develop covert modes of seeking sensation and may confuse sensation with vital truth.

Developmental implications of falsification: the case of hamlet

"There is nothing either good or bad but thinking makes it so," declaims Hamlet (Shakespeare, 1603/1961, II, ii, 255–257), whom we may consider as an archetype of late adolescence. The adolescent may shift, permutate, combine, or reverse points of view, leaping mental boundaries from one affective view of reality to another, and from reality to fantasy, morality to immorality, narcissism to mutual recognition and concern.

Perhaps *Hamlet* describes the predicament of all adolescents, in danger of prematurely recognizing disconcerting truths concerning parents and the adult world. Hamlet was haunted by dream thoughts—ghostly, dissociated realizations concerning his parents and was afraid to trust and act on his convictions. "With thoughts beyond the reaches of our souls" (I, iv, 56), adolescents are not quite prepared "to be," rather than "not to be." No longer unquestioningly loyal to the Establishment of parents, schools and other institutions, and the prevailing culture, they are not sufficiently experienced or solidified in their identities to trust their consciousness and unconsciousness to guide their behavior. They must depend on others—peers and adults—to enter into trustworthy dialogues.

Hamlet dramatizes how parental falsity inflames the adolescent and sets the course for intergenerational conflict. *Hamlet* longs to find and communicate the truth about an Establishment that he suspects deceives and, through its deception, attempts to "pluck out" his independent spirit:

> You would play upon me, /you would seem to know my stops, you would pluck/out the heart of my mystery, you would sound me/from my lowest note to the top of my compass—and there is much music, excellent voice, in this/little organ—yet cannot you make it speak.
>
> (III, ii, 379–385)

Because Hamlet cannot quite believe what he knows to be true, he provokes and embroils the adults to reveal themselves: "Players cannot keep counsel; they'll tell all" (III, ii, 151–152). He defensively commits himself to counter-falsification, behaving like a crazy adolescent, putting "an antic disposition on" (I, v, 172). He speaks and acts purposely to confuse. Under the protective cover of an abrasive self-presentation, Hamlet attempts to "catch" psychological reality, to confirm his cynical but accurate view of the corruption of the adult moral authority. "The play's the thing/Wherein I'll catch the conscience of the King" (III, i, 905–906).

However, increasingly bitter and alienated from adult support, Hamlet cannot sustain constructive role-playing. Disregarding the prudence he offers to the professional actors—"Suit the action to the word, /the word to the action" (III, ii, 19–20)—he abandons truth and reason. In his self-falsification, Hamlet has become his own enemy, as well as the Establishment's.

My treatment of Simone, a falsifying adolescent

Simone, an attractive and physically mature 15-year-old girl, appeared for her first appointment, accompanied by her mother. I introduced myself to both, and since Simone seemed to have no trouble separating, I indicated that I would see her alone. Following me into my office, Simone arranged herself easily, and with a lackadaisical "hi," she waited. I felt immediately that she anticipated being bored.

"So?" I asked, expectantly.

"So," she repeated. Her confident, carefree attitude informed me that she had been here before and knew what to expect.

I continued: "So, I'm supposed to ask you why you are here, and you're supposed to tell me."

"I know—I've already seen my guidance counselor and the school psychologist. They think I have problems and need therapy. I don't. I saw my mother's therapist, she didn't say anything, are you going to be silent, too?"

"Are *you* going to be silent, since you don't want to be in therapy?" I responded.

"I didn't say I didn't want to be in therapy. I said I had no problems and no need of therapy."

This was to be the first of Simone's many corrections for my failing to get right her presented version of the truth. I had the distinct sense—common with an adolescent patient—that I was being provoked and also tested to see how I would respond, such that Simone could "catch" on to me, and that she did not herself fully believe what she said. I looked at her quizzically, expecting that she would feel and think further about our communication. But she merely waited for me to continue, as if we were in agreement that she had answered sincerely and had made perfect sense.

"Mmm," I said with a slightly sarcastic edge. "This might be interesting. A person with no problems, no needs, but willing to come to therapy."

"That's right," she responded, ignoring the nuance in my response. "I have lots of study halls and my mother's driving, or I'll take a cab. It will break up a day."

So there would be perks in this unneeded therapy, I thought. Simone could vacate a portion of the school day and spend special time with her mother, or at least get her attention. With adolescents, I have often been impressed that a benefit of treatment has been the increased family contact imposed by the necessity of transportation to and from my office.

It was my turn to correct Simone: "Several days, if we decide to work together." Simone's mother had advised me that Simone was failing in school and was listless and "out of it." If I were to make some inroads, analytic and otherwise, two sessions per week would be minimal.

"Several days," she echoed, unruffled.

"Why does everyone think you need to be in therapy?" I asked.

"My grades suck," she replied sheepishly. "Oh, also, my parents are going to get a divorce, and everyone thinks that might have something to do with it—maybe, but I don't think so. Most of my friends' parents are divorced. I'm used to it."

"Then what's going on?" I continued, noting inwardly the falsity in her omission of the indications of depression and drug taking, my inferences from her mother's report.

"With…?"

"With you, that you're having difficulty completing schoolwork."

"Nothing. I can make it up when I want to."

"You don't want to?"

"I guess not now." (Pause.)

"So what's with your parents' situation?"

"Their problem, not mine." (Pause.)

"I see what you mean; you want me to talk."

"I'll talk. But you have to ask me questions."

I was confused, for I had been feeling that Simone was finding my questioning intrusive and was turned off by it.

"I just did," I said, hoping for clarification, perhaps direction, but she responded with a sweet smile that left me with neither.

"I guess not the right ones," I added.

I would discover, through trial and much error, a jarring but ultimately clarifying disjunction between an aspect of Simone's transference and my countertransference: What felt right for Simone were the therapeutic equivalents of "where are you going?" and "who are you going with?" But whenever I attempted to move the conversation in the direction of her feelings, she accused me of "getting psychological" and diverted the interrogation. However, often when I felt I was being mundane, unimaginatively concrete, or pushing farther than most adolescents would like in asking personal questions, she revealed selective and often important bits of confidences. For example, her ground-floor bedroom—separated from the parental suite—had an easily accessible window that became a nightly portal for a small clique of party-minded friends. Thus, in time, I learned about different ways she acted and acted out, but what did her behavior mean? She offered no hypotheses and showed little curiosity in mine.

Unruffled and blasé, Simone was a late-20th-century adolescent version of *la belle indifference*. She was surreptitious and deceptive, lying to her parents, shoplifting, copying homework, and cheating on exams, but she was not false when divulging these aspects of her life. Her falsity lay in her "antic disposition" (Shakespeare, 1603/1961). Her pleasant—if superficial—personality, represented by a bright smile, served as a barrier to psychological insight. Even when she was being honest, as in acknowledging her dishonesty and sharing her exploits with me, she resisted thinking or feeling about what she was communicating. No matter how alarming I found her situation, to Simone, everything was "good," "fine"—"it doesn't bother me, why does it bother you?"

After an unproductive go-round, in which I presented the risks in her behavior and got no affective response, I might ask: "Does it bother you that it bothers me?" "Not really" was her typical response. And then, occasionally: "This is what you do, you're doing what you're supposed to do." [Explain?] "Your job." [Explain?] "You don't know what your job is?"

I heard an insinuation that I was play-acting "being bothered," and, therefore, I was a fake. Simone could seem vaguely disdainful, but when I attempted to check out my impressions about her critical feelings about my job, our relationship, or me, she would clam up and look at me vacantly. Particularly unappealing to Simone was an admission of annoyance or an expression of dislike, much less of anger. She expressed a genuine, if unfocused, care not to be malicious or purposefully hurtful. She was not going to be angry with her dispirited mother or callous father, who precipitously abandoned the family, and she would not be angry with me. If she appeared blank, sleepy, or mildly stoned on marijuana or Quaaludes, her parents seemed not to notice. But I did notice—and, unperturbed, she agreed that she habitually "tuned out," with or without drugs. Like Hamlet, she professed little interest in "all the uses of this world." I expressed concern and struggled to find the "right" questions that would awaken her and give us access to her defended-against emotionality.

Simone derailed my therapeutic efforts by imputing an aura of falsity to our interaction. To give another example, when we talked about her mother and how sad her mother seemed, Simone's eyes clouded. I commented that Simone seemed sad, too. "Of course," she remarked gently, "she's my mother." She was sad for her mother, but not for herself, she explained. When I called attention to her eyes and their incipient tears, she granted me only: "Maybe, but maybe you're seeing things, saying what you want me to say."

"My eyes can't be trusted, or I can't be trusted?" I asked playfully.

"Same thing!" she retorted.

Simone seemed not the slightest bit annoyed by the proposition that I might be trying to get what I wanted by putting words in her mouth. She accepted without question (even with some pride) that she could be manipulative, a user, and a role player. It took me a while to realize that she expected the same behavior from me.

I had to learn to accept—even embrace—this role without offense or challenge, just as she did. The following segment from one session represented a turning point in my understanding and therapeutic stance. We were discussing the Thanksgiving weekend that had just passed, the first in which her family was no longer together.

SIMONE: My father wanted us [the children] to have a second Thanksgiving with him. It was supposed to be on Friday, then he changed it to Saturday night, because Elaine [his new live-in woman] was going to be away, and he could hook up [with another woman].

BILLOW: [I dramatized an aghast reaction. As my empathy seemed not to register, I continued with the following.] Don't you feel pushed aside?

SIMONE: I guess so.

BILLOW: You're not mad?

SIMONE: I don't know. I don't like having to sleep at his house, because I can't go out with my friends. Besides, I don't like Elaine that much. I don't think my father does either.

BILLOW: Oh. What don't you like?

SIMONE: I said I don't like her that much.

BILLOW: [I was not going to give up a chance to explore an affect.] What don't you like about Elaine that much?

SIMONE: She's kind of a phony.

BILLOW: Mmm? [Here I dramatically cleared my throat.]

SIMONE: [Smiling.] No, not like me. I don't pretend to like someone when I don't. Elaine thinks she might become my stepmother and she smiles too much. You don't say I smile too much. You say I smile so I don't show my feelings.

Whereas I might not have said that Simone smiled too much and could be phony (and I believed I *had* said both explicitly), I certainly had implied both, and I thought we had agreed. In response to Simone's distinction without a difference, I felt misunderstood and as though my therapeutic efforts had been betrayed. Yet I thought it best not to contradict or ask her to explain.

BILLOW: I see what you mean; go on. [Not for the first time, I participated in Simone's self-misrepresentation, taking solace in Samuel Butler's maxim: "Truth does not consist in never lying but in knowing when to lie and when not to do so."]

SIMONE: Nothing. She's okay. She means well. She dresses a little young. You wouldn't know the label: "Betsey Johnson" [a women's clothing store]. If you knew it, you would know what I mean. Hippy-dippy. It's kind of cute, but not really my father's style. He's sophisticated. He got my mother a lot of expensive jewelry, even though she doesn't wear a lot.

BILLOW: Did she appreciate it?

SIMONE: What?

BILLOW: The jewelry.

SIMONE: I think so....[dead pause]. What?

BILLOW: What?

SIMONE: Nothing.

BILLOW: Whenever we begin to look at your parents' relationship, you tend to get quiet.

SIMONE: We're talking about jewelry.

I again found myself tangled and near a therapeutic precipice. If I continued to play along, saying, "Yes, of course, we're talking about jewelry," I felt I, too, would be a phony, and like Elaine, I would be humoring Simone in an effort to win her over. Bion (1970) described predicaments like this: "The analyst is challenged to accept them [the patient's falsifications], at the risk of showing himself unmindful of the truth, or to reject them and assume the role of being the patient's conscience" (p. 98). The therapeutic goal, which did not seem reachable in the immediate future of my relationship with Simone, was to cut through the dissimulation. But I felt it was essential not to cut her down, punishing her for obdurately refusing to think and feel psychologically, such as by unduly confronting her defensive inconsistencies, denials, and rationalizations.

However, it was difficult not to feel super-egoish, as well as not to behave in that manner. I could do little at the moment, other than appreciate Simone for her unconscious ability to put me in the predicament that Bion described. She had not merely a "blind eye" (Steiner, 1985), a capacity to avoid her unconscious (even conscious) knowledge of the parental relationship. She could be blindingly, enchantingly concrete and dumbfounding. The situation was hopeless, but not desperate.

BILLOW: Okay, I'll play. We're talking about jewelry; before we were talking about dresses.

SIMONE: Yes.

BILLOW: And before, Thanksgiving dinner.

SIMONE: Yes.

BILLOW: And your father.

SIMONE: My father's girlfriend. You're interested in my father's girlfriends.

BILLOW: I sound pretty shallow. More of a gossip than a psychologist.

SIMONE: You said it. I didn't say it....

BILLOW: I can see how this fits into your theory that this is a waste of your mother's money.

SIMONE: [She corrected me.] My father's. See, you don't pay attention. [Simone could be quick at catching me at any imprecision, petty or important. This lent weight to my suspicion that, under her antic cloak, she had interest in truth, and was assessing my capacity to represent it.]

BILLOW: You caught me. Now you know, I don't pay attention.

SIMONE: You do enough. [Here she relented.] I don't care if you get his money.

BILLOW: You sound a little bit spiteful.

SIMONE: [She spoke flatly.] You're being psychological. [And then, she wearily preempted my interpretive response with embarrassing accuracy.] No, I'm not angry at you, or at him.

BILLOW: I'm so predictable—a good enough useless psychologist. [I smiled, as much to myself as to her. Simone, of course unfamiliar with the Winnicott allusion, assented with a nod. She seemed neither amused nor interested in pursuing the topic of my therapeutic conventionality, which she appeared to take for granted. We returned to talk of her busy Thanksgiving weekend.]

I doubted that Simone fully believed her characterization of my sham professionalism, but we continued as if she did. To link up effectively with Simone's falsity, I had to get on better terms with my own.

The analyst's falsity

Bion argued that any interpretation involves a theory *about* the therapeutic experience, but because interpretations are intellectual, they interfere with what he called *becoming*, which involves the analyst's empathic identification with the patient's difficulties: achieving the sense of being or becoming those aspects of the patient's problematic self to which attention has been drawn. To "reduce" the level of falsity in the analytic interaction, the analyst must attempt to "see the column 2 [*psi*] element in his thoughts" (Bion, 1965, p. 168), as well as in the patient's.

The truth of Simone, as I came to infer and patiently accept, was too painful for her to bear and put into words. Simone could not tolerate confronting the reality of parental neglect and evasiveness, but she herself came to represent these characteristics and to projectively identify them with me. In introducing traumatic themes and illuminating their symbolic currency, I had to consider when and if my interpretations were given in the service of protecting and relieving myself of Simone's insistent projective identifications and putting my own back on her.

Rather than merely or primarily talking about it, I had to be a part of the narrative and live with the emotional consequences of that. To a significant extent, Simone gave me no other choice but to *become* her projective identification. Smith (2000) identified one source of the analyst's anxiety in such a situation: "The patient allows no room to negotiate his or her image of us, a negotiation that we call interpretation of the transference and that inevitably helps analysts reestablish their own sense of themselves" (p. 114).

Simone arrived with an intuitive notion and active distaste of the analytic screen (Jacobs 2001). However, her notion of Establishment falsity was much larger and included authentic psychoanalytic activity. She found intolerable most of what defines our work—not only transference interpretation but also construction and reconstruction, character and dream analysis, discussion of family dynamics, and free association.

To *become*, I had to share in Simone's particular form of mental disaster and willingly suspend many psychoanalytic prerequisites. This involved being more inquisitive and well informed regarding the superficialities of her life, and less interpretively active and confrontational. Here are some typical interventions and follow-up questions: "Really! You're kidding—you partied all night!" [Who with? What did you do?] "Aren't you having a Spanish test today?" [What grade did you get? Oh my! How did your friends do?] "How did you like Aspen?" [You got a new jacket—so, what color? Which trails did you go on? Did you try X restaurant? Who'd you see there?] "What's up for the weekend?" "Who's in that movie, should I see it?"

I gradually relaxed into my degraded relational and clinical status, with less self-recrimination and remorse. I confess that I came to look forward to Simone's confidences regarding the failed marriages of her friends' parents, the rumors regarding the shops and shopkeepers in our suburban town, and, of course, her own intrigues. I became genuinely curious and well informed about her tastes in clothes, vacations, celebrities, cars, movies, music, and so forth, and offered my own opinions. My interest in thinking and formulating waned, as did even my ironic rejoinders (e.g., "okay, I'll play") that attempted to call attention to her bald falsities. So, Simone had found—or "co-created"—a therapist for someone who had no need of therapy.

To my confession, I add that, to the extent to which I could cease and desist trying to function as a "real" analyst, partnering Simone in "wasting" our time, I felt more genuine as a person relating to another person and re-aler as a professional. Said differently, in functioning with increased awareness of my clinical dilemma, I crossed over a barrier of professionalism that to some extent was self-protective and thus false.

Simone relaxed as well into our gossipy relationship and, by our third year of work, she ceased calling attention to its failure as "real therapy." Our mundane conversations seemed to reawaken interest in Establishment endeavors, and she began spending her nights sleeping rather than partying. Chatting about the daily activities of an increasingly normal high school life took up more of our time. It went almost unremarked that her grades improved sufficiently for her to say goodbye shortly before leaving for college. Her major and career interest? I doubt it will surprise the reader who has endured long-term therapy of adolescents: psychology!

Falsity and the relational levels of the container-contained

Bleandonu (1994) suggested that Bion's appellation *psi* likely refers to *proton pseudos*, the "first lie" that Freud (1895) located at the heart of hysteria. Indeed, Freud understood the etiology of neurosis as related to one's lying to oneself. Cure was achieved by catharsis: the patient's finding and accepting the traumatic truth. Freud first attempted to uncover the archeology of his patients' truths through hypnosis, which he later abandoned in favor of free associations.

Bion's extension and important modification of Klein's seminal idea of projective identification has provided a conceptual vehicle for understanding disavowed associations (inter)subjectively. Associations may be inferred from gathering in or *containing* the patient's projections. As the analyst considers his or her countertransference, they may come to understand how they function as "a particular kind of person" in another's fantasy, without necessarily offering interpretive opinions. In registering the patient's projective identifications, and in responsively modifying the therapeutic stance in relationship to them (Mitchell, 1993, p. 177; Sandler, 1976), the analyst offers him- or herself as a transmuted, milder version of the projective identifications. Thus, the analyst's *becoming* allows the patient to detoxify and work through pathological projective identifications (Grotstein, 1995, 1999).

Containing is thus not only a vehicle of empathic understanding but also a way of being with the other and asserting influence.

Bion's model of the *container-contained* describes three forms of relatedness: destructively *parasitic*, benevolently *symbiotic*, and *communal* (via a shared language system) (see Chapter 7). It aids the therapist in understanding disavowed associations, expressed via projective identifications, and the uses to which these ambiguous and subterranean communications are put in the psychotherapeutic situation to advance or interfere with truth seeking. Moreover, it provides a way of thinking about and working with the needs of many patients for noninterpretive activity conveyed via preverbal and paraverbal communication, symbolic play, and certain forms of enactments.

Moving the treatment of Simone from parasitic to symbiotic relatedness

Simone's parasitic assaults on my authenticity could be indirect and not immediately identifiable. An early clue was her detached, nonchalant disposition, which did not match her exigent situation and reason for being in my office. Like the endangered Hamlet, in critical impasse, she could "speak daggers but use none" (Shakespeare 1603, III, iii, 414). Simone threatened to starve me emotionally and numb me intellectually, transporting her projective identifications via bland affect and vacant speech. Thus, there was method in Simone's seemingly nonconfrontational manner of interviewing the interviewer.

Her description of prior clinical contacts was revealing: "I've already seen my guidance counselor and the school psychologist. They think I have problems and need therapy. I don't. I saw my mother's therapist, she didn't say anything, are you going to be silent, too?" So, one danger was that I would talk too much—or too little. She did not "need" that kind of therapist.

I decoded an ambivalent invitation in her initial exchanges. As Simone put it: "I didn't say I didn't want to be in therapy. I said I had no problems, and no need of therapy."

Whereas I understood Simone's distrust, her refusal to let me "play upon" her, I attempted to communicate that I knew she was playing on me. I aimed to establish at the outset that I was not hoodwinked into believing that Simone felt and thought as little as she conveyed. It would have been disastrous to be lulled by the patient into an inauthentically affable posture and to ignore her misleading and subtly provocative behavior. In my experience, even the most cynical and unforthcoming adolescents yearn to break through their silence and establish symbiotic connection. They grudgingly ally with a therapist who addresses their antagonistic falsity and the predicament that necessitates it. Hamlet's yearning for dependable communication echoes throughout the drama, expressed in his mournful final words: "The rest is silence" (V, ii, 368).

I met Simone's noncommittal smile with a humorously skeptical attitude. She was not going to be co-opted by the Establishment, and I was not going to be co-opted by her. My suspicion and distrust mirrored hers; I could be friendly, but not entranced by her friendly posture into assuming that we had or could establish a positive communicative link. My intended goal was to reciprocate an ambivalent invitation. Whereas I did not believe her, perhaps I could come to believe *in* her.

Simone herself had to take a similar journey from skepticism to trust. She did not want someone who would presume to define her, her problems, or her needs. She did not trust the reality that an adult could thoughtfully care and respond to her, and hence, why would she believe in the reality of a "real" therapist? My empathic gestures and interpretive forays were met with bland indifference. I was a member of the psychotherapy Establishment, not truly "bothered" by her unacknowledged anguish but rather emotionally indifferent: "This is what you do, you're doing what you're supposed to do....Your job."

I could not "pluck out" of Simone that which she chose to hide and protect; I could not make her speak (Shakespeare 1603, III, ii, 379-ff). To engage in something approaching a meaningful dialogue, I would have to come up with the "right" questions, yet veer away from anything that smelled too much like therapy. I would have to find a way to represent moral principles without being moralistic and therapeutic principles without being unduly or relentlessly therapeutic.

I grasped that it was essential to call attention to her parasitism: her unstated wish to have me participate in her falsifications. I had to learn to show her—and to accept emotionally—that to further a symbiotic bond, to some extent, I would participate. This entailed relaxing my psychoanalytic conscience and becoming a (seemingly) superficial object of Simone's internal and external worlds. For, when I was being sincere and doing my job, as traditionally psychoanalytically defined, I was reinforcing her belief in adult falsity, and most often she blocked out those who did this. When I submitted to her pressure not to do my job, not to be "psychological" or a real psychologist, but to exchange small talk and gossip, she became less guarded, livelier, and affectively more available.

It was not easy to modify my professional stance. I could not and would not withhold feedback when Simone responded to my questions with tales of risky behavior. I remained openly troubled by the recurrent incidents of parental hurts and disappointments. I felt the seriousness of Simone's disavowed agony regarding her father's affair and philandering, and her loyalty conflict as she observed her mother's situation. Hearing the metaphors of displaced interpersonal and internal conflict, the idealizations and losses, tried-on identities, and so on that were embedded in Simone's accounts of peers, boyfriends, and would-be stepparents, I had to control my commensal urges—that is, my wish to interpret, to be helpful, to clarify, and to inform. In drawing attention to her recurring dilemmas and their meaning, I had to consider that I might be trying to relieve my own agony, whether or not I would succeed in relieving hers.

The window of interpretive opportunity with Simone would open but briefly. With humor, sarcasm, nonverbal as well as verbal acknowledgment, I attempted to bring to the fore—to our mutual consciousness—the reality of her negative feelings. These feelings and related fantasies about me were often expressed via her projective identifications of my mental vacancy, insincerity, or rigidity. I felt encouraged that the therapeutic relationship offered something new and valuable whenever Simone tentatively or explicitly criticized me—"You don't listen," "You're [just] doing your job"—or when she protested openly, "You're being psychological." My "kingly conscience" may be sullied with falsity, professional, and otherwise, but unlike Hamlet's adversaries or Simone's parents, I was not averse to bringing this view of me to our mutual attention, putting this perspective into words, and accepting without protest that it could be right.

In other words, to contain Simone and to move her from parasitic to symbiotic and then to commensal levels of relatedness, I invited her projective identifications and encouraged her to stay with them mentally and linguistically, rather than merely to discharge them and withdraw. However, these exchanges, lively and important as I believed they were, were intermittent and short-lived, marked by retractions, denials, shifts of emphasis, and sudden and frequent withdrawal of interest and affect.

Simone effectively blocked commensal communication. There was no progressive, insight-oriented, verbally articulated exploration of transference-countertransference configurations. She rebuffed entry into areas of her mentality, particularly when it threatened her with a realistically ambivalent view of the figures in her life, leading to an open acknowledgment of her anger and disappointment in them.

However, the therapeutic relationship was not without meanings. Our interplay, her vacant nonchalance, and her subtle and not-so-subtle put-downs expressed symbiotically (i.e., enactively), the disavowed emotional experience in which we alternated in roles of truth seeker and deceiver, abandoner and abandoned.

To unblock development, the adolescent patient may need to reanimate early emotional involvements and ego positions, including fantasies, as well as pathological coping and defensive patterns. At times, the analyst must join the patient in the reanimation process, such as by engaging in what Blos (1979, p. 295) referred to as "guided acting out."

While Simone refused to participate in a conventional psychoanalytic dialogue on the communal level, in which unconscious and preconscious meaning was gradually revealed and understood, she came to participate symbiotically. To some extent, this provided the basis for her treatment to be considered a successful analytic experience, wherein developmental arrests are unblocked, pathological acting out is decreased, and constructive social participation is resumed. We may infer that Simone began to utilize her capacity for commensal relating, as evidenced by her significant improvement in school performance, evaporating interest in antisocial thinking and behavior, and age-appropriate life choices and goals.

From symbiotic to commensal relatedness: treatment of Simone, ten years later

"Hi, this is Simone," she said on the telephone, nearly ten years from our last conversation. She was unhappy and did not know what to do, and her mother suggested that she call. Could I see her soon? She was working for her father's business and commuting to New York City. He had married Elaine and had a child whom Simone enjoyed. She wished to be on her own; becoming a school psychologist or guidance counselor remained an option. But her immediate problem was her husband, William, a young stockbroker whom she had married shortly after college. "All my friends were getting married, and I liked Will. I still do." She started to cry. "I don't know if I love him, and he complains about me. I don't want to hurt his feelings. He loves Mookie [her dog] so much."

Although sad for her, I was pleased that she could feel feelings—for herself and for another person—with a depth that I had not previously experienced in her. Apparently, she had not either, for she reported that she had not cried or spoken about what was on her mind, not even to herself. But there was little pretense in this consultation or in the twice-weekly individual sessions that followed, as Simone began to explore what she was feeling, mostly in relation to William. Why had she married him? Who was like him in her past? What made her happy/unhappy with him? Were there other men she felt different with? One of her high school friends made her laugh—maybe him, she was not sure, and she felt guilty when they phoned each other.

Intermittently, William joined us. He was pleasant, if rather humorless, and only vaguely interested in his own psychology. More important to him was correcting the marital problems, for he wished to buy a home and start a family. These were Simone's professed goals, too. William felt Simone was not interested in him or in being with him. "She lights up when she is with her friends from high school, but not with me." Simone acknowledged that he was correct. She could not or did not explain further, and instead proffered for the first time the falsifying smile from her adolescence.

Simone remained quiet, which I assumed was due to the newness of the marital consultation, but she continued to sink into the background in subsequent joint sessions. In our individual work, we began to explore how and when she hid and avoided being herself, and how it replicated her childhood and adolescence, as well as mirrored her mother's marital nonresponsiveness. We touched on her father's abandonment, and she agreed that she did not want to do to William what was done to her. But, to a striking degree, in the second therapy as in the first, Simone seemed uninterested in the possible effects of her parents' breakup on her development or present situation. However, rather than accusing me of being psychological, she politely gave nodding acceptance to my interpretations and directed us back to her pressing concern: "What should I do?"

Again, I had to readjust my analytic orientation and goals, relax, and first allow her to define the relationship. Then I could consider how she wished to use me and why, and the extent to which I would "play." Simone now could feel some of her negative feelings, but they caused her confusion, pain, and guilt, and she wanted me to make her feel "nicer" (her word) and to repair her marriage. While I sympathized with her wishes—and respected that she could state them so directly—I offered no hope that, without her participation, I could fulfill any of them.

Whereas in the earlier therapy, I had to accept my being an untrustworthy object, in this therapy, I could challenge her desire to put all her trust in me. That is, I did not predominately accommodate her symbiotic wishes by taking on a role defined by her projective identifications. I offered interventions that encouraged her to function commensally, that is, to put her emotional experiences into words, such that we could both think about them. I affirmed that when she would come to articulate her own feelings, which she could no longer pretend not to feel, she would make constructive decisions. "But I don't seem to feel anything for William," she countered, quite sensibly, "that's my problem." How different this was, I reflected to her, for now she knew and could communicate that her lack of feeling signaled the presence of problems, rather than their absence. It became clearer to Simone that she wished to separate.

"You tell him," she pleaded. "I'm afraid to hurt him."

"But why would it hurt less if I told him?" I inquired.

"I can't do it."

Simone's unresolved conflicts around aggression, apparent in her need to protect William as well as herself from her negative feelings, had contributed to an increasingly false marriage. As she became more confident and emotionally expressive, and certainly less depressed, William began to assume that they were progressing with shared goals. He listened to Simone's feedback and genuinely tried to respond to her tentative offerings of dissatisfactions and complaints. But the therapy was producing a false impression. While Simone expressed interest in addressing her marital difficulties with me, she reported no desire to continue to do so with William. We now knew that she was living a marital charade. Once again, I was entering into a deception orchestrated by the patient.

I explained the dilemma to Simone, and she was concerned, for she did not wish to mislead William. "That's why you have to tell him," she begged. We compromised: we would tell William together. "You begin," she insisted.

At the following marital session, I shared my concern that William might be getting an unintended message about where the marriage seemed to be heading. I reiterated the obvious, that the couple did not communicate clearly or directly with each other, and that it would be harmful if Simone did not do so now.

William made it easier for the three of us, for he asked Simone if she was thinking of ending the marriage. She replied with a timid "yes." William bristled and expressed annoyance that Simone had not let him know sooner, and he turned angrily to me. I explained that it took Simone some time to become clear, and what made it so difficult was that she did not want to hurt him.

"I want to be your friend," Simone interjected. They both began to cry, and in short order, they began to discuss how to proceed. For the first time in the marital therapy, they were working together.

Conclusion: two treatments on different relational levels

Blos (1963) differentiated between two types of acting-out adolescents, distinguished by different developmental levels and the therapeutic techniques they responded to. In both, the adolescent's sense of reality has been disturbed, due to parents who "falsify by word or action the reality of events to which one of the child's senses was a competent witness" (p. 261). In the more primitive type, which characterized the younger Simone, the adolescent denies ambivalent feelings toward primary objects and seeks re-merger via magical control (i.e., projective identification) of the external world. The adolescent remains concrete, does not respond to interpretive activity, but requires a therapist-inspired "guided acting out."

In the second type, which came to characterize the older Simone, the individual is more compulsive and conceptual, and is capable of establishing a sense of historical reality, temporal ego continuity, and meaning. As the adolescent remembers and puts memories into words, he or she no longer has to repeat (Freud, 1914). In terms of the concepts advanced in this paper, Blos's two types correspond to the respective parasitic-symbiotic and symbiotic-commensal ends of the container-contained relational spectrum.

Throughout Simone's first therapy, I periodically offered interpretations, and while I cannot say what effects, if any, they might have had internally, Simone would not engage verbally. Therefore, it was necessary to think differently about how to advance the therapy. What proved effective was my thinking about our communications in terms of notions of the container-contained, in helping her progress through the three levels—from parasitic to symbiotic and finally, commensal relatedness.

Simone entered therapy with the belief that all adults are false. It was necessary for me to become a sham in behaving as a psychological therapist, and thus an ironic personification of adult falsity. But by not insisting on my Establishment-sanctioned or professional-role prerogatives, I was able to become a good enough "bad" object that Simone became engaged in the process between us.

Thus, my falsity allowed access into her world, such that we could proceed from a parasitic relationship to a symbiotic one. In this therapy that preceded her college years, Simone established a preverbal foundation of trust, allowing her to retire many of her parasitic tendencies. My containing Simone involved efforts to intuit what she was feeling, to verbally formulate her emotional thinking (and mine), and to accept her evacuations and falsifications of these thoughts and feelings, expressed symbolically via enactments by both of us.

We developed a shared language, but we did not clear an analytic path leading to an ever-more-direct communication within the therapeutic relationship about Simone's disillusionment and distrust. We progressed close to a "Dear-Diary" or best-friend sort of relationship, openly embracing concrete but not abstract meaning-making. Simone remained uncomfortable during the few instances when she acknowledged positive or negative feelings about the therapy, our relationship, or me.

I believe our first interlude of psychotherapy succeeded because Simone and I created and tolerated a benevolent balance of truth and falsity. She had learned what Hamlet could not: that not all Establishment falsity is toxic. She had built up a sufficient mental representation of me as a trustworthy symbiotic partner to respond unambivalently to her mother's suggestion to call me when she found herself in trouble again.

While she had bonded sufficiently to me and other Establishment figures to participate constructively in college life and her endeavors thereafter, Simone had difficulty thinking for herself and being on her own. There were consequences to her remaining symbiotic and failing to establish secure commensal relations. She married a man whom she did not talk to nor think with. This type of empty emotional relationship caused her sufficient pain to return to treatment.

In the first therapy, a blasé Simone conveyed the impression that she was doing me a favor by tolerating my presence and responding to my questions. She falsified, and I had to play along. In initiating the second treatment, an anxious, sad, and needy Simone questioned me: "What should I do?" She entered therapy feeling guilty and paralyzed, which seemed partially a defense against her aggressive impulses, which were not being directly expressed in any open exchange with her husband.

To some extent, Simone's helplessness falsified, by keeping her from connecting deeply to her husband or herself. At the same time, her unguarded impatience and frank desire for me to do her thinking and feeling were refreshingly different in their emotional honesty, and thus encouraging. Simone was openly immature and dependent at this inauguration of therapy, providing us both with a clear and realistic view of who and where she was in her development.

Simone began her second psychotherapy ready but not quite willing to function commensally, that is, to contain her thoughts and endure the process of self-conscious emotional thinking. She did not need me to think for her, although she attempted to make me feel that she did. Simone did not relinquish symbiotic wishes easily, as when she requested that I do her work with William, but she could tolerate my challenging her wishes. As she released me from her projective identifications—in which I was the object of all her trust—she discovered that she was able to find her own truths, make rational decisions based on them, and tolerate the painful consequences and unavoidable psychological turbulence that accompanies a responsible marital parting.

I felt a pang when Simone announced that she wanted to stop treatment and try it on her own in New York City. She seemed clear in her mind, speaking without much apprehension. Certainly, she knew that our work was not complete, and I wondered if, once again, I was going to be left to contain what Simone did not want to feel. During the following weeks, she took comfort from the truism that her life would involve unknown risks as well as possibilities, but I did not share this sense of comfort and continued to express my concern. "I know where you live in case I need you," she commented warmly at the end of our last session. I then felt reassured, for I believe a mark of successful therapy is reached when containing is reciprocated. Simone addressed my separation anxiety gracefully, without rubbing it in my face. Her parting words represented sophisticated commensal communication, then sparing the two of us from confronting all the truth that was at our disposal, without being false. To my ears, Simone was also acknowledging that there was much unsaid meaning in the room that remained to be articulated and analyzed, should she appear for a third analytic interlude.

An intersubjective approach to entitlement

In this chapter I consider a particular emotional aspect of the analytic experience: the sense of entitlement or the feeling of being special. I conceive of entitlement as an irrational but not necessarily pathological mode of experiencing psychic reality, one which belongs to both analyst and patient participating in the intersubjective matrix (Billow, 1997, 1998).

This understanding differs from most conceptualizations of entitlement, which emphasize its pathological nature and largely locate it within the patient, while neglecting the therapist's dynamics and contribution to the interaction (Coen, 1988; Grey, 1987; Levin, 1970). In contrast, the basic premise of the intersubjective approach is that psychoanalytic data are mutually generated, co-determined by the organizing activities of both participants in the reciprocally interacting subjective worlds of patient and analyst (Stolorow, 1997). Thus, many factors are important to consider before concluding that the patient is exhibiting an exaggerated, even pathological, sense of entitlement: the analyst's level of tolerance for perceived entitled behaviors in others, their authoritarian and regressive tendencies, their diagnostic and technical biases, and other countertransference manifestations.

It may seem to be a curious imaginative stretch to place the empathically inclined, dedicated psychoanalyst in the clinical domain of such characters as Shakespeare's villainous Richard III, whom Freud (1916) considered as the embodiment of malignant entitlement. However, I contend that patients frequently make this association, experiencing their analysts as grasping for power, insisting on their way, and likening to seek revenge when thwarted.

Freud (1916) himself implied a symmetry between patient and analyst when he candidly acknowledged the universality of entitled beliefs: "We all demand reparation for early wounds to our narcissism, our self-love" (p. 315). Thus, in this essay on the "exceptions," Freud briefly considered the analyst's entitlement, a particular aspect of what is usually referred to as countertransference.

I also wish to illustrate how in some instances there can be a conflict between the analyst's and the patient's values concerning entitlement, quite apart from transference and countertransference per se. It is given that analyst and patient each have a view of what constitutes legitimate—or illegitimate—entitlements. But neither view is necessarily invalid, or even transference dominated. What one individual may consider special, such as the analyst's wish to analyze or the patient's wish to be accommodated, may feel antagonistic to the other's sense of security and well-being. Clarifying the difference in values may sometimes relieve impasses and stalemates in treatment.

The analyst's vulnerability to irrational entitlement

Many aspects of the analytic relationship suggest the analyst's vulnerability to irrational entitlement. Traditionally, he or she is the special one with exceptional power and moral authority (see, for example, entire issue of *Psychoanalytic Quarterly*, 1966, 65, No. 1). As Michels (1988) has emphasized, the asymmetric nature of the therapeutic situation tends to promulgate the analyst's "rights" over the patient's: "Both metaphorically and actually the therapist sits in the most comfortable seat, controls the time and place of meeting, receives payment, and is protected from discomfort" (p. 55).

Michels takes for granted that the analyst sits in the seat of the expert and is legitimately entitled to protection from discomfort. I disagree and have elsewhere suggested the opposite (see Chapter 2). The analyst's view of reality, like the patient's, is affected by "irrational emotional involvement" (Renik, 1996, p. 392), anxiety, and discomforting ignorance, all of which may contribute to, as well as interfere with, a successful psychoanalysis (Bird, 1972; Racker, 1968; Renik, 1995). Bion (1973) advised that "in every consulting room there ought to be two rather frightened people: the patient and the psychoanalyst. If there are not, one wonders why they are bothering to find out what everyone knows" (p. 13).

At times, the analyst may be unwilling or unable to tolerate not being special, feeling his or her expertise rejected or ineffective. The analyst may experience the patient as malignantly not caring about or understanding his or her therapeutic ministrations, and perversely blocking efforts to love and to be loved. This was indeed the situation which Freud (1916) described. The "exception" was the individual unresponsive to the analyst's insights, "one of the components of love" (p. 312).

Freud did not consider that the analyst, feeling unjustly deprived of love and narcissistically wounded, may respond to the patient's perceived entitlements by evasively drawing upon entitled attitudes of his or her own. Instead of mentally processing subjective pain and anxious confusion, the analyst may resort to rigid thinking and illusion, transforming the analysand's thoughts and feelings into fixated ideas of transference, defense, or resistance. The psychoanalyst's treatment of entitlement may come to represent an illusory path to omnipotent Truth. When "truth" itself becomes "special," employed "with a big T...this gets people into a frame of mind in which they become unable to think" (Russell, 1927/1970, p. 265).

Psychoanalytic ideas, put into therapeutic action, may potentiate a patient's rebellious entitlements, since the patient may feel—quite correctly—misunderstood and uncared for. The literature on entitlement has not adequately appreciated how the analyst, believing to be properly utilizing theory and technique, may behave like the "exception," and thus contribute to the often-reported escalating dramas and negative therapeutic reactions characterizing certain treatments.

The patient experienced as pathologically entitled may make the analyst particularly vulnerable to not thinking, and hence to counterentitlement. Coen (1988) characterized entitled individuals as using sadistic demandingness and projective identification to promote sadomasochistic bonding. They "mandate" empathy, experiencing the therapist as a self-object who must be omnipotently coerced to give, rather than one who gives out of genuine love and caring (Shabad, 1993). Ladan (1992) described the entitled analysand's inveigling the analyst to indulge the patient's secret fantasy of doing something else and not being in analysis. Attempts to control the other's mind, and to resist or counter such control, may be, then, important aspects of an interaction involving entitlement. One of Richard III's joyous triumphs was his success in seducing Anne's mind, and not Anne herself, whom he promptly discarded. An unfortunate fate of seduction and abandonment may await the analyst whose mind is overwhelmed by the patient's irrational entitlements, or by their own.

In each of the following case examples, I attempted to analyze what I experienced as the patient's (or supervisee's) excessive or inhibited attitudes of entitlement. I also volunteered and encouraged an analysis of my own entitlements, positive and negative, excessive and inhibited, as I came to understand their possible roles in the interaction. I tried not to assume a position of superior knowledge and judgment, or to assume that my perceptions were necessarily correct, or more correct, than the patient's. In each situation, I found the interaction to throw a fresh and unexpected light on the psychoanalytic experience.

Case I: exploring righteous indignation

"I can't work now," one individual regularly reported during our first months of psychoanalytic therapy. "I'm so angry I need to ventilate." He would fume silently, becoming quite flushed, sullenly not complying with my encouragements to speak. Soon I no longer needed or wanted to encourage him. He occupied many sessions angrily denouncing his customers, supervisors, and fiancée, all of whom treated him unjustly. My precursory efforts at exploring feelings, transference, character, or genetic patterns were impatiently and rather harshly rebuffed. My attempts to bring attention to his responses only seemed to aggravate him.

When what I perceived to be righteous indignation emerged, I most often adopted a respectful, interested silence. However, this stance felt seductive, manipulative, and inauthentic to me, given my own quickly mounting feelings of indignation. I experienced him enslaving me in his narcissistic fantasy (Kernberg, 1975; Kohut, 1971), inhibiting my healthy entitlements to think, feel, and respond as I wished. I rationalized my inactivity as empathic accommodation, respecting his fragile ego defenses, in the service of building a positive alliance in which he would feel cared for and understood. But I wondered whether my concern was for my own faltering ego defenses, rather than his (Billow & Mendelsohn, 1990), my fear of betraying my ambivalent feelings, and my wish to end a session in which I felt particularly ineffective and helpless.

I often felt tempted to identify and explore his unquestioned right to explosive anger, and occasionally ventured to ask why talking calmly and trying to understand his anger did not supply adequate ventilation. Unfailingly this provoked indignation, a disgusted sigh, and a comment such as "I can't understand why you would say that! You're supposed to be a sympathetic professional!"

Gedo (1977) has described how the therapist, in responding to "infantile claims" of patients, by necessity must maintain "maximal tact and empathy... any failure in this regard is inevitably followed by humiliation and outrage" (p. 792). This patient's claim, I decided, was for me to understand and accept his view of reality, his emotions, and his use of me.

Blechner (1987) has characterized two strategies for treating entitlement: the "frustration" and the "gratification." I prefer the terms "interpretative" and "accommodative." The first, originally promulgated by Freud (1916), emphasizes maintaining traditional psychoanalytic boundaries and recommends analyzing dynamic, genetic roots of entitlement. Michels (1988) advises not

> to placate or mollify the patient by gratifications that grow out of a desire to dilute the patient's resentment and disappointment or bribe him into pseudo compliance... the therapist must be sensitized to the patient's response to it, accepting and tolerating anger or dissatisfaction and interpreting resistances to expressing, or even experiencing, the frustrations of the treatment.
>
> (p. 56)

Winnicott and Kohut, in contrast, view entitlement as expressions of need and attempt to adapt the environment so that the underlying desire, aim, and object may be discovered and experienced. Analysts influenced by their theories have stressed the importance, and often the inevitability, of living through a lengthy period in which the therapist provides a holding environment before the patient is ready to tolerate interpretative activity (Gedo, 1977; Stark, 1994). The analyst, so as not to iatrogenically encourage the patient to "forfeit" a trust-building stage of healthy entitlement, must distinguish a period of "normal and necessary omnipotence (specialness, uniqueness) from pathological omnipotence" (Grotstein, 1995, p. 6). At times, manifest wishes are therapeutically gratified without analysis.

The patient implicitly adhered to the gratification theory of therapy in which he considered ventilation and automatic confirmation to be a right, and also a method of cure. He found me to be unsympathetic in even introducing the frustration-interpretation theory.

I was disheartened by his disappointment in me. He had named a truth about my entitlement, while I was trying to name his. I was *supposed* to be a sympathetic professional, but other feelings predominated, including my perhaps irrationally based wish to follow my theory of cure rather than his. I felt guilty for not behaving more sympathetically, in addition to feeling guilty for not helping him get a better understanding and control of himself, even though these were not his goals.

Chastised but still not willing to renounce my right to maintain a frustration-interpretation technique of entitlement, I took the opportunity to extend the discussion to include his implication regarding my deficient capacity to love and understand him. I acknowledged that, as he had discovered, I was not that sympathetic a professional. Judging from his tone, I continued, he seemed to be morally offended by me, and I could understand why he would feel superior and indignant.

I braced myself for his disapproval, which I received, but something in his tone seemed markedly different. It was softer, and I detected a gleam of new interest in me and curiosity about what I had to say. "What do you mean, I feel superior?" He said he had never considered himself as superior. He acknowledged that he became angry when anyone would be insensitive and inconsiderate, as I sometimes was, but he never considered himself above or better than anyone else. Again, his tone as much as his words implicated my failure in moral and professional judgment: "I can't understand why you would say this about me."

Feeling emboldened, I continued the dialogue: "You may not be aware, but you are sounding superior right now. You say that you can't understand, but I believe you are saying that I don't understand, and that I should." He looked flabbergasted, but he did not explode. In fact, his anger turned into the first warm smile of our relationship. This he countered by shaking his head, as if to say I had done it again with my latest unsympathetic intervention.

All in all, the interaction seemed a success. I believe my acknowledgment of the validity of his indignant feelings, of his "right" to be entitled as a response to my perceived entitlement, relieved a pressure to retaliate by excluding all other thought and behavior. I somehow succeeded in helping him establish some distance from what I diagnosed as his thought controlling, "super[ior] ego" (Bion, 1977). A mental space now existed in which he could tolerate the frustration of considering the reality of someone else's ideas, my ideas of me, my ideas of him, and my ideas of what constituted a thoughtful analytic interchange.

Mixed with his anger was what I took to be gratitude for my active interest and persistence. In now perceiving that he cared for me and what I had to say, I felt more confident that I could care for him, and for the first time, I felt truly sympathetic. I found blessed relief from my own guilty feelings of superiority. As we have continued our work, I have found it easier to accommodate his indignant mode of processing frustrating experience, while he more easily accommodates my lack of sympathy, that is, my pressure to identify, discuss, and interpret his righteous indignation. Thus, we mutually recognize certain entitled elements in each other's subjectivity.

I suggest that our interaction illustrates the existence of entitlement "thresholds," a reflection of personal limitation in capacity or willingness to function in a relatively relaxed and creative manner when confronted by perceived entitlement from another. Individuals feel entitled to their entitlement, but often do not extend the same privilege to others. A patient may respond to the analyst's inquiry with indignation and recrimination, and further may attempt to make the analyst feel malignantly entitled when he or she attempts to analyze entitlement. As in this example, the patient does not merely project and provoke, but may quite accurately identify irrational, even pathological entitlement in the analyst's personality and use of theory and technique. And as others do, the analyst may reach a personal threshold, a limited toleration for such exploration, and may contribute to the irrational entitlement in the consultation room while attempting to analyze it.

Certain claims of entitlement may lower the analyst's threshold, such that his or her own retaliatory counter-entitlements are more obviously brought into play. The analyst needs to be aware of characteristic responses to pressure to "do something that he feels he should not, or ought not, or doesn't want to do" (Blechner, 1987, p. 249). To avoid his or her own experience of impotency and submissiveness in the face of a patient's aggressivity, the analyst may collude, circumventing reality and creating an illusion of peaceful coexistence (Ladan, 1992). Not analyzing entitlement may be a narcissistic defense rather than a necessary technique, indicating the analyst's irrational entitlement. On the other end of the interpretation–accommodation continuum, an analyst may precipitously intrude upon a patient's psychic readiness, demonstrating an entitled disregard of the intersubjective reality.

Cases 2 and 3: working with manifestations of inhibited entitlement

In a situation of restrictive or inhibited entitlement (Levin, 1970), the individual feels "not entitled" to a feeling or an attribute of specialness which is believed to exist within someone else and which may be feared as well as envied. The individual feels without rights, or powerless to assert rights, in a world of powerful others, and may exhibit self-effacement, social with-drawal, and masochistic mental activity, fantasy, and behavior. In the following case anecdotes, the individuals felt restricted in their rights, par-ticularly when comparing themselves to me and my rights. They attributed certain entitled psychologies to me and treated them as my inalienable "per-sonal possessions." In the first example, it is "feeling like a real analyst"; in the second, it is a "critical attitude." I attempted to focus on the rigid fantasy constructions by taking a previously unexplored look at what my psychol-ogy and clinical presence were possibly contributing to the other partici-pants' persistent beliefs in my specialness and their lack of specialness.

Case 2

My patient, an advanced analytic candidate at our institute, expressed dif-ficulty in setting fees adequate to his level of considerable experience. "I guess I'm not ready to accept a regular fee; I'm not a regular analyst, a real analyst. I don't have it yet."

"What's 'it'?" I asked.

"I don't know, a certificate of authority. Am I certifiable?"

Was he saying, I asked, that one has to be crazy (certifiable) to be a real analyst, and had he anyone particular in mind?

"Not you—you're a real analyst and you're not crazy. You can relax and rest on your laurels."

"What laurels?" I inquired.

"You know, your age, accomplishments," and then, with hesitation, "thinking you deserve it all, thinking you are a big, hot shit. I don't think you think of yourself that way—maybe I do. I do. I don't think I would want to be in treatment with somebody unless I thought he was a big, hot shit."

I said, "But maybe I do think of myself that way, too, and what is worse, that I haven't been aware that I do." I asked him to expound on his assertion regarding my possible overblown view of myself.

He said it was not healthy to think you are "something"; that was being delusional. His father, in a related professional field, "always acted like the certified professional, even with us kids." Apparently, the patient needed to see me as professionally important, but was afraid of the consequences to our relationship if I also saw myself as important.

I agreed that if one acted only as a professional, as in being a professional analyst, and not also being a person, one would be delusional indeed. I sug-gested that he did not seem to be sure whether I acted like a person or was a person. He conceded that maybe he did wonder whether the spontaneous, human qualities he saw in me were simply techniques mastered in analytic training, "like in a course, 'Basic Techniques in Realness.'"

I asked what gave him the impression that I might be adopting a role. He said he was touched that I permitted him to question my behavior. I replied that I could not stop him from doing so. Then he realized: "I've stopped me from questioning your behavior, or from admitting to me that I do it all the time. In fact, that's probably all I do!" He then continued with an association linking me to his father. He spoke of his fear of his anger toward his father, his father's possible envy of him, Oedipal rivalry ("having it all" included mother), his desire to be like his father, and his desire not to be like his father.

This all made sense, of course, but in a rather intellectualized way. I felt that we needed to get back to his belief that my sincerity camouflaged an underlying grandiose self-involvement. At a moment which I took to be opportune, I interrupted him and asked: "Who are you associating to, a big, hot shit, delusional analyst?"

He smiled broadly, through tears. "This is like before, when you asked me why I thought you might be role-playing. I can't believe that you are really interested in my opinions, and that you respect them, particularly if they're about you, no, about anything. I'm always waiting for the subtle put-down that never comes. It makes me nervous, like I can't trust you. With my father, I could count on feeling bad. It's kind of a secure feeling."

We made much analytic mileage analyzing the transferences described here. But his experience also reflected realistic and quite important dimensions of our relationship. Regarding my contribution: in the little analytic pond of our institute, I am "special," entitled by status, authority, and even age. Moreover, in our institute's corridors, I do maintain the role of "the analyst" and would feel uncomfortable relinquishing it. Regarding his contribution: he would be naive not to expect put-downs from his teachers, I being one of them. Worse yet would be his situation with faculty and peers should he relinquish his "real person-hood" acolyte status. With some humor and irony, we acknowledged the legitimacy of his perceptions of my entitlement and his non-entitlement. The discussions have released us from our rigid positions on the entitlement–non-entitlement continuum, as we move towards a mutuality and equality in our relationship.

Case 3

In a second case example of manifest inhibited entitlement, an analytic candidate under my supervision tended to swallow her control case's stream of complaints and dissatisfactions. The patient was free-associating, the therapist reasoned, and therefore her spontaneity should not be challenged. Further, since there were grains of truth in everything the patient said about her, the novice analyst felt she would be hypocritical to criticize the patient's criticisms.

The candidate volunteered that she had a mother who felt it was her privilege to criticize her daughter, since it was for her own good. I asked her to consider whether being critical was a privilege and to consider how her mother and her patient possessed a privilege but she did not. I then inquired whether such a privilege existed in the supervisory relationship. It did. Criticism in supervision, as in her relationship to her mother and to her patient, was a one-way street. I teased her a bit. Could she not challenge me since, I presumed, I did not spend our time spontaneously free-associating? She replied with humorous recognition, "True, but you're supposed to criticize me, it's part of your job. Okay, I get it, I'm a hypocrite after all! I don't want the power to criticize. I don't like doing it, but I guess I like getting it."

I said that I didn't like her privilege very much, my having to criticize her. She replied, "Don't worry, I criticize me for you, so you don't have to do it." I said I was still worried, because no matter which of us played out "critical me," I would not get a chance to be anything else. I reminded her of the old saw of who controls whom, the sadist or the masochist? The enactment of her restricted entitlement, left undiscussed, threatened to overpower and control me. I suggested that her patient, like me, might not like feeling special all the time and might feel burdened and alone in being the sole critical one, and that the patient might find relief in addressing this unbalanced aspect of the interaction.

In these examples, I did not, and could not, renounce my right to be special, which included a right to be an authority or to be critical. The goal was not to cure or banish all expressions of forthright and restricted entitlement but to transform what was being mutually enacted and defended against into emotional ideas—some realistic, some not—which could be thought about and developed in the intersubjective context.

Case 4: segment of an analysis

After a long period of the patient's distrust, a productive relationship ensued with a woman with a history of maternal deprivation. Although capable of doing psychoanalytic work, she developed a predilection for bringing to her hours' physical possessions, such as photographs and mementos, to "share" her life. She brought in food, such as two pieces of cake, to celebrate her birthday or the occasion of an anniversary of treatment. She paid the most cursory attention to any interventions I made around such behaviors, such that I realized that despite my efforts, these were incidents of accommodation and gratification.

When I suggested that she consider sharing her life without bringing in "the evidence," she compromised on "picture sessions." In these hours, or segments of therapy hours, she detailed her trips, children's projects, new interests, progress in sports activities, and so forth. I soon realized that she was following the letter but not the spirit of my mild injunction. I brought this to her attention, and she agreed, unenthusiastically offering one of my own, uninspired formulations, "I guess I want you to care for me the way my mother didn't."

I concluded, from her habit of parroting my interpretations, that she had decided that I needed to be considered special in the "analytic" way that I periodically insisted upon. I was extracting attention and taking it away from her. She was going to have to put up with my tedious need to discuss the meaning of her behavior, our relationship, and so forth, before I would be able to return to her caretaking. The patient seemed to confirm Bromberg's (1983) observation that certain individuals found interpretations to be empathic disruptions and processed them as a sign of the analyst's narcissism.

We had, then, each been experiencing the other as excessively entitled and had responded with an unacknowledged, characteristic interactional mode: I confronted and interpreted her entitlements, while she accommodated mine. When I tentatively offered this opinion, she interrupted, beginning to cry. With a newly found freedom of expression, she turned her eyes to the ceiling of my consultation room and asked rhetorically of it: "Yes! Why do we always have to analyze?"

I had no difficulty considering her complaint regarding my timing and pacing, and I felt willing to discuss with her how to modify my technique. But she did not want to talk further about the situation between us. She had transformed herself into a picture of "relentless woundedness," to paraphrase Stark (1994) who described a character type of "relentless entitlement." She was a sensuous image of hurt and distress. Again, those pictures! I thought. I felt clumsy and guilty for imposing my subjectivity over her developmental need. I made a tacit agreement with myself not to always analyze.

It was an agreement I apparently could not keep, for I found myself asking in a subsequent session, what did she want to do if not analyze? I had stumbled on the right question, for she put into words what much of her behaviors were about. She wanted me to look at her and to treat her and everything she did as special. We then came to understand how her demandingness camouflaged her underlying sense of inferiority. She felt that I could not really care for her but, rather than ignore her felt need, she attempted to control me by acting hurt and arousing my guilty compliance. I asked her whether it was merely an act, or whether she found it genuinely hurtful when I pressured her to have analysis the way I wanted, rather than the way she wanted.

My willingness to acknowledge my own entitled demandingness released a flood of memories concerning her willful mother's bossy and entitled behaviors, and her own desperate need to acquiesce to them. These sessions were often painful to her. But she also evidenced much pleasure, describing the analysis as a "haven" wherein she truly felt special, cared for, and understood. I did not challenge, interpret, or disrupt these emerging pleasurable feelings. I assumed that the patient was basking transferentially in what Bromberg (1983, p. 459) described as a curative period of undisrupted "core fantasy of entitlement." I believed that I was providing an environment in which she could build or rebuild a stage of hallucinatory, idealized, symbiotic objects.

I did not comprehend a quality of her pleasure until, after a year in this phase of our work, she confessed that even in the sessions in which she did intense grieving, she often became sexually aroused by being in my presence and hearing the sound of my words. She admitted that in several sessions she purposely brought herself to orgasm. I realized that she had been sexualizing our sessions, taking in my words as phallic objects to be enjoyed. The pictures, once again! Words functioned on the level of sexual hallucination.

I wondered aloud: "Are we having sex now?"—acknowledging to both of us my sincere confusion. She sheepishly replied that we were not and asked if I were angry with her. I replied quite honestly that I was too surprised to be angry, and that I was trying to understand the situation between us.

I thought of her plaint, "Why do we always have to analyze?" Perhaps the woman was speaking for every patient's hatred of analytic entitlement. The patient wants to be a special person, and not simply a patient. The analyst wants to be an analyst, and not simply a special person. Even now, I wanted to control and construct the relationship in my way, putting experience into words, clarifying, and interpreting, all of which called attention to me and my understanding of the patient's clinical reality. In her hallucinatory sexuality, she could construct the relationship in her way and could both retaliate against and enjoy my control.

I have described two approaches to the treatment of entitlement, between which there is some tension. To simplify, one difference between the technical approaches is not *whether* or not to analyze but *when*. The accommodative and interpretive techniques converge on the belief that when the underlying dynamics come to be clarified, the manifest claims of entitlement may lose their urgency. In practice, each clinician finds his or her own compromise between gratification and frustration, accommodation and interpretation (Blechner, 1987). But on what basis is the compromise reached? How do we know when the patient is ready to move on and can tolerate the frustration of non-accommodation? There is, of course, no definitive or purely objective method of assessment. The analyst must rely on what we once called "clinical intuition," and now subsume under "subjectivity."

I had believed I was sensitively accommodating to, and perceptively analyzing, the woman's regressive entitlements. From one point of view, I was. But from another, I had been enacting a fantasy treatment, missing crucial aspects of the woman herself, and her use of me. She did not disturb my gratifying fantasy of our relationship, and I did not succeed in disturbing hers. Our interaction has demonstrated to me how little the analyst knows, or can know, about him- or herself, much less about the other person in the consultation room. It is a measure of the analyst's illusionary entitlement to believe otherwise.

Conclusion

The analyst's entitlement to assert professional prerogatives, such as intervening, making interpretations, or remaining silent, may be influenced by
a realistic consideration of technique, by perhaps unavoidable limitations
in understanding another person or oneself, and by irrational attitudes and
behaviors, all of which may affect the interaction. Thus, many subjective
factors within the analyst play a significant role in assessing whether a patient's perceived entitlements are appropriate or inappropriate, intractable
or readily analyzable. The technical challenge involves, then, deciding how
and when the analyst may "share" his or her subjectivity (Aron, 1991) concerning (what the analyst experiences as) the patient's entitlement. A controversy may arise, since the patient may reveal decidedly different opinions
about the types and distribution of entitlement in the consultation room.
It is quite possible that the patient has formed such opinions not only on
the basis of his or her representational configurations but by a realistic,
if previously unrealized or unpublicized, assessment of the analyst's own
entitlements.

As so often happens in psychoanalysis, controversy breeds opportunity,
for now the analysts may encourage a dialogue. The focus enlarges to include the mutual consideration of the analyst's perceived entitlements and
their effects on the analytic relationship. To the extent to which the dialogue
may be meaningfully sustained, the dilemma of accommodation versus interpretation is partially resolved. Entitlement becomes a topic of thoughtful
conversation rather than a mode of processing experience. Both parties may
begin to understand how they have been accommodating to, and reacting
against, the other's perceived entitlements, as well as their own.

I have used myself as an example of an analyst who initially believed he
was constructively analyzing treatment-resistant entitlements. The course
of the work in each of the four cases involved identifying expressions of
entitlement in myself, as well as in the patient or supervisee. I came to
understand that such distinctions as normal or pathological, entitled or
counter-entitled, often become irrelevant. The focus of the work shifted towards uncovering the bidirectionality of entitlement experiences, revealing
the varying elements of entitlement, and discovering how they function in
the therapeutic relationship.

The analyst may achieve greater freedom to participate in a lively, appreciative, even humorous manner, when he or she owns personal entitlements
as part of the ongoing action. This entails the analyst accepting that, like
the patient, he or she needs to feel and to be treated as special, and that,
when threatened, characteristic defense patterns are likely to emerge in the
interaction. The patient may quite accurately perceive aspects of the analyst's psychology of entitlement and may use and abuse such knowledge in
the therapeutic relationship. At times, the positive trajectory of the work

may seem to dissolve in a heated exchange of views regarding perceived entitlements. This dialogue may be expressed in a reactive vocabulary of unacknowledged entitlement: denial, protest, rationalization, indignation, recrimination, appeasement, hallucination, accommodation, and even interpretation.

I have attempted to demonstrate how these different expressions of entitlement and reactions against perceived entitlement may become constructive building blocks in a working, mutually empathic relationship. I have suggested that progress is more likely to occur when the analyst acknowledges subjective and interactive aspects of entitlement as they emerge and are discovered in the ongoing clinical work. As always, when the analyst is receptive to the patient's view of reality and is relatively non-defensive and non-authoritarian, interpretative activity is more likely to be respected and integrated into the psychoanalytic work.

The goal is, of course, to get beyond labeling, judging, submitting, rebelling, and retaliating, to the experience of mutual recognition. Ironically, as the psychoanalytic dyad learns to mutually confront the interpersonal realities of entitlement, each participant may realize that attitudes of entitlement are universal, and that his or her entitlements are no more special than the other's.

Section V

Doing our work

Editor's note

Early in his career, Billow enjoyed attending Harold Searles's controversial live interviews of psychiatric patients. During one of the interviews, Searles said something along the lines of "I wish I could see things through your eyes." Without skipping a beat, and to the utter surprise of Searles and the audience, the patient removed his glass eye and motioned for Searles to take it. As a showman, Searles recognized that he was outshined and tipped his hat as a sign of respect. In thinking about this moment, which Billow relayed to me years later, I believe that it speaks to several elements in Billow's work, as well as to the reasons he was inspired by Searles. First, it provides a symbolic illustration for the desire to know (K) the other's experience and its limitations, as we can never really see things through the other's eyes, or as they "are." Second, it suggests inevitable, symbolic groupishness in every dyadic interaction: besides helping and being helped or asking questions and answering them, Searles and his interviewee were also paying attention to the witnesses in the audience (and elsewhere), conscious of their impressions and judgments. Third, the element of surprise allowed everyone in the room to review previously-held assumptions. And finally, for both Searles and Billow, in order to learn the art of psychotherapy it is important to witness seasoned clinicians as they do the work, as a way to initiate a honest dialogue about what actually happens in the consulting room.

In this final section, the reader is invited to witness Billow as he is *Doing the work* and thinking about it, in his most recent contributions. Building on Bion's metapsychology, Billow maps out a unique way of working analytically in and with the therapy group. As the reader will notice, each intervention, assessment, or conjecture begins with the therapist's interrogation of his emotional reactions, with an emphasis on what seems novel and fresh. At the same time, Billow is always attempting to enlist group members to think and collaborate psychoanalytically. This is most apparent in the vignettes with his long-standing groups, where members exhibit sophistication, as they too tune into their emotional reactions, provide feedback to fellow members, and push for less falsity, pretense, and superficiality.

Surprisingly, the title of Chapter 16, "Doing our work: words, deeds, and presence," lacks a subject. Who, one might ask, is doing our work? For Billow, whether the leader's presence is obvious (as in "It's all about 'Me'") or not, it is always central to the kind of work that gets done in group. Two words, seemingly contradictory, come to mind when thinking about the quality of presence he is advocating for: patience and passion. Patience allows the group and ourselves to experiment without overly defined goals in mind. If we are not unduly anxious, we can utilize binocular vision (Bion, 1961) and gaze inward as well as outward, locating unformulated thoughts and new dimensions of ourselves and our group members. When successful, patience leads to new discoveries and enhances the creative dimension of the work. At the same time, the therapist's passion (see also Chapter 6) needs to convey an emotional investment in the work of the group and in the lives of its members. If an intervention is any good, it underscores a meaning that the therapist urgently needs to express. As Billow reminds us, our passion and convictions (including the conviction that we can never be certain) give vitality to our words.

That said, our subjective convictions are not—and should not be—the ultimate source of authority in the group. In Chapter 17, referencing the work of French philosopher Jacques Derrida, as well as other deconstructionists (e.g., Barthes, 1967), Billow develops the idea that the group's discourse should continually be subjected to *Deconstruction*. By this he refers to the search for ambiguities, hidden meanings, and hierarchical positions in the group's "text," and in its speakers' sociocultural-historical contexts. As with all references to French post-structural philosophy, this requires much clarification, beyond the scope of these remarks. I will therefore limit my commentary to Billow's concepts.

For Billow, deconstruction both honors the group's "text" and seeks to add new and different layers of meaning. In this respect, deconstruction is a reaction to the modernist emphasis on progress, at the expense of tradition, as in "out with the old, in with the new." As a part of the modernist tradition (in philosophy), Freud (1923) used metaphors like **destruction** and **demolition** to prescribe what, in health, ought to occur to one's infantile wishes. In contrast, therapeutic deconstruction tries to imbue the text with fresh meaning without necessarily getting rid of old ones: at times by suggesting preferable meanings, and at times by simply raising doubt about fixed narratives. Billow defines three types of deconstructive interventions: transformative, reflective, and diversity.

Transformative deconstructions challenge speakers to reevaluate their testimonies, consider a change of emphasis, or revise their meaning. In one of the examples, a group member angrily reported how wounded she felt by her daughter's lack of generosity. Deconstructing the term "generosity," Billow and the group challenge her "generosity" towards her fellow members, suggesting that being receptive to and reflecting on others' input are broader and preferable dimensions of generosity than the concrete way she was using the term.

Next, Billow defines reflective deconstructions, which do not explicitly suggest preferred meaning, but instead suggest that each word, or signifier, can have different meanings, especially for different people. Through casting doubt about a member's—or a group's—certainty, new vistas for exploration are created. For example, in one of the case examples, Billow works with a group member to deconstruct her unequivocal rejection of "blame." "What's wrong with accepting blame?" he asks, challenging her certainty regarding the others' intentions (to hurt her) as well as her assumption that blame must induce shame. Such interventions may be aimed at expanding one member's characterological boundaries, but are always also directed at the rest of the membership, suggesting an open-minded, open-ended attitude to learning, one that likely involves criticism and even disapproval.

The third type of deconstructive intervention addresses diversity, and more broadly power. More so than the transformative and reflective deconstructions, diversity deconstructions focus on the cultural-societal meanings assigned to communications. While still attending to the spoken words of the clinical hour, this type of intervention considers the speaker's, and receiver's, respective positions of power while shedding light on hierarchies and on our inevitable embeddedness in language and cultural assumptions. An apt example details various group members' reactions to a male member calling his girlfriend "a dead fish" who he wants to "bring back to life." While amusing to the men in the group, this communication seemed crude and offensive to the women, bringing forth associations of being seen as an object to be consumed or manipulated, as well as the trope of the frigid woman.

As should be clear by now, all three types of deconstructive interventions pertain to the therapist as well as the patient or group member. Like others, the therapist's ideas are only true (with a capital T) until they are contained by other individuals (Bion, 1970). Once shared with the group, all ideas are inevitably altered and subject to deconstruction. And as Bion (1970) highlighted, the willingness to entertain and alter thoughts is itself conducive to mental health.

Chapter 18 in this section deals with the related concept of witnessing. Whether vocal or silent, each member of the group is at once *witnessing* others and being witnessed, and through this process expanding and layering their views of self and other. Billow's account of witnessing, and its unique significance for the group situation, was first developed in response to his invitation to present the annual Louis R. Ormont Lecture at the 2018 AGPA conference. Although he does not say this explicitly, and while admiring Ormont's showmanship and artful use of humor, Billow challenges the Modern Analytic emphasis on immediacy, the discharge of emotions, and the fast-paced use of "bridging." When witnessing and being witnessed, in the sense that Billow develops the concept, group members are "in the moment," while simultaneously turning attention elsewhere, associating to recent and distant memories, and images of the future.

Through this multifocal process members enhance their reflective capacities, tolerate speculative formulations and criticisms, and loosen the grip on some of their long-held beliefs. However, as Billow notes, due to trauma, some members initially require—or even demand—witnessing, without yet being able to be compassionate, sophisticated witnesses themselves. Time, patience, instruction, and beckoning (Karen, 2012), from peers or therapists, may help them grow into the role of witness, which in turn advances the group's truth-seeking, truth-bearing culture.

We end this volume with a chapter that describes a personal journey of Billow's and a topic ubiquitous to all groups—the need for attention and the maladaptive, self-defeating ways people go about getting it. As with many of the ideas presented in his writings, Billow's process begins with a desire to make meaning out of something curious and not sufficiently understood, most often related to behaviors and feelings aroused in the dyadic hour or group, and in him. In this instance, Billow observed how members could become dramatic, abrasive, insistent, and so forth, without getting their needs met. His initial formulation suggested that, while many of the group members suffered from what one member playfully labeled as "an attention deficit," they would rather disingenuously withdraw than have their efforts shunned. Only after the group concluded, and he was left dissatisfied, could he conjure a personal memory of his father's hurtful term directed at him as child, AGM (Attention-Getting Mechanisms), which captured something important about the group's process. He went on to amend his formulation, now believing that being shunned did not extinguish AGMs, but in fact exacerbated the urgency to be seen.

In remembering and reconsidering his childhood experiences of attention seeking and his unextinguished tendencies to repeat such behavior, Billow achieved a better understanding of himself and of the different group members' struggles that he shared. It was a reminder of just how difficult it is to unlearn maladaptive behavioral patterns and one's tendencies to repeat, regardless of the anticipated mistreatment. Nonetheless, as the group members reflected on their attention-seeking patterns, inside and outside the room, they were better able to describe and take ownership of their respective AGMs. Along with their therapist, they shared a commitment to do better.

Chapter 16

Doing our work

Words, deeds, and presence

Alas, groups do not happen and run on their own. We generate, structure, and monitor a group, and while every group is different, they all bear the imprint of our words, deeds, and presence.

Bion (1961, p. 143) asserted that "Every group however casual meets to 'do' something," and that well-functioning groups share a "common purpose." More precisely, individuals come together with different constructive purposes in mind, although they share many goals, such as wanting to feel better, get closer to people, resolve ambivalence and confusion, and solve problems. Our work is not only about such common purposes. It also involves a type of creative motive that has been described with many metaphors: "move the needle," "push the envelope," "break through," and "transform." *The work is done while we are also doing something else.*

The binocular vision

In Stephen Sondheim's (1984) musical *Sunday in the Park with George*, George Seurat describes the subjective duality of an artist's work: "However you live, there's a part of you always standing by, mapping out a sky."

While George participates in the manifest world before him, he also lives separately to "map out" his subjective experience. Like the artist then, the therapist utilizes "binocular vision" (Bion, 1961), which provides two different views of the same phenomena: one directed towards the group's process and the other towards the therapist's personal discovery.

Sondheim's George exclaims: "Look, I made a hat/Where there never was a hat." The work is not the act of applying brush and paint to canvas, or of making good interventions. George's palette has produced many hats. George utilizes his internal experience to emotionally visualize this new hat where there was not that hat before, although it may look like many other hats.

Just as two of George's brush strokes are never the same, and never identical to those of another painter, each clinical intervention is unique and ours alone. We find ourselves in a group situation that may look like many others, but we are in the midst of a creative endeavor, or could be, if we intend it so.

We start with the purpose(s) of why the group has come together and what the members seek. Common purpose comes first and drives the work. However, the work seeks to actualize the uncommon. We aim to take our groups to places that they have never been before. But we have to get there, too.

Executing the work: the performance art

George qualifies that "Having just a vision's no solution/Everything depends on execution." How do we best go about performing the work? It is not only what we say but who we are and how we say it that influences the group. In using ourselves, our words cannot be easily separated from our rhetorical deeds, and these from our very presence.

The tools of the work

Words

The group functions as a discourse community, under the direction of its leader. Words matter, and "put it into words" is the implicit and explicit operative. While appreciating the importance of play and nonverbal interactions, we try to place them within the system of language.

The putting-into-words process functions best when we are able to condense and refract meaning, promoting reflection rather than resolving discourse. However, to open things up emotionally and provide mental space, we also nail down discourse, especially to the group's here-and-now. We clarify, interpret, and even offer definitive answers, which can resolve unnecessary confusions, end fruitless debates, and provide room for fresh directions.

We want to make sure that others—and we ourselves—are listening and responding in a manner that is relevant and respectful to what is said, yet challenging too. Incongruities and discontinuities should be interesting and sufficiently agreeable to stimulate curiosity.

To practice what we preach, we speak publicly, not only in mind. Speech "communicates aspects of intrapsychic experience that can be made conscious only in action ... [we] locate aspects of ourselves, and hence of the patient, only after hearing ourselves speak" (Smith, 2000, p. 120).

Binocular vision requires verbal participation, which gives shape to our "unformulated thoughts" (Stern, 2009) and "thoughts unknown" (Bollas, 1989). Inevitably, we stimulate resistances, rebellions, and refusals (Billow, 2010b) and participate in their resolutions.

Deeds

The therapist draws from one's unique and characteristic modes of playing, speaking, listening, and gesturing. Communicative play begins at birth, as the parents vocally and gesturally greet their child. It remains within the relational repertoire of therapeutic discourse, and if it is not, it needs to be (Winnicott, 1971).

Through this array of rhetorical deeds, we generate a group culture attuned to verbal, paraverbal (e.g., tone, pitch, pacing, sighs, etc.), and facial and bodily expressions of meaning. The therapist's use of indirection, ambiguity, emphasis, humor, sarcasm, and irony calls attention to the nuances of self-presentation and self-other recognition—to the metapsychology of what is said and what could be meant.

Presence

Presence relates to LeBon's concept of prestige (in Freud, 1921, p. 81), which describes the emotional power of the group leader by virtue of "being," but also by function and reputation.[1] Individuals come to group—and stay—because of our importance. Our position increases in intensity, depth, and meaning—as in the course of any serious psychoanalytic therapy. And the group and its members come to mean more to us, too.

Arguably, more than words and deeds, presence speaks the loudest. Presence adds tenor—layers of impacted meaning—to what is said, as it is said, and not surprisingly how we are perceived and our work received. Individually and collectively, the group senses the therapist's presence, and the therapist senses being sensed. Our mood and expression fluctuate in interaction with the group's relational currents. Try as we might, we cannot control tropisms of attraction and repulsion. Our body speaks, as in smiling, nodding, and looking towards and away. The dilations of our pupils, the movement of our eyebrows, and the tone of our voice convey varied combinations of empathy and understanding, curiosity, perplexity, and challenge. Like other members, we tense in enduring mental pain and relax in prolonging mental pleasure.

Binocular vision is not "20/20." We do not see ourselves as do others. The therapist's "me"—a complex of feelings, thoughts, fantasies, and action tendencies, many of which remain out of self-awareness—affects how we relate to our groups and how they relate to us (Chapter 3).

I bring three related performative meanings to the term "presence": presence of mind, being present, and presentation of self.

PRESENCE OF MIND

The work rarely rolls out smoothly, nor should it. No matter how mindful, every choice exposes our own "conflictual network of associations" (Smith, 2000, p. 124). Presence of mind always involves tolerating anxiety and always involves compromise between opposing forces, conscious and unconscious, rational and irrational: pleasure and unpleasure (Freud, 1900), aggression and reparative love (Klein, 1952; Segal, 1957), and truth and falsity (Bion, 1965). These compromises lead us towards and away from understanding the member and the group situation, towards and away from the work.

BEING PRESENT

Presence does not mean being hyper vigilant or overly task focused. In maintaining binocularity, we listen actively, treating the group's discourse and behaviors as associations (no matter how seemingly mundane), while receptive to our wandering feelings, thoughts, and reveries. If we allow ourselves to be moved to action by the knowledge of what stirs us, we will more likely be directed to the work.

PRESENTATION OF SELF

Chapter 11 delineates four interrelated modes that describe the therapist interactionally and that supply conceptual references to our self-presentation: diplomacy, integrity, sincerity, and authenticity.

Further discussion: word, deed, and presence

The more work we do as leaders—the more we risk in feeling and idea—the more the group members do independently of us, and the more likely it is that the work will be a collaborative enterprise.

Whether sitting quietly or actively participating, turning inward to my own reveries, or coping with a difficult group interaction, and whether anything gets said or done, I am aware that I have work to do. I have work to do with each member, with the whole group and—separately and conjunctively—with myself.

I feel my way around this question: What work is being done, or should be, or is avoided? I monitor communications for their sincerity and emotional openness. I think about whether I can or need to do something to actualize growth potentials. At the same time (and when I have the wherewithal), I relax, let my mind wander, enjoy my curiosity, and follow the press of my emotions. Usually, that leads me to what I might do next. If I feel I have something to say that could add emotional depth and understanding, I do not mind interrupting or diverting from whatever else is going on. When I intervene, I attempt to affect the group-as-a-whole. But my target remains the mind of each individual.

I encourage attention to the psychological impact of each person on every other, and of group itself. During some intervals, the group leads and I follow. No matter, as long as each group meeting becomes a living event with a potential to change the psychology in the room. Something needs to happen; fresh experience needs to emerge that we witness in common and can respond to.

The psychic truths that emerge should become relevant to all of us, including me. The work happens to us: we evolve as a person as we do the work.

Clinical example: the work happens to us

In the midst of an impassioned exchange with John, Irma casually mentioned a "private" session in which John had been discussed. A third member of our long-standing group, Max, broke in and addressed me (agitated): "I have my doubts about you, Rich. You talk about your individual sessions with other patients." I waited, nonverbally encouraging him, or others, to say more about this possibility. Only Max continued, shifting the ostensible topic of grievance. "Your policy of charging for missed sessions. I wonder if you have different rates for different patients."

GROUP MEMBERS (PROTESTING): What if he did? Why does it bother you? Maybe it isn't all about the money—the way it is for you.

IRMA (TO ME): I feel so bad for getting you in trouble. (To Max) Rich didn't say anything. I just knew that he knew what I was saying about John and agreed.

BILLOW (REASSURING IRMA): I'm not in trouble. You don't have to explain.

Several members—including John—expressed confidence in my keeping confidentiality. Now a fourth member, Carl, burst out angrily to Max: "If you can't trust your therapist, you should go somewhere else. You need to own what you're doing, and not lay it on Rich."

MAX (UNPERTURBED, RETURNED TO ME): I know this is my issue too. I don't trust people, and my wife doesn't trust me, and for good reason. But when I asked you in individual about charging people different rates you said you wouldn't answer until the end of the session so that I could explore what I was feeling—I thought that was patronizing, but helpful.

I again received support: "What's wrong with what he said?" "Why is that patronizing?" "Rich can never win with you."

"Don't listen to them," I advised Max, with a conspiratorial smile. "They are a bunch of puppies. 'Yip yip yip.'"

MAX (ONLY SLIGHTLY AMUSED): They protect you, all the time. And you don't need protection.

BILLOW: Maybe they love me.

MAX (SOFTENING): They do ... I loved my last therapist.

BILLOW: Could you love me?

MAX: It's a distinct possibility. But I wouldn't trust you. This is all from my mother, I know that. She said not to trust anybody.

BILLOW: But you trusted her to take her advice, and you trust me enough to say you don't trust me.

MAX: Yeah, she would have killed me if I challenged her.

BILLOW: Well, you did it pretty good. No pot shots—you seemed to be careful not to purposely hurt me.

Max blushed, and when the group pursued what he was feeling, he smiled sheepishly and brushed aside their efforts.

"A small step for humanity, but a giant leap for Max," I offered. The group laughed.

Max flashed me an appreciative smile: "Thank you, you got me off the hook," A faint flush reappeared before he turned away.

The group had expressed anger about how Max spoke to me and criticized my work, and they needed to review. "It must have been difficult when your integrity is challenged." "I would have felt humiliated." "I would have told him to go fuck himself." "I still feel guilty when accused, even if I know I didn't do anything wrong. And then I get pissed." "I can feel guilty when anyone is accused! I am a bad person and must be responsible. I usually don't say anything."

I responded: "At one time, for sure. All of what you are describing. Now I think about why someone would want to put me down—maybe I did something too. No one likes paying for missed sessions. [to Max] You took a chance with all of us, not only with me."

Discussion

Max was the ostensible target of intervention: His "blush" was Seurat's "hat." But I made another "hat" too. At one time, I might not have encouraged Max to continue. Under the guise of clinical tactic and "correct" technique, I might have "analyzed" him, directing energy away from his attack, and from my anxiety about being exposed. I might have called attention to Max's characteristic arrogance, likely with a slight, contemptuous flare of my nostrils. I was close enough to the "old me" to monitor myself for any disapproving taint—any whiff of counter arrogance. I recognized with relief that I had not succumbed to the talion principle, the eye-for-an-eye cycle of aggression–counter aggression.

Oscar Wilde described his work: "A writer is someone who has taught his mind to misbehave." I had to protect group process from my protectors, Irma, John, perhaps the whole group, and moralizers, such as Carl, who instructed Max to "own" his behavior. In actuality, in modifying his more typical unreflective antagonism in our exchange, Max had begun to do just that.

My ironic humor supported Max's claim—which he himself only partially believed—that his compliant group cohorts, "a bunch of puppies," like their leader, could not be trusted. "Dog words" ("yip yip yip") signaled the group to consider that they were being anxious for me, and that they could calm down. As Max said, I did not need safeguarding. I could trust myself to keep one eye on his aggression and the other eye on mine.

The work, while interior, is also intersubjective, stimulated by and responsive to group experience. Leading a group with less secure positive alliances, I would have been in a different frame of mind: cautious with irony and metaphor, and distant from thoughts or assertions of "love." I might not have made any hats, done the work, or done it as effectively. The supportive members lessened any vestigial need for self-protection. I could run interference for Max, blocking and countering the group's attempts to shut him down.

Notice that the weight of my construction, while using language, was carried mostly by rhetorical deed—humor, expressive discourse ("yip yip yip"), and blatant irony ("don't listen to them, they are a bunch of puppies")—and by an unthreatened and hospitable therapeutic presence that encouraged Max's creative co-participation.

Clinical example: benefitting from the authority of the group

Helen, a spirited, older woman, joined our group of eight members and quickly became a center of interest. After a while, we became aware that it was difficult to engage Helen to reveal herself. My quizzical smile or puzzlement over her elusive responses could be greeted with: "Don't be so impatient with me." If I tried to slow her down to clarify or elaborate: "Ok, you want to hold me to the fire."

She volunteered the basics: early loss of her mother; raised by a distant father and older sister. "But what has gone on since?" members inquired. "Should I bring in my resume?" she retorted. When questioned further, she would ask: "What are you getting at?" Not wanting to be unduly pressuring, members learned to be careful and not pursue. But one member, Joe, would not quit easily and took delight in engaging her. A dapper dresser, his compliments on Helen's stylish wardrobe led to a lively weekly repartée that all of us seemed to enjoy.

After one of these exchanges, Suzie, also new and our youngest member, said with amusement: "Maybe I'm wrong, but I think all the men have a crush on Helen!"

When no one picked up the theme directly, Joe continued. He ruefully compared Marci, his live-in companion, to Helen "She insists on dressing like a slut and sometimes I'm embarrassed to go out with her. But she doesn't want to go out anyway. She feels I 'abandon' her if I am not glued to her side. She gets crazy and has a fit, even throws things. [to Helen] You would dress great!"

I had assumed that Helen would be flattered by Joe's attention. Still, I asked.

HELEN: Joe likes me, I think. But when he says these things, he throws me off center.

"He's flirting with you," I said, echoing Suzie's insight: "Joe wants to bring you more into the group, not always in the best way, but who else has succeeded?"

JOE: I bring dead fish to life.

When Helen winced, Joe said he was not talking about her: "You're an alive one! And I don't mean fish."

Helen shook her head: "Are you sure you aren't trying to get at me? It feels sadistic."

There seemed to be little to be gained from explaining or reengaging the pair, and members moved on. After several weeks, Suzie returned to the theme of Helen and the group's relationship to her, now with a different emphasis: "I was thinking about you, Joe. If you treat Marci the way you treat Helen, I could see why she goes crazy and throws things. You probably go over the line with her."

HELEN: Thank you [Suzie].

She addressed me critically: "I know you can't pick up everything, but you really missed that Joe can be sadistic."

Several of the men buttressed Joe, who reassured Helen of affectionate feelings. But another woman, Joan, supported Suzie. "Joe doesn't do it to the men, or to the other women. I wouldn't let my husband beat me down, although he still tries sometimes."

SUZIE: I don't think Joe wants to hurt Helen, he is always looking after her. My ex-husband just ignored me. I realize now [since joining group], he was always very "nice."

JAMES (TO HELEN): I admire Joe for taking a chance. I am always careful of how I speak to you.

HELEN: Why?

JAMES: You seem so easily offended.

HELEN: You are very kind.

BILLOW (RHETORICALLY): Is there anyone here who is not kind to you, even Joe?

HELEN: Joe throws me off my game. I feel beaten down.

Feeling some risk, I pursued, referencing Suzie's description of marital neglect: "Would you rather be treated 'nice'?"

"Yes, I want to hide! Group is very difficult for me, scary. Ok, I am paranoid."

I brushed aside Helen's unconvincing self-diagnosis: "Well then, you are brave to stick it out with us!" I assumed that Helen, or others, would catch the word play of double meaning: Helen was brave by "sticking out"—staying and also calling attention and engaging us. She seemed to enjoy being part of the group, despite her denial.

However, the group went in another direction, acceding to Helen's demand to be treated "nice"—taken at her word, rather than mine. A sympathetic chorus attested to the plight of new members: "It took me a year to open up"; "Me, more than that to figure out how group works"; "You should have seen me at the beginning, I thought I would be drummed out." Like James, everyone was being "kind."

That ended the work with Helen for that session. My words were un-heeded, and my rhetorical deeds unappreciated. Because of my symbolic importance as a combined parental figure of mistreatment and neglect, my very presence made me not nice and unkind. Deprived of my repertoire of therapeutic tools, I too felt thrown off my game, beaten down. There seemed no way for me to right myself with Helen.

Discussion

The French essayist, Montaigne (1685/1958, p. 499), described the dual fo-cus of his artistic process: "I turn my gaze inward I fix it there and keep it busy … I continually observe myself, I take stock of myself, I taste myself." Still, his capacity for "sifting truth, whatever it may amount to" was "estab-lished and fortified … with the authority of others."

The group was one source of authority, offering opinions that "fortified" my own, even when at the same time validly challenging or differing from them. Suzie first called attention to the male "gaze" (Simons, 1992). "All the men have a crush on Helen!" And at a later session, she gave voice to the female "gaze": Women could experience Joe as going "over the line" and making them go "crazy." "Joe doesn't do it to the men, or to the other women," Joan reiterated.

Further discussion: the work

"Don't be so impatient with me," Helen had protested, with justification. For even when I did not speak, my inventory of rhetorical deeds betrayed myself. My facial expressions and body movements conveyed more than therapeutic curiosity, but therapeutic ambition, and what lay behind it.

Evading the male "crush," which at the same time she stimulated, Helen served as the unavailable female: mythic, transferential, and actual. "All that I seeke is to eternise you," the male poet universally laments (Drayton, 1594/1896, p. 56).

In wanting "to bring dead fish to life"—a combined reference to his de-pressed mother, girlfriend, and Helen—Joe, arguably, spoke for all men in all groups.[2] "Now call her goddess, then I call her thief … Now do I curse her, then again bless her … Some men by which like my method well" (Drayton, 1594/1896, p. 50).

Certainly, Joe spoke for me. Helen stuck out as an "exception," which Freud (1916, p. 312) defined as an individual unresponsive to the therapist's insights, "one of the components of love." She deadened my efforts to love and to be loved—in the manner that I desire and expect, no matter how un-realistic. So I too was an exception, feeling entitled to reparation for any felt deprivation in female love and attention (Chapter 15).

Therapist and members operate as material presences and as complex "relational images" (Migliorati, 1989, p. 198). The roles we play and those we assign to others obscure binocular vision. To do the work, we must find our way out of hall-of-mirrors narratives. I could not rush Helen out of her complex of relational images, and I had to expand my own. Male and female relational images had provided a synergism of starkly different but complementary perspectives. With this realization, I was able to revisit the situation and offer an integration:

> What Suzie said related to Joe's work, and what I said related to yours, Helen. If you (Helen) could believe that people like you—you would not be so quickly off balance. And if you, Joe, could recognize that your humorous "thrusts" are not always "kind," or taken that way, I don't think Helen—or Marci —would be thrown off balance.

When we are able to access it, binocular vision allows us to "re-view" (Bion, 1961) the group situation and rebalance the work.

Clinical example: from common purpose to the work

Maxine's tortured monologue opened our session:

> I just got off the phone with my mother. I can't take it. "Ma, I have to go. Is there anything you need now?" "No, there is nothing anyone can do." This is what she does, she pulls me in and then makes me feel useless.

I intervened to address both Maxine and the group: "Maxine is describing how controlled she feels, really, out of control."

"Yes, it feels awful," Maxine continued, until Ben broke in impatiently, "I want you to relate to us. You need to use your own executive function to take charge with her and with yourself."

Several members protested: "We let you talk—no matter how long you take." "Maxine is hurting."

I supported both Maxine and Ben: "Maxine is 'channeling' her mother, Ben is letting us know how it feels to be under her spell."

Maxine nodded, taking my remarks as encouragement. Ben leaned forward, and we sensed that he was preparing to pounce.

"Are you going to create a commotion here and call attention to you?" Elliot challenged Ben. "You're not going to like this either, but I have my own story to tell." Maxine invited Elliot to continue. "My ex-wife feels like my mother. Both whacked the hell out of me, one physically, the other emotionally."

Elliot's voice grew louder and intense:

> I can't get her to sign divorce papers. She looks dreadful, hoarse and bloated. "Elliot, could you help me a little now. I haven't been able to work in a few weeks." I felt terrible. Of course I would help her, but I took it to another place, questioning my decision, deciding that I had been unfair and would chuck the whole divorce. I had to realize that this is just how I felt as a little boy. My mother could abuse me, whack the hell out of me, but if she was upset, I felt I had to totally abandon whatever I was doing and take care of her.

Members seemed sympathetic, and when one member, Susan, shook her head with a dramatic sense of alarm, I assumed she was too.

SUSAN: I feel 'whacked' by you, Elliot, your anger seems so violent.
ELLIOT: Can't I express myself here without being accused and guilt-tripped?

Susan retreated, with a wounded expression. While directed at Elliot, I thought to myself that Susan's guilt-inducing posture was itself a whack, an effective punishment for all of us for not protecting her from Elliot's freedom of expression.

Another member, Michael:

> I never understood how my parents wouldn't listen to anything I had to say until "this guy" (turning to me) made me realize it. My father would put me down: "You became a lawyer? How did you do that." (In the same sarcastic tone) Thanks a lot, Rich!

Michael's humor had the effect of consolidating a group theme: How could parents be so oblivious, even cruel? The group process had common purpose, but I doubted that it represented the members' share of the work.

Discussion: the work

As I had listened to the familiar narratives of parental mistreatment, disconcerting snapshots appeared in my mind's eye, superimposed over the group's elaborations and mutual support. Memories of how and when I replicated the worst of my parents—and not their best—colonized my mental space (see also Chapter 13 on psychic nodules). The group members were caring individuals. Each had been a better parent than I, or so I imagined. I suffered what seemed an endless interval until a relieving realization: My visualizations refracted *any* parent's history—not only mine. I addressed the group:

"As distressing as it is to recollect how we could be treated by our parents, it feels worse to realize that we act like them sometimes. Even here," I underscored.

No one spoke up. I wondered if the members now experienced me as a critical parent—theirs, my own, or a past "therapist me." But there was no turning back, retreating to an inauthentic neutral presence. I chose my words and delivery with care not to be unduly accusatory.

"Let's look at what just happened with Michael. Even though you were teasing, you put me down with the same sarcastic delivery your father used with you."

"Well I know I don't do that to the children," Michael protested. "Maybe to my wife, sometimes. But not like my father—a real Archie Bunker." (A reference to television's *All in the Family*.)

I went on to review other interactions, first addressing Maxine: "Ben yearned for you to relate to him, the way you yearn for your mother to relate to you." I paraphrased her words: "He didn't want to be 'pulled in and useless.'"

MAXINE: I want to. I hate feeling like a victim. I lived that way too much of the time—even in my marriage, useless to do anything about what was happening to me. That's how my mother behaved in hers.

"And you, Ben, all set to start a 'commotion,' anything not to be pulled in by your mother." At earlier stages of group work, any maternal reference would enrage Ben, but he smiled in recognition.

Elliot joined Ben:

I have a "commotion-mama." Never thought I was one too. (And in a friendly tone, to Susan) I started a commotion; I've been told I've done it here before. But really, Susan, you can be so melodramatic. It really gets me confused and feeling guilty when you say that I whacked you.

Further discussion and conclusion

The balladeer Leonard Cohen (1992) counseled: "Forget your perfect offering/There is a crack in everything/That's how the light gets in." No therapist makes a perfect offering. We are creators of cracks, whacks, and commotions, and are not merely subjected to them by others. Members of this group had been self-pitying, impatient, dismissive, short-tempered, melodramatic, accusative, and guilt-inducing—imperfect dimensions of "me." To do the work, I had to make sure I did not whack the group—both for denying their culpability and for painfully rousing my own.

Ray Bradbury (1992, p. xv) captures something of our creative process: "Every morning I jump out of bed and step on a landmine. The landmine is me. After the explosion, I spend the rest of the day putting the pieces together."

We "jump" into the clinical experience, and however familiar, we are greeted with landmines—emotional irruptions of the unwanted or unexpected. Some of them arise from without, but some must arise from within. We suffer smoke and pain of personal recognition, and hopefully reach interpersonal and technical coherence. The work entails observing what is in front of us: the exchanges that are publicized in group discourse. At the same time, we also concentrate and self-reflect, and enter into it too. Maintaining binocular vision, we gaze inward, tolerating the "cracks" that appear in our own mind while attending to the therapeutic situation. Our distress throws light on that which is not being adequately felt, thought, and talked. We cannot truly reach others without also doing this kind of work with ourselves.

Notes

1 In my first supervisory session, Bion frankly acknowledged: "It helps to be famous."
2 In poetry in general (particularly but not only in the Western tradition), the male serves as lover and subject, and the female as the desired and often reviled "other," defined by phallocentric ideology and imagery (Hullah, 2016).

Chapter 17

Deconstructive interventions

When we say "stay in the room," redirect attention to a disregarded or unnoticed interaction, play with words and metaphors, or even raise a quizzical eyebrow, we are making a deconstructive intervention. In this chapter I will distinguish among three types of deconstructive interventions, all aimed at expanding meaning and therapeutic growth.

Transformative deconstructions refer to how individuals—singly or collectively—set out to dismantle one set of conventions to supplement or supplant with another to create new meaning. *Reflective deconstructions* aim to enlarge the range of thinking by mining for and analyzing alternative meanings behind conventions, which may involve words, conceptions, and interactions. *Diversity deconstructions* direct attention to social and political meanings— and consequences—of specific narratives, based on power relations and point of view, such as gender, sexual orientation, age, race, or ethnicity.

Why deconstruct?

In order to preserve a well-working group, or attend to the difficulties of an ineffective one, the therapist wears two faces: being constructive and deconstructive (Billow, 2005). While serving an important function as a normalizing communicative matrix (Foulkes & Anthony, 1964), groups breed like-thinking and conformist perceptions and behavior (Bion, 1970; Freud, 1921). To aid the group to reconsider the familiar, to expand categories of thinking and being, and to give voice to the disempowered, we disturb the very status quo that we work to establish. We contest characterological boundaries, falsities, social prejudices, and collusions that obstruct or preclude emotional learning and growth.

To deconstruct the other(s), we must make efforts to deconstruct our self, too. We need to counter tendencies towards a facile leadership style— relying on theory and technique to avoid tolerating doubt and confusion. Therapeutic relationships foster ritualization, in which we foist on ourselves or accept a too-comfortable persona as the "expert," "container," or "one who knows." It is the never-ending process of deconstructing ritualized roles that establishes the conditions for authenticity: for self/other awareness and for mutual growth (see also Hoffman, 1992).

We self-deconstruct when we tolerate seeing, hearing, feeling, and thinking of ourselves from the perspective of others—each of our group members represents a source of difference. We have our experience of the group and its members, and they have theirs. If we listen to each other's perspectives, every group meeting both deconstructs and increases understanding and mutual involvement.

Freud: our premier deconstructionist

While brought to the vernacular by the writings of Jaques Derrida (2005), deconstructionism existed before Deconstructionism. Parents are one's first deconstructionists, as they introduce novelty and surprise, and gently tease and defy cognitive expectations. Parent–child interplay is *transformative*, aiding the development of a new platform of "basic trust" (Erikson, 1950/1993); is *reflective*, expanding the infant's range of thinking and potential meaning; and respects *diversity* by empowering the infant's perspective.

Along with other great late 19th- and 20th-century thinkers, Freud is a prominent forerunner of deconstruction: "I was one of those who have 'disturbed the sleep of the world'" (Freud, 1914, p. 21). We are following Freud when we "stir up contradiction" (p. 8), imputing alternative or diverse motivation and meaning to clinical discourse and enactment.

Psychoanalytically oriented theory and practice may be conceived as a series of deconstructions of Freud's work. Many of his ideas, diagnostic formulations, and methods have been modified (such as drive or instinct theory, frequency of sessions, and use of the couch), rejected (the "death instinct"), supplemented (child analysis and group treatment), or reformulated with different emphasis (e.g., ego psychology, object relations, interpersonal or self-theory).

Nonetheless, despite proclamations and revisions, many of Freud's ideas, principles, and procedures remain intact and recognizable. Examples include the primacy of unconscious influence, the study of the therapeutic participants' interactional patterns (transference-countertransference), the relevance of the past and sociocultural influence, and the reliance on verbal communication and exploration.

I turn now to three types of deconstructive interventions.

Transformative deconstructions

Transformative deconstructions privilege one form of thought, feeling, or behavior over others, redefining or prioritizing what is real, true, or most meaningful. The therapist offers what he or she believes to be a healthier, deeper, fresher, or more unified perspective. By disrupting, challenging, and interpreting an individual's (or a group's) repetitive, internal dramas—and the accompanying defenses and enactments—people come to experience themselves as beings capable of change. Something new or the possibility of something new is created in clinical situation.

Clinical anecdote: deconstructing character and group defenses

Mark reported missing the last session because he had ear trouble. "It's related to TMJ—jaw locking. I get it when I feel anxiety that something bad is going to happen and it is my fault. I'm trying to become aware when I feel that way, before I start clenching."

ANNA: Listening to your pain makes me want to reach out and give you a hug and say, are you okay?

MARK: I try to focus on where my bad feelings are coming from—why do I feel this way about myself?—and sometimes that helps me relax my jaw.

ANOTHER MEMBER: When I get self-critical, my back tenses.

Several others pick up the theme of being self-critical and engage in parallel processes of self-analysis.

At one point, I interrupt the process (addressing Mark): "You seemed to have difficulty relaxing into Anna's hug. [Ironically to the group] No one seems very relaxed right now."

MEMBERS: You moved away from Anna and got intellectual. And then we all did.

ANNA: I'm a hugger, but I thought maybe Mark isn't, and that I went too far. I became self-critical about what I said.

DISCUSSION

I repeated forms of the word "relax" to implicate what was not happening, but should. Mark's preoccupations and obsessive defenses had spread to the whole group. I asserted a truth claim, deconstructing one mode of thinking and acting, and encouraging what I defined as a more enlightened and disinhibited mode for both Mark and the group.

Clinical anecdote: asserting a truth claim to influence behavior

MOIRA: I'm upset. My daughter accused me of not being a generous mother. I wanted to be reimbursed for a $35 purchase I made for her. She always manages to forget to repay me and I resent it, and my daughter resented having to go upstairs to write a check. She said: "I'm generous to you, I put you and dad up for three weeks after Hurricane Sandy." I didn't think it was generous. It is what you do. I would have done it for her and her family. In fact, we have, and I told her so.

I intercepted Moira's dispatch of her motherly and grandmotherly good deeds: "It is not just what you think and what you do, it is learning about what the other person thinks."

MOIRA: Yes, but she is wrong. I had to defend myself.

JOHN: That went well…

Ignoring John's sarcasm, Moira launched another round of self-justification; I interrupted (with affectionate sarcasm): "You're being generous with your opinions!"

Moira (to me, challenging yet softening): "Well, you're not [being generous]!"

Group members (referring to group behavior) joined in, supporting us both: "When it isn't about you, Moira, you are incredibly generous." "Very helpful and right on."

With mild refusal, Moira surrendered to the consensus: "I'll think about it, but I still resent how she [my daughter] treats me."

DISCUSSION

The repetition of "generous" was not to contrast alternative meanings (as with reflective deconstructions, see below) but to make a truth claim. My goal was to influence and enlighten the member's thinking and influence a change in her behavior, and to free the group from the grip of a "monopolizer" (Yalom, 1995, pp. 369–375).

Shakespeare's *Julius Caesar* provides a dramatic example of the power of sarcastic irony, implication, and word repetition in making a transformative deconstruction. Mark Anthony's "Brutus is an honourable man" deconstructed a truth claim ("honourable") by contrasting it with an unstated antonym ("dishonourable"). Transformative deconstructive rhetoric swayed the group of Roman senators and citizens to take a new path, switching allegiances and inciting war.

What happens to the group member's words when the therapist deconstructs them to foster transformation? Repeating the group or a member's words with an ironic tone, or a different emphasis, does not necessarily take away the original meaning. Rather, it grafts an alternative or expanded communication, often with the implication that it is preferable.

In both clinical examples, the combination of communicative devices—repetition, emphasis, humor, and irony—pushed the member and group towards something new, from what was not happening, but could and should happen.

Reflective deconstructions

Reflective deconstructions highlight and unearth alternative perspectives and meanings behind words, conceptions, and interactions. Unlike transformative deconstructions, reflective deconstructions intend to communicate that there is no one truth, or a superior truth, only perspectival truth, and hence, multiple truths, multiple psychic realities.

Clinical anecdote: a stating and negating intervention

In the midst of a discussion on various attitudes towards work, a member asked me why I decided to become a group therapist. Taken aback, I answered quickly: "I like people." And then, a moment later, I added: "Or, I used to." The group laughed, and our focus returned to other members.

DISCUSSION

My purpose was not to insult the group but to counter what I feared was a misleading communication, fostering idealization. To say "I like people" belied the complexity and ambiguity of my relationships and, by extension, of all our relationships in group and outside of group. I wished to unsettle any assumptions that I was different from other people—unambivalent and pure of heart.

Reflective deconstructions often challenge or undermine their truth claims at the same time they are making them. In Magritte's famous painting, a simple picture of a pipe is accompanied by the elegant script: "This is not a pipe." The painting pictorially asserts meaning while verbally negating it—a painting of a pipe is not a pipe. The artwork deconstructs the notion of a single truth claim, making us reflect upon context and perspective.

In my clinical example, adding the clause "or, I used to" fostered reflection of the whole communication—it contained its own negation. It was not meant to be a purely declarative statement—"I used to like people, but now I don't"—nor was it taken that way. If the members of this long-standing group and I had not built a mutually affectionate and trusting relationship, such a remark could have been misinterpreted, and hurtful.

Clinical anecdote: challenging a truth claim

In a demonstration group run by the invited presenter Jerry Gans (2016), one member said to another, somewhat flippantly: "I wish you would just shut up now." Gans nonchalantly asked: "Shut up now, or do you mean forever?"

DISCUSSION

I understood Gans's metacommunication as undermining the casualness of the speaker's delivery, suggesting that likely the speaker—and the intellectualized demonstration group—was hiding a more intense array of "true" feelings, including frustration and anger.

Gans's "either/or" phrasing was rhetorical; the implication of "now" and "forever" invited reflection on something likely wished for and not: the irritating member's presence and absence in the social reality of the group and in the psychic space of the speaker's mind.

Clinical anecdote: questioning truth claims

Betina, approaching 40, explained her unhappy single status as not yet having found "the right one." When members quizzed her on what she meant by the term, she teared up. "I feel you are blaming me." The group had attempted to examine her assumptions, words, and actions, but she had shut them down. So I continued:

BILLOW: What is so bad about accepting blame?
BETINA: It makes me feel like a bad person.
BILLOW: Well, how bad are you?
BETINA: It hurts to be criticized.
BILLOW: You don't want helpful criticism either?
BETINA: Just praise (with a self-aware smile).

DISCUSSION

So often, our interventions may be challenged as not being the "right ones," but who's to judge? The member's conscious or unconscious? The group itself? You? Me? I felt I had a choice: leaving the individual in her own solipsistic world, or deconstructing it. A number of words and terms were reexamined in this interaction and left open for further reflection—the truth values uncertain: "right one," "blame," "bad person," "bad," and "criticism."

Clinical anecdote: deconstructing the role of leader

In a recent American Group Psychotherapy Association (AGPA) Open Session, the demonstration group got off to a slow start. At one point, a woman turned for help to Earl Hopper, the leader, referring to him as the "group facilitator." Hopper retorted: "I am a group analyst, not a group facilitator."

Hopper's remark, or perhaps also his mode of delivery, seemed at first to have confused or intimidated the members, who spent some time debating possible meanings before turning attention to the speaker himself. The longer lasting effect of the communication, while difficult to ascertain, seemed positive, for the group pulled together and many of the participants—the men particularly—enjoyed testing and, finally, movingly connecting to its leader.

DISCUSSION

Part of the value of indirection, negation, metaphor, and other implicative acts is to draw attention to the multiple and ambiguous meanings of words and their relationships to each other. Hopper's definitive "I am a group analyst" called attention to the indeterminate nature of the leader and the group's relationship to him or her.

Anything that has meaning gets its meaning from the context of other words related to it—similarity or difference. Hopper's group now had two terms to think about and make denotative and connotative links. What do the words mean when they are juxtaposed? How do they illustrate the varying truth values and expectations of this group in formation?

I saw Hopper's intervention as potentially transformative as well as reflective, an effort to deconstruct the collusion around concrete thinking and to move the group to the psychic and social unknowns involved in analytic thinking and feeling. The term "facilitator" has become jargon, and Hopper's intervention had the potential to counter the clichéd argot that often accompanies demonstration groups and move the group to something new.

The members first banded together and refused, pressuring Hopper to facilitate their version of group process. A useful tension evolved as Hopper held onto his constructive-deconstructive principles, such that Open Session became a learning event for the observers as well as the participants. Hopper made us reflect on ourselves. Do we as leaders want to facilitate—and make things easier?—or do we want also to analyze, which may seem to make things more difficult for all of us?

Diversity deconstructions

Spurred by the writing of Jacques Derrida (2005), deconstructive theory (and related postmodern movements) emphasized that it is impossible to approach material naively, but always through preexisting lenses, such as cultural, ethnic, racial, gender, or sexual orientation. Derrida stressed the sociopolitical nature and consequence of meaning. He asserted that the dominant discourses of a society contain implicit hierarchies by which an order is imposed on reality and which suppress, exclude, or subordinate other potential meanings.

Diversity deconstructions assist individuals in discovering and asserting their individuality and authenticity, while bringing to awareness their cultural and historical embeddedness and its intersubjective effects. One of their goals is to better understand where we each stand in the pecking order of privilege with regard to power, status, and influence.

Clinical anecdote: cultural diversity

Taking seats for debriefing—it was the last half hour of a two-day workshop at a Southern regional group conference—a participant complained that there was no seat for him within the large, two-ringed circle. Someone had taken his seat, or his seat had been removed along with the seats of those who left. Finding no satisfaction in the group's response, he began to interrupt the proceedings with provocative comments: "How come no one owns [taking my seat away]?" "Does no one notice or care—why not a provision for me?"

After a few minutes, one of the seasoned professionals said: "You know, I can't say this to patients, although I wish I could. But I can to you: 'Get over it!'"

I heard the remark as sardonically amusing, and I assumed that there would be sufficient good cheer between the spoken to and the speaker to end the issue. But the remark offended the listener and, more surprisingly yet, turned the whole group against the speaker, who was morally condemned. I began to formulate some hypotheses as to what might be emerging symbolically in lieu of an orderly debriefing. Was the complaining member the mouthpiece for the dissatisfied and insufficiently nurtured? I registered my confusion.

A woman explained: "This is not how we talk to people in the Deep South. We don't insult people to their face… we smile at you, and you don't realize it until later that you've been stabbed in the back."

DISCUSSION

Members of a different subculture had heard the same words differently, driving different clinical sensibilities. To my Northern ears, "get over it" was music; to my Southern colleagues, the phrase was noxious and discordant.

Educated by my introduction to cultural diversity, I closed the conference with reference to the "insult" of termination, given that we are "unseated" from fantasies of—and desires for—uninterrupted connectedness. I thanked the group for how much I learned from the workshop, to its very last minutes.

Clinical anecdote: challenging diversity claims

In the midst of a demonstration group, Marty, an African American woman sitting next to me, broke in. She said that she felt "invisible" and that the other black people were the only ones who made eye contact with her. Marty acknowledged that she tended to focus on race and was the one to bring it to attention at meetings. She always checked out who was black or might be black. Several Caucasian members protested that they were not racist; they felt connected to Marty and looked at her as much as at anyone else. But Marty insisted, extending her contention to our sponsoring organization and clinical settings in general.

Marty drew only modest interest and emotional support from the other black members. The youngest in our group qualified: "It is important for me to be identified as a woman of color." From the mix of domestic and foreign accents, it was not clear who identified as African American. No one seemed to want to be conscripted into Marty's subgroup, as she defined it.

I turned to Marty as if having a private conversation, complimenting her for bringing forth issues of race, but suggesting that we let other people get a chance to express themselves and see where the group goes. I explained that, as the leader, I wanted to keep our new group from breaking down into black and white. If we had time, racial issues would assert themselves, but in a more personal, group-related context. Not entirely satisfied, Marty reengaged with the group and carried on.

DISCUSSION

In a new group particularly, all members (including the leader) are faced with Marty's problem of "invisibility" and must deal with the desire for recognition. Some people turn attention to themselves. In referencing race, Marty took the opportunity to define and test her ideas of relationships, to both the leader and the group at large, by mounting a protest and invoking a race polemic. In my enactive tête-a-tête, I supported and demonstrated what I took as her legitimate "selfobject" (Kohut, 1976) needs for connectivity without submitting to her potentially explosive agenda of racism.

Sometimes, the leader harmonizes by supporting the members' efforts at being experienced in their own terms. But the leader must also be willing to decenter members from their customary and often stereotypic self-presentations and perceptions of others (see Agazarian, 2012, on stereotypical vs. functional subgroups). Social signs and signifiers may encourage or prolong stereotyping, narrowing the range of potential emotional experience and the likelihood of a vital group.

Diversity deconstructions: further considerations

Gender, ethnic, religious, sexual orientation, or racial references, expressed via interaction, slang, irony, or even pejorative language, may be utilized effectively as a rhetoric tool to call attention to difference and perspective, and to break down defensive boundaries and prejudices. Or, they may be hurtful and counterproductive. In an example from Chapter 16, a member's use of the phrase "I bring dead fish to life," while an amusing metaphor to some (the men), confirmed the women's view of the speaker's derisive sexism.

Clinical anecdote: deconstruction gone astray

In a recent AGPA Open Session, a naïve use of the racial term "brothers" by the white demonstration group leader in reference to two African American employees who had set up audio feeds inadvertently created uproar. In calling attention to the role of technicians, the leader had intended to deconstruct concrete notions regarding group boundaries, beginnings, cultural influence, and membership.

However, many of the group participants and audience members could hear only a racial slur. A subgroup of the attendees walked out of the debriefing session, some of them proclaiming that the demonstration group should have been suspended. The incident reverberated throughout the whole conference and afterward—despite the speaker's multiple apologies, reiterations of intention from a theoretical and personal point of view, and participation in the subsequent Large Group sessions.

DISCUSSION

The French post-structuralist semiotician Roland Barthes (1967, p. 2) famously declared that the key to a text is not to be found in its origin but in its destination: "The birth of the reader must be at the cost of the death of the Author." Communications do not have invariant meanings, but depend on the cultural complex and state of mind of the listeners as much as (or more than, according to Barthes) the mind of the speaker.

The phrase, "two brothers," resounded in a particularly sensitive relational space. The AGPA Conference occurred a few months after the presidential election of Donald Trump. Many of the attendees were dispirited, even traumatized by the unexpected turn in political life and its ongoing divisive effects. It is possible that the incident—while regrettable—became a vehicle for expression of the hurt, anger, and despair towards that which was occurring in the larger group, the United States.

Conclusion

Derrida (2005) insisted that deconstruction was part of a living dialogue rather than a superimposed method. Yet one wonders whether deconstruction is possible without a coherent perspective—a notion of what we are deconstructing and an awareness of our therapeutic motives. When applied to the treatment situation, deconstruction implies a sensibility, value, and therapeutic action orientation.

The clinical anecdotes have illustrated how the group leader's use of or receptivity to certain words and phrases may further or interfere with leadership goals. To review: "relax," "generous," "used to like," "shut up now or forever," "right one," "blame," "bad," "dead fish," "facilitator," "group analyst," "get over it," "black," and "brothers" all served deconstructive purposes, but not all successfully or in the same way for all participants. Things fall apart in making deconstructive interventions, and we risk that they may not come together again.

Sometimes deconstruction leaves unmoored that which needs to be anchored or asserted as a pragmatic constant. In a new group, particularly, the participants may not understand the intentions of deconstructive interventions. Group process stalls, or wanders away from feeling, and the members may engage in an intellectualized debate about words. In any group, our discourse goals must be perceived as caring and helpful. We want to deconstruct certain thoughts, without attacking the thinker or the group itself, to call attention to and stimulate deeper connections—mental and interpersonal.

We heed this caveat attributed to T. S. Eliot: "It's not wise to violate the rules until you know how to observe them." Truth may be questioned, of course, but not all truths abrogated, such as standards of conduct (e.g., regarding physical contact, violence to person or property), payment of fees, time boundaries, and respect for the therapist's (and other members') privacy.

Yet, to function with integrity, we heed this point of view, so well described by Bob Dylan: "To live outside the law, you must be honest." When they work, deconstructive interventions break apart static patterns of thinking and relating, providing space for unconscious, irrational, or suppressed levels of experience. A "truer" and richer mode of being emerges—less conventionally "lawful," with greater access to fantasy, feelings, and creative thought.

Deconstructive interventions may disturb us therapists as well as our groups. When our empathic immersion in an individual or group's point of view is disrupted, we risk being experienced as unsupportive or uncaring. In my opinion, deconstructive interventions work best when they present ourselves as empathic thinkers: confident hypothesizers rather than as assured "knowers."

Group psychotherapy by its very nature is deconstructive—arguably more powerfully so than dyadic therapy—if the leader fosters a democratic process in which all voices are respected and, rather than reaches for closure or consensus, celebrates diversity. The therapist is not the sole designer or arbiter of deconstruction, of course, and we cannot be sure whose voice— the therapist's or the members'—resonates most deeply and when.

A danger of any movement is believing in itself too much. For nothing is truly destroyed in deconstruction, except a belief in certainty. One idea builds upon what came before, and what seems to be the "last word" is merely the latest or next word, convention, discovery, formulation, or conclusion. While we may consider our brand of deconstruction transformational, others may not (see Mills' [2005] critique of the excessive claims of the relational movement as "revolutionary" [as in Mitchell (1993)]). Despite our beliefs and best efforts, the revolution may be delayed—or not arrive at all.

Chapter 18

Witnessing

The axis of group

> Trippers and askers surround me,
> People I meet, the effect upon me of my early life or the ward and city
> I live in, or the nation....
> My dinner, dress, associates, looks, compliments, dues,
> The real or fancied indifference of some man or woman I love,...
> But they are not the Me myself.
> Apart from the pulling and hauling stands what I am,
> Stands amused, complacent, compassionating, idle, unitary....
> Looking with side-curved head curious what will come next,
> Both in and out of the game and watching and wondering at it....
> I witness and wait.
>
> [Walt Whitman, *Song of Myself*, Section 4]

We enter the group and make choices regarding what we observe and focus on, and how we participate. Unavoidably, we are thrust into a public position of the witness and the witnessed, faced with an outcome over which we have limited control: How do we make our presence known?

I call attention to an essential feature of group psychotherapy: *Witnessing*. While not unique to our modality, the social intensity of group gives witnessing special status. I consider it a central axis of personal growth and transformation. We therapists are always trying to be witnesses. One of our tasks is to draw the group to a similar mode of psychological functioning.

Inspired by Whitman, I put forth witnessing as a state of mind, an existential stance, and a mode of relational engagement. To witness, one is "in and out of the game," part of the social enterprise, but willing to stand alone to declare a "Me myself." The influences of "early life," social pressure (the "pulling and hauling"), and self-postures and affiliations ("my dress, associates, looks,") all must—to the extent possible—be acknowledged, yet put aside. *Song of Myself* depicts a continually evolving and expanding self. The witness exists within, yet is capable of transcending social, temporal, and spatial boundaries—compassionate and sufficiently detached to produce independent testimony and free enough to contradict it.[1]

Witnessing transcends observing and participating

The Athenian historian, Thucydides (c. 460–400 BC) concluded that "Most people, in fact, will not take the trouble in finding out the truth, but are much more inclined to accept the first story they hear." No clear line demarks observation from participation. Witnessing, when operative, subsumes both. Witnessing gets closer to truth by extending the psychic field beyond perceptual registers and manifest behaviors. The "compassionating" witness "listens to listening" (Faimberg, 1996) and sees through one's own eyes, and others' too. In resonance and dissonance with others, the witness participates spontaneously, but also with forethought and afterthought.

Individuals enter group with certain intentions, bringing and expressing motives and goals, both conscious and not conscious. However, a much wider psychic field envelops all participants. As John Lennon (1980) put it, "Life is what happens to you while you're busy making other plans." Witnessing deals with the impact of embracing experience beyond observing and participating: the uncertain consequence of coming to know and becoming known.

Witnessing exists in the public domain

In everyday (and legal) usage, the so-called dependable witness is one who observes reality and participates by attesting to truth. However, even when intending to be forthright and objective, witnesses can offer only subjective testimony. I should say, intersubjective testimony; witnesses—expert and not—are also influenced by the setting, the milieu, and by being witnessed.

Testimony necessarily involves reconstruction, framed within the Procrustean iron bed of culture, context, and conformity; the interplays of unconscious processes; and the dynamic constitution of memory itself (Tulving, 2002). Even when within the grasp of objective knowledge, a person still decides how—and how much—to offer testimony. We assert control of the data by adopting roles, appearance, and manner of self-presentation. Knowing that we are being observed, and as we experience validation and invalidation, we make reciprocal adjustments to what we allow ourselves to hear, see, offer, and respond to. Social forces may seem "invisible," but they are unrelenting and to some extent define and delimit observations and participation. George Orwell (1946/1968), ever aware of social pressure and the erasure of individuality, cautioned that "to see what is in front of one's nose needs a constant struggle."

In striving to witness, the group member asserts agency and will (as much as he or she is able) to overcome excessive social and intrapychic constraint—from self-censoring and conformity. To go "naked and undisguised" (Whitman, 2004, Section 2), one must unclothe the pain-avoidant emperor who rules from within, declaring, "Ignore what is in front of your nose. Don't speak to me about me." The axis of witnessing tilts towards psychic pain. It arouses what Bion notated as "K," the "truth motive," a felt need to grasp life with curiosity and to think about and make meaning out of experience, even when this process arouses anxiety—arguably, which is always.

The witness waits

Being both "in and out of the game," the witness "waits." Witnessing develops over time and intersubjective space, during and after the session. Freud (1912) got to this crucial dimension when he cautioned, "It must not be forgotten that the things one hears are for the most part things whose meaning is only recognized later on" (p. 111). While not named as such, witnessing has been in the psychoanalytic lexicon since its inception. The concept harkens back to Freud's (1896) early formulations regarding "nachträglichkeit" (or afterwardness), the belated understanding and continual resignification of events and their effects on behavior.

Witnessing develops later, which may be after a few moments, a session, or years. It can be—and ideally is—life changing, but it cannot always be explained in words, or ever fully. "Approach to meaning" includes that which is not targeted into distinct images or verbal language—"memories in feeling," in Melanie Klein's term—the subsymbolic, procedural, and implicit modes of processing information and learning, which are associational, subterranean, and continual. We hear about its transformational effects from group members: "I don't think about group, but it is with me all week." "I've changed, but I don't know what you [the group] did." "My daughter didn't want me to come, and now she reminds me of group day" or "I never could have said this to you before."

No activity in group goes unfelt or unobserved. However, what one sees, hears, and feels is just a first impression, albeit valuable. The witness controls urges for focus, formulation, or action, all of which may lead to a narrowing of psychic range and premature closure. Witnessing tolerates the tentative pause, uncertainty, a mental and temporal space between the immediate and the mediated. Bion (1974, p. 101) referred to this process of waiting as involving "binocular vision—one eye blind, the other eye with good enough sight." The "blind eye" allows for something else to emerge in the psyche that remains open to experience. According to Bion, the something else—undiscovered meaning—first develops in the mind of the psychoanalyst. In my opinion, there is no predetermined first. Witnessing develops from the nucleus of a group as it engages in the search for meaning and is subject to mutual influence. Often, other group members come to perform this type of transformative work.

Therapeutic witnessing challenges the dichotomous distinction between the there-and-then and the here-and-now. Birksted-Breen (2016, p. 5) underscores that "here and now always refers to that which is not apparently there, the unconscious, the lost connection, the absent other, the non-represented." Meaning deepens with social and private reference, and evolves—or it doesn't. When individuals "get in touch with their feelings," "bridge" to others, subgroup, consider, or make an interpretation (about an individual, the group, the social unconscious, etc.), they are observing and participating and attempting to make meaning. They may be functioning along the transformational axis of witnessing, but this may not be so. We cannot be sure of how enduring the meaning-making process has been for a person, in a particular group session, or for that matter, over the course of the entire treatment.

A group revolving around the axis of witnessing mutually creates and revises testimonies. Given therapeutic time and space, members see through and see more in the narratives of others (if not always their own). The group comes to challenge a member's testimony and reveal what may lay behind it. The objective of therapeutic witnessing is not merely group validation, or consensus, then, but revelation, as new psychic gestalts inform and impact the life of all members.

Case example: from testimony to witnessing

MARSHA (*DISTRESSED, OPENS SESSION*): My father's leg swelled up and he's in the hospital [describing medical condition]… He said he didn't want visitors, only my mother. When he saw me he yelled: "Don't let her in." He always treats me like that, pretending he doesn't want to see me or know who I am.

LINDA: Does he treat your brother the same way? When I gave birth, my father traveled from Florida to be there for his grandson—he knew it was a boy—but not when my daughter was born.

EDDIE: Well, at least you still have parents. My father worked all the time, and died suddenly. I was in school; the principal said I had to go home. I met the priest there, and he said "now you are the head of the family." And I was. From ten [years of age], I had to take care of my mother.

While Eddie had presented the nub of this narrative before, he still stirred the group's empathy: "What an unfair burden!" "No one comforted you." "Where was your mother?"

EDDIE: She cried—all through my childhood—I didn't have one. I had to comfort *her*. Always about missing my father and not wanting to live. That's when Rich says I became numb and cut off my feelings.

Several members reported feeling sick in their stomach, and others were close to tears.

EDDIE (*CONTINUING FLATLY*): I cried a lot, but always alone. I used to wait for him to come home…

ALANA: How old was your mother when your father died?

EDDIE: Forty-six.

ALANA: What! She reminds me of my mother—in her nineties. When my father died it was all about her, her loss, her pain, and still is thirty years later. I've said to her, "Ma, I lost my father, I miss him too" [she tears]. But she's oblivious to my feelings, always.

We had heard Alana's narrative before, as well as Eddie's alibis for maternal limitation and failure that, predictably, followed: "They were from the old country. My mother spoke Italian. It was always the same. I had to take care of my sister too."

ALANA: Bullshit! She was still a mother. I also was in charge of my sister, and still am (now an invalid). Both of them exhaust me and take away my life.

MEMBERS TO EDDIE: Where's *your* anger? What are *you* feeling?

EDDIE (*IGNORING HERE-AND-NOW REFERENCE*): Never got angry. What good would it have done? My father wasn't around; my mother wouldn't listen [continues]....

BILLOW (*IGNORING HERE-AND-NOW REFERENCE*): "You don't need to explain, you already have. Try to listen to what people are saying; they are giving you something to think about."

FROM MEMBERS (*FRUSTRATED*): "Yes, stop and *listen*." "*Feel,* don't rush into words."

EDDIE: "I go numb, frozen."

BILLOW (*PROTECTIVELY*): "So give yourself some time to thaw out!"

EDDIE TO GROUP: You all are very caring. You have a level of understanding that I don't, I'm still new at this.

MEMBERS (*IGNORING HERE-AND-NOW REFERENCE*): You're still talking rather than taking time as Rich suggested. Come on, you're not that new.

Another well-worn apology followed: "I'm not that evolved."

I was about to intercede again, when Eddie turned to Alana, with some caution: "I think I feel the same way the group feels about me when you speak about your mom. Like before, how you *have* to rescue your mother and sister. You act like you have no choice and won't listen to anything we say about how they manipulate you."

We had on occasions gingerly attempted to impress these ideas, only to be met with sanctimony and reiteration, but Alana received Eddie without challenge.

JOSH: I have to say that I had the same reaction to you, Marsha. It was hard to give you anything when you were talking about your father. You talk around your subject before getting to you. Like you spent a lot of time telling us about your father's condition in gruesome detail, but not about how you feel.

MARSHA: Isn't it obvious that I feel upset.

LINDA: We were trying to open you up to other feelings, to how he treats you differently from your brother.

MARSHA: But I know that already.

JOSH: Exactly, so why repeat the story?

MARSHA: I guess I'm hurt and I needed to tell you.

JOSH: Tell him.

BEN: I would say "fuck it." My parents don't listen to me, and I've given up.

LINDA: That's your fallback [Ben]. You don't allow yourself to be tender, show how you are hurt.

BEN: True, but why should I? They might even make fun of me.

JOSH: You're cautious here too, afraid to be direct.

BEN: I've heard that from you since you joined the group.

LINDA (REFERRING TO HERSELF AS WELL): Ben doesn't believe anyone really cares how he feels—even if they "hear" him.

Linda narrated an ongoing conflict with her "tone deaf" husband; others connected Linda's narrative to their own stories, historic and present.

An interval has been spent assessing the prevalence of fixed testimonies and their defensive function both personally and in group, but now discourse seemed to move in a different direction. However, at several intervals, the speakers paused and reflected on themselves. Were they telling stories, being indirect, hiding, or listening and being vulnerable? And how did that relate to their relationship predicaments? A nascent *nuclear idea* had emerged from the collective process: *witnessing*, although unnamed as such. A series of individuals had spoken without bringing dynamic meaning to their individual monologues. Now, members were mutually addressing what they had been enacting, here and elsewhere.

Discussion: witnessing and being witnessed in group

The group process illustrates the human tendency to use familiar narratives as "fallbacks," to move away from something nascent, something tender that may "hurt." We anchor ourselves in place and time, shaping experience into stories, or what Spence (1982) referred to as "historical truth." And then, we come to tell stories about stories. In this group session, in which members came to understand their use and misuse of narratives, Eddie initiated the witnessing process. Referencing his own behavior too, he hesitantly confronted Alana's blinkered testimony: "You act like you have no choice and won't listen to anything we say." Josh directed Marsha to her father: "Tell him [and not merely recite to the group]." Linda offered Ben alternatives to fallback testimony: "Allow yourself to be tender, show how you are hurt." In each of the transactions, members encouraged members to see beyond their stated narratives, such to spur transformative potentials.

Witnessing addresses but does not obviate hurt, which in this session radiated literally and figuratively to the bodies of the empathetic. To the extent that the group could "hear"—listening to their own narratives as well as others in new ways, enduring the temporal process of feeling and understanding psychic pain—they could witness.

The traumatized individual suffers disturbances in witnessing

An extensive clinical literature addresses disturbed witnessing from the perspective of the traumatized (e.g., Herman, 1997; in reference to group see Klein & Schermer, 2000). The deeply traumatized person cannot witness (in the sense I use the term), but requires witnessing. For even in telling one's story, he or she has difficulty in believing it. Describing the terrors of Auschwitz, Primo Levi (1958) expressed profound self-doubt: "As I sit writing at the table, I myself am not convinced that these things really happened" (p. 161). Traumatized individuals such as Levi have suffered experiences that are truly "unthinkable." They testify in bodily, cognitive, and behavioral disturbances—in the all too prevalent manifestations of post-traumatic stress disorder (PTSD).

Group members attempt to understand the testimony of trauma by allowing their minds to resonate with it and by expressing feelings and showing they are moved. In validating both its subjective and external realities, therapeutic witnessing may succeed in gradually releasing the traumatized individual from overwhelming identifications with his or her story. While a profound and often nonverbal communication of recognition, such witnessing does not imply total congruence or blanket acceptance of the other's point of view. A sense of communion must be absorbed but abandoned too. No one can ever fully understand or communicate another's pain. In the "otherness" of witnessing (Poland, 2000) are opportunities for healing and growth.

At times, the therapeutic witness needs to disrupt testimony, narratives that express established patterns of "victimhood" (Meissner, 1976). Inhabiting a fixated self-state, the traumatized individual may maintain an attitude of passivity and helplessness, yet also dominate the group and demand special recognition. Healing progresses as the individual transforms an identity from "victim" to "survivor" to "thriver"—not forgetting the traumatizing events but coming to some understanding about what the events mean and the impact made on one's life. The witness forgives what can be forgiven, mourns, and moves on as best one can (Karen, 2001).

Case example: witness suppression

Marvin, a successful engineer, introduced himself and effortlessly joined the casual give-and-take that could briefly begin a session, particularly with a new member's entry. However, such protracted good-natured exchanges began to become a norm, petering out to silence. Marvin came to suspect (as did I) that our slow starts, labored pauses, and lulls might have to do with him: "Is the group always like this, or is it me?" "Apparently, you have known each other for a long time and I'm disturbing long-standing relationships." "I feel like an intruder."

JOEY (*WHO TENDED TO TAKE THE LEAD OF GROUP REASSURANCES*): Don't worry about it. We need new blood. This happens sometimes, we usually figure out what's it's about. I used to feel like a disturbance too. The sluggishness continued, and in the midst of what seemed to be an unproductive pause, I asked, dubiously: "Is Marvin such a 'disturbance'?"

JUDY (*WITH TREPIDATION*): Marvin didn't say why he's here. He seems a lot more normal than the rest of us [humorously].

JOEY: Yeah, spill your guts.

MARVIN TO JUDY: Well, since you asked. I'm not exactly semi-retired, but I have time to do things I haven't done before. My wife is in a group and thought it would be a good idea. So why not try it?

THE GROUP PURSUED: Are you always so agreeable? Why did your wife want you to join?

MARVIN (*IRONIC*): Well, she doesn't think I am agreeable. She thinks I'm difficult. I think she's difficult.

GROUP: What's difficult about you?

MARVIN: She thinks I get moody and withdrawn, "depressed," but no one else seems to think so.

Several members shared their positive impressions: "I can see why no one thinks so." "You have a nice way of connecting, when you do." "Very friendly, and you seem interested in others."

He nodded: "I am. But I don't understand how this group works. I'm not privy to your history; apparently you get a lot from it [the group]. I'm not sure what I'm going to get, although I do find it interesting." During the following session, Marvin realized that he recognized another member, a man who had been invited to Marvin's tennis club several times by a mutual friend. Judy volunteered that her husband also played at that club, and although she "hated everything about the place," Marvin might see her there occasionally. He blanched, and she said gently, "don't worry, we don't have to talk to each other."

Despite the members' attestations of the value of group and assurances about our confidentiality, these revelations did not sit well. Certain subjects were now "off limits." Marvin had hoped the group would offer anonymity, and now that was not possible. I then received an email regarding the upcoming session. "I'm taking the night off. I'm not sure I'm getting enough out of group to continue and want to think about it over the weekend."

I informed the members, who were concerned but not surprised. "He seems in and out." "Can't tell if he likes us." "Not well enough to commit." "He's a nice guy, not everyone is into therapy that much, look at me." I emailed back the next day and encouraged him to "come and discuss, so that you can get enough." I added that his email had mirrored an unhappy pattern of "withdrawing, going along, or giving up," something we discussed prior to his group entry. He did not respond, but appeared the following week, about ten minutes late.

The group turned to him expectantly, and when I said I had shared the gist of our email exchange, Marvin responded with a faint smile: "I didn't say I wasn't going to come, I said I would think about it. I'm willing to give group more of a chance, if they will have me. Besides, I would feel too guilty to quit."

I said that the question seemed to be whether he would have us. He brushed away my comment: "I'm sure the group went on fine."

"You're friendly but you're a fuckload of work," Joey ventured, never shy about the use of expletives.

"Wow, you shoot from the hip!" Marvin responded with a disapproving edge. Others tried to soften Joey's insight: "We still know very little about you."

MARVIN: Well, what do you want to know?

MEMBERS: Perhaps it would be better to say why we know very little.

MARVIN: My family kept our distance from others. Perhaps my parents didn't trust people, after [having been interred during] the holocaust. We were told never to tell people 'our business', which was 'private'." He paused, and with feeling: "I agree. Even now I have one close friend; my wife tells me I should get some others.

MEMBERS: What about kids?

MARVIN: I wouldn't say we're "friends." They're closer to my wife.

MEMBERS: And? Does that bother you?

MARVIN (IRRITATED): A lot "bothers" me.

JOEY (REGISTERING SOME EXASPERATION): My kids are the most important part of my life. I am sure they are to you too, although they may not know it. Maybe you treat them like you act with us. I can imagine what your parents must have been like, very controlling and not too friendly either.

MARVIN (TAKING OFFENSE): Not really, I think I had a lot of freedom. I know you aren't supposed to like your parents in this group. But I like mine. My parents never fought, and never complained—and if you did, they would say that we have so much to be grateful for. I respect my parents a lot.

JOEY (APOLOGETIC): I don't know you that well. I guess I'm way off.

Attempts to enlighten Marvin with a nuanced view of mixed feelings flagged, but stimulated personal reflections regarding demanding parents, whom they compared unfavorably to their own democratic parental behavior. Towards the end of the session, I noted that Joey had become quiet. Joey: "I'm listening. In my family, respect didn't go two ways, just like some of you were saying. It was my father who demanded respect, but he didn't offer it, not even to my mother... Maybe I'm feeling quiet for hurting Marvin, being like my father again. What do I know anyway?"

MARVIN: I'm not hurt. You made a comment and then said nothing.

FROM THE GROUP: A "comment"! Joey was never more articulate! He took a chance with you. You're angry at what he said.

MARVIN: I don't think so, I just don't agree.

And then, adding parenthetically: "My sibs have a very different view [of their parents]—they got away from them as soon as they could." While attributed to his siblings, Marvin had offered a promising fragment of a revised testimony, in line with Joey's version. We would wait for later sessions—which now had returned to their characteristic intensity—for Marvin to begin to take emotional ownership of why others saw him as they did.

Discussion: a pattern emerges

The traumatized individual reveals a fragmented self, "frozen in a developmental time when self-experience was traumatically arrested" (Bollas, 1984, p. 210). The witness tolerates the emotional buildup of experience "without reaching for fact and reason until a pattern evolves" (Bion, 1970, p. 124). Fragments of Marvin's dissociated internal drama played out dramatically with Joey, and substantiated that which had intermittently stifled group process. An atmosphere of inhibition had enveloped the group since Marvin's entry, a pattern marked by repetitive intervals of gaps, disjunctures, and ruptures in communication.

Marvin's reliance on intellectualization, repression, and dissociation broke down in the irruptive interactions with the provocative Joey. A psychic *nodule* (Billow, 2016) asserted influence on allowable testimony. A vigilant parental presence lodged within Marvin, monitoring allowable expressions of feelings and ideas, and punishing transgressions. In fealty to his traumatized parents, he rebuffed those who trespassed into guarded areas of his mind—his "private business." Hence, his ambivalence to group, vigilance against social exposure (as with social contacts at the tennis club), minimizations of Joey's insight, and hostility to Joey himself. There seemed to have been two choices in Marvin's family: mental submission or flight. Marvin had opted for the first, and his siblings, the other.

Marvin's pattern came to make sense to many of us, but not yet to Marvin himself. We had been subjected to some of the testimony's constitutive elements—self-justifying oppositionalism, punitive distancing, and veiled threats of abandonment (as in his email). Characterizing such behavior as depression, his wife directed her "difficult" husband to our care. Sequestered within a fixed narrative, Marvin severed forms of self-consciousness, recognition of others, and gratitude towards them. His interpersonal maneuvers could quiet the group and specifically, undermine Joey's capacities to observe, participate, and witness: "I guess I'm way off", "I'm feeling quiet for hurting Marvin... What do I know anyway?" Joey had begun to witness, but he had trouble maintaining that stance in the group. Marvin's status as witness was fluid but uncertain.

Therapeutic witnessing involves "recognition from the inside, that which comes from a coexperiencing" (Grossmark, 2010, p. 90). Aligning his personal history with Marvin's, Joey had led our group in unraveling some of the familial ties that wrapped Marvin within: "I can imagine what your parents must have been like, very controlling and not too friendly either." Joey displayed "figurability" (Perelberg, 2015), describing substitutive scenes that could function like screen memories. While Perelberg ascribed this mode of participation to the analyst, any therapeutic participant may exhibit this creative function, which is also an aspect of witnessing.

Witness protection: further discussion of the two groups

The way out of social embeddedness is not to escape from the group but to participate differently, a learning task often defined and set in motion by the group itself. The first group exhorted Eddie to listen empathically and not rely on a cache of preformed opinions and suggestions. Other members too had to become more experimental, freer to try new behaviors and new narratives, rather than rely on stories treated as sacred texts. In the second group discussed, Marvin had to separate from one group (his family of origin) sufficiently to understand its impact, so that he could become a working member of other groups, and also more of a separate individual.

The two groups illustrate how a member evolves from a traumatized individual to a psychologically informed witness. Eddie and Marvin both contended that they did not "get" how group worked. Eager to adapt to the culture of our group, Eddie benefitted and expressed gratitude when confronted. "You all are very caring," Eddie declared, and I understood from his words and behavior that the group could establish boundary and educative functions—all within the purview of the empathic witness (Grossmark, 2010). Eddie did not need much protection. He did not seem unduly hurt by confrontations and challenge, but recognized and inspired to take chances in how he observed and participated.

In contrast, the ambivalent Marvin initially repelled influence. I had to protect a space for Marvin's frozen parental idealizations to thaw out, such that he could link to others and embrace our culture. I trusted that if Marvin endured, our very presence could alter the original traumatogenic situation that he replicated. Utilizing a "holding" position, I took in good stride or ignored his aspersions about our group, and did not attempt to argue him out of his condescension about its questionable suitability. While he declaimed that certain subjects were off limits for him, I observed how he respected the chances other members took. He was fascinated by transference explorations, intently following how members linked our here-and-now to their outside and past behavior. Realizations began to emerge in Marvin's associations. His siblings did not "like" their parents either, he repeated, now resonating with the group by elaborating with some depth their reasons, while still disowning his own.

Marvin declared himself an intruder in the group; in actuality, the group was intruding into Marvin's mind. And successfully, for he has become a committed member, acknowledging without fully elaborating that he "gets a lot. Besides, my wife actually seems to like me." In retrospect, even the lengthy casual exchanges of the early sessions had a constructive purpose, providing time and space for bonding (Chapter 8), establishing a foundation of safety and mutual interest in what would follow.

Reis (2009) emphasized that to occupy the essential position of the empathic witness, the analyst must understand "that performative and enactive features of traumatic experience are not to be simply translated or transduced into symbolic form, and that a part of the integrity of the experience of trauma is itself its wordless registration" (p. 1360). However, what is wordless to the traumatized individual comes to register on other group members who are less patient, are willing, or adept than the therapist in moderating the witnessing process. As with Joey, they forge ahead. Ideally, they provide what Bromberg (2006) referred to as "safe surprises." Yet inevitably, they create irruptions (Billow, 2016). Therapeutic witnessing disrupts the patterns that have emerged in the group, loosening the fabric of dissociative structures that secure the "felt stability of selfhood" of the traumatized individual (Bromberg, 2006, p. 182).

The therapist reserves the right to intercede in interviews that threaten to become interrogations, protecting all members from the effects of brash confrontations or premature interpretations. Yet we can never be sure that group occurrences are sufficiently safe, or too safe, to be therapeutically efficient. Certainly, too much therapeutic doing—structuring, bridging, confronting, interpreting—and too narrow or intense a focus, jeopardizes the witnessing process. Undue striving for understanding or being understood represents a dissociation of subjective experience. Life "happens" and is never without risk.

Summary and concluding remarks: being a witness

It has been important for me to write about this subject. I have been both commended and criticized for being active, interactive, and self-referential, in my clinical theorizing, case reports, and leadership of demonstration groups (Billow, 2013c). Some considered me too relational while others, not properly so (see *Group Analysis*, 2017, Issues 1–4). Here I emphasize the witness function, which provides mental space for the therapist to reflect upon the here and now—to recalibrate one's mode of observing and participating—to recenter the therapeutic "Me myself." Witnessing gives second and third opportunities, and many more, to review, to think, to find significant patterns, and, as I do, to write about the evolving therapeutic journey, all of which has led to my personal and professional development.

In reference to theory and technique, witnessing describes a therapeutic model of group process: an implicit basic rule that the therapist attempts to instill, partially by the nature of interventions and partially by the example of his or her own reflective behavior. Witnessing directs the therapist to the creative work involved in stimulating psychic growth—to the work we do while we are also observing and participating. Groups operating on the axis of witnessing focus and concentrate, yet tolerate and benefit from interruptive play. Complex views of self, other, and reality emerge, which may be challenging, contradictory, and unresolved, sometimes painfully so. Still, the group coheres, with a relief in meaning that that is "beyond happiness." In appreciating the transformational properties of witnessing and being witnessed, and accepting our limited ability to capture, nail down, or cognize this process, the more likely we therapists can relax, wait, and let group happen.

Some members arrive as witnesses, while many grow into the role. Confirmed by a sense of "being" rather than "being right," witnessing declares: "Right, or not right, this is me—my take on experience." Within the therapeutic frame, the witness takes no testimony as fixed, or at face value. Even one's own. It is not a bad attitude to bring to life.

Note

1 In Section 51, Whitman writes:

> Do I contradict myself?
> Very well then I contradict myself,
> I am large, I contain multitudes.

Chapter 19

Attention-getting mechanisms (AGMs)

A personal journey

Since Freud's discovery of the talking cure, psychoanalytic theory and technique have concentrated on the modes and mechanisms of *paying* rather than *receiving* attention. Freud (1912) stressed the importance of a mental attitude removed of preconceptions and self-censoring; to make available for thought and feeling whatever comes to mind, via "free association" (the patient) and "free floating attention" (the therapist). It is not easy to pay attention. One must control urges for focus, formulation, and action, all of which reduce anxiety and uncertainty, but narrow psychic range and behavioral options. To join a collaborative process of exploration and scrutiny, therapeutic participants need to feel and believe that the other is there too, attending to the relationship.

Needs and bids for attention infuse all realms of human behavior. We start out needing attention and need it until we depart. Wired into our biology are mechanisms that elicit human contact (Thiele & Bellgrove, 2018). Spurring the infant's cry, they are physiological and behavioral, guarding against the physical and psychological damage of isolation and neglect. The loner, performer, scientist in the lab, and scholar in solitary pursuit—aloof or friendly—all cope with needs and wishes to make their presence known.

This final chapter is an example of how I "do the work" and records the evolution of my thinking about dilemmas in getting attention and the self-defeating attempts at their solution. Individuals center attention on getting attention, including therapists of course, and those of us who write and seek publication. Motivations are complex, often beyond mental reach (Dijksterhuis & Aarts, 2010), and at times unsatisfying or even dismaying. A group member put it this way:

> I talk in group partly to contribute and partly to be seen as contributing. But I really don't know what to do with attention, it makes me feel uncomfortable. I'm better at performing than at listening to what comes back to me.

Pursued or conspicuously avoided, pleasing or displeasing, attention-getting features in people's narratives, the enactments they play out, and the tactics and techniques that we therapists employ.

I describe segments from two sessions of a stable, psychoanalytically oriented group. The first alerted me to the topic and, unexpectedly, stimulated personal associations and remembrances, which centered on a cumulative childhood trauma. I approached the second session, which occurred several months later, better equipped to understand the proceedings and to connect my ideas to current diagnostic criteria, technical considerations, clinical research, and metapsychological theory.

The first group session

BEN (*SPEAKING TO THE FLOOR*): I'm a stock market addict…. I've lost a lot of money day trading.

The group had struggled with Ben regarding risky fiscal behavior that undermined his successful small business. Balance a portfolio, diversify? He knew better than the several investors in attendance. When his favored stock market segment turned against him, he telephoned for individual appointments, before confessing to the group. Over time, he lost well over a million dollars. Analogies to intoxication, alcoholism, or addiction infuriated Ben. He would be a successful trader if not distracted by business! We could only register concern and fear, which seemed to sooth him and end discussion. While once again sympathizing with his latest series of losses (in a robust stock market), several members voiced their encouragement. He had finally acknowledged "addiction." We paused hopefully, expecting Ben to explore his insight, but Shaun broke in with amusement: "I think you are a performer. You love to dramatize!"

Shaun's interruption riled Dwight: "And, how does that relate to our topic? How does that help?"

"He's dramatic, he loves to perform." Shaun explained by repeating himself in reverse order, irritating more members. Once again, Shaun was out of synch. The group's disapproval seemed not to register on Shaun, who blithely continued, until Dwight's loud protest redirected members to Ben: "Can't you stop?"

BEN: I don't want to stop. I can't stop.…I need money, I know I could do it if I could devote myself to the market.

Ben's retreat from acknowledging to justifying his behavior stimulated a rehash of familiar group remonstrations and my pedestrian intervention: What were the members feeling? The chorus of "helpless," "pulled in," "pulled down," "invisible" "frustrated," "worried," and "angry" did not move Ben. Neither did my reflection that he seemed to be smiling to himself with a sense of satisfaction. Ben had removed himself mentally, and rather than respond or encourage response to this new provocation, I turned to the unresolved tension between Dwight and Shaun.

DWIGHT (*TO SHAUN*): You do this all the time, being a step behind or off topic. Like you're not listening. It really pisses me off.

While resonating with Dwight's annoyance, several members were alarmed by his harsh delivery.

As if to justify himself, Dwight reiterated: "It's like you're oblivious! You don't listen but carry out your own agenda. This is just how I felt with my mother."

SHAUN: How don't I listen?

Dwight reddened in an effort at self-control; others rushed in protectively, imploring Shaun to think and not respond so quickly. Dwight's anger was scaring them.

"Why *so* angry?" I asked Dwight, who was still combustible. "He doesn't fucking get it. And he doesn't get that he doesn't get it," he replied. "I know, I'm too much, too angry too often," Dwight conceded sorrowfully, "I've heard it all my life."

"And?" I pursued, inviting further self-examination that did not follow. Others: "I know how Dwight feels, you can't get through." "Useless." "You feel you don't count."

"I just space out when you talk, Shaun," Josh volunteered, with some disdain.

Shaun offered a familiar mantra of not being as evolved as other members. His parents were immigrants, he reminded us, and he did not speak their language, or the language of the group. He was grateful for the feedback, for he wanted to learn. Shaun's declaration met some sympathy and much disregard.

JOSH (*UNMOLLIFIED AND CLEARLY ANNOYED, ADDRESSING THE GROUP*): I've been struggling with this feeling of not counting too. No matter what I do, my parents always make it about them, just like you, Shaun. When I became a baseball star in high school my father took credit for being the coach. I couldn't wait for him to get off the sideline and shut up. Same now, I take our family on a foreign adventure, my mother tells me about her trip and how we could have done it better. I just seethe, I don't always realize it, but my wife does and, when she's not intimidated, calls me a 'downer' and tells me to stop moping.

DORIT: I often feel invisible to my husband, like with my father who ignored me. I tell him what I want and he ignores me, does what he wants, mostly, nothing. Same thing with my son; he's a good kid but "no" is never "no." I just give up and seethe, like Josh.

Ben joined in, as if he had not been a major force in this chain of events. "My parents tried. They were so tied up in their own conflicts, with themselves and each other, they couldn't attend to us [the children]. I was like a wild child, doing what I wanted."

Addressing Ben, I took a chance with an idea that Shaun—of all people!—had introduced earlier and met with rebuff. "Do you think you became 'dramatic', as Shaun suggested, as a way to get their attention?"

Ben registered no recognition, flummoxing the group. It fell on me to refresh his memory with some of his often-repeated past exploits, beginning with school truancy. "You've been carrying out risky 'performances' since you were a little boy...."

Ben defended his parents and himself: "I had an attention deficit disorder, and my parents didn't know about it, no one even knew the term then. [humorously] Had it been invented?"

I returned his humor: "You're being inventive now.'"

DORIT: I withdraw when I feel invisible, I did that as a lonely child. I feel like I have no other choice, and you, Ben, get dramatic, and pull us in.

"No other choice?" I echoed dubiously, to the room as much as to Dorit.

Several women took this opportunity to address Dorit.

JENNA: Maybe you scare them and they shut you out. I used to do that with you.

KATHERINE (*TIMOROUSLY*): When I first came to group, I either was going to leave or hide to protect myself from your hostility. I went home with a stomach upset and a long bathroom visit. Even my husband could figure out what was up, and felt sorry for me. You seemed displeased with my very presence. Even when you didn't say anything, I knew you didn't like me. Now I love you.

DORIT: I love you too. Both of you. I don't feel that you are going to shut me out and make it all about you, as Josh said.

The expressions of mutual love among the three women were all well and good, except that Dorit had turned away from further exploration of her formidable behavior, her projective identifications spurring them, and their alienating social effects as described by the other women. Everyone seemed willing to ignore the unresolved tensions in the room. I did not want to remove the group from developing what I perceived as the germ of an expedient idea, one that I could not quite formulate. How to get to it?

I tried to capture what a number of members were saying: "You don't want to be visible, if you're going to be displeasing and shut out. So Ben isn't the only one suffering from an attention deficit." The group laughed in agreement, but I left group feeling unsatisfied. I needed a word, a concept, something that I suspected existed that would explain more fully what was happening in this group, in all groups. I found it in my past.

Attention-getting mechanisms: some painful recollections

"A-G-M, AGM mechanism," my father would say knowingly to whatever adults happened to be around. I came to know at an early age what he meant: *attention-getting mechanism*. He applied it to my frequent displays of obstreperous behavior. Attention-getting mechanisms (AGMs) explained everything. I do not remember anyone inquiring about the term or being dubious about my father's diagnostic authority, which he had earned as an outstanding physician, but extended to the psychiatric domain, without concern for its effects on me. I shucked off his characterization of my behavior, which grated, but toward which I eventually felt familial affection, not admitting to myself that my father's disloyalty hurt.

Even to a young child, the implication was clear: AGMs were not something to be proud of or displayed. I grasped the derogatory undertones, but not my motivation and interpersonal dilemma. Perhaps if he, or somebody, had withheld censure and asked me about my experience, I, and we, would have come to a more satisfying resolution of a situation that pleased nobody. I got the message from my parents that I should not call for attention (although they did), which goes against the grain of active, inquisitive children—arguably, against every living soul. Irritated by my father's denigrating label, and not understanding the larger social context and my predicament, I did nothing with my unquieted feelings other than what drew unwanted disapproval and disrespect.

Following my recollections, I pursued clinical and research literature. Imagine my surprise that after 65 years I discovered that no standard term existed for what I had assumed to be common psychiatric parlance. I found one scant reference (Dreikurs & Solz, 1964). The initialism, AGM, hardly existed! I honor my father's memory by reviving it here.

I have come to understand how my parents' marriage—perhaps all relationships and certainly those in groups—could be described in terms of the coordinations between competing needs for attention. Self-defeating AGMs arise as social protest. When unfulfilled needs meet unfair and excessive competition, neglect, or punishment, desperate measures may be resorted to and persist even when unsuccessful. Without knowing it, I had been initiated and actively participated in our family's dysfunctional AGM system. It took me a long time to find better mechanisms for pursuing my needs for recognition and attention. Still, according to my groups (and others), I have not yet perfected this skill set.

Connecting self-defeating AGMs to diagnostic and research findings

It is likely that my father had heard or read about the concept of *attention-seeking*, as interest and research in child development became popularized in the 1950s (e.g., Gewitz, 1956), along with child-rearing bibles (e.g., Spock, 1946). *Self-defeating attention-seeking* officially entered the literature as a personality disorder in 1968, with the publication of the second edition of the *Diagnostic and Statistical Manual of Mental Disorders (DSM-II)*. *Self-Defeating Personality Disorder* (also known as *Masochistic Personality Disorder*) was discussed in an appendix of the DSM-III in 1987, but was never formally admitted into the manual due to controversy regarding gender bias and concern over blaming the victim. The current edition, the *DSM-5* (American Psychiatric Association, 2013) places *attention-seeking* in the *dramatic* cluster of personality disorders (subcategories: antisocial, borderline, histrionic, and narcissistic) and emphasizes its excessive qualities in behaviors and emotions.

Adopting a psychodynamic rather than symptom-based approach, the *Psychodynamic Diagnostic Manual (PDM-2*; Lingiardi & McWilliams, 2017) revived the category of the *Masochistic (Self-Defeating) Personality* to describe the types of relationships, feelings, and coping strategies of individuals who undermine their success and sabotage interpersonal relationships. Associating self-esteem and closeness with necessary suffering, the *PDM-2* attributes to these individuals a sense of moral superiority conveyed through their altruistic submission to others.

One might suppose that, since it is adaptive to protect oneself and self-regulate, individuals would modify behavior in response to bad outcomes. However, the draw of the "bad is stronger than [the] good" (Baumeister, Bratslavsky, Finkenauer, & Vohs, 2001). Children more readily and clearly come to understand and define themselves in terms of bad rather than good self-referents supplied by important others, such that self-destructive behaviors emerge and endure into adulthood (Baumeister & Scher, 1988).

To conclude this brief review, self-defeating, attention-seeking patterns figure in diagnoses and descriptions of character, personality, and pathology. All point to critical relational disturbances of attunement and mutual recognition (Benjamin, 2018), typically originating in childhood. I am proposing that such disturbances in interpersonal relationships and self-regulation are often memorialized and expressed symbolically and publicly by self-defeating AGMs.

Self-defeating AGM: definition and formulation

A self-defeating AGM refers to a repetitive interpersonal style or particular behavior or constellation of behaviors that one adopts and displays publicly that is unhealthy, repetitively counterproductive, and ultimately harmful to self and/or others. Such AGMs vary from the subtle and seemingly inhibited to the blatant, excessive, even pathological. They arise in response to trauma and psychological disturbance and, as such, are the outcome of enduring deficits in getting appropriate and sufficient attention. They are expressed through tone, words, gestures, and short- and long-term behavioral actions. These repetitive behaviors reflect desperate attempts to cope with and resolve emotional tensions that remain partially or fully out of self-awareness. Intrapsychic relief is temporary; interpersonal problems remain, while aggressive feelings turn against the other, as well as the self, which has relinquished capacities for reflection, anticipation, and self-control.

Given an ideally responsive world, there would be no reasons to cross a threshold into the self-defeating realms of AGMs. Yet, and as testified by my own memories as well as by members of our group, recurring experiences of felt or actual failure of the social environment to adequately respond persist. Infantile protests are often insufficiently understood or responded to, leading to a buildup of tension, frustration, and expression of aggression towards loved ones and needed caregivers. Parents neglect, reject, dominate, or overindulge their children, sometimes all in a single day, and adults treat each other similarly.

Quiet or clamorous, calm or agitated, our calls for attention often are fated to be inept, ill-timed, maladaptive, or improper, and we resort to self-defeating AGMs. We get attention not in the best ways, or the best kind, and avoid attention too, just when we could really use it. *And sometimes, even when we know what we are doing, we do it anyway.*

Review of the first group session

Equipped with a refined concept, a term, and increased empathic understanding, I reviewed the group session that I have described. I had ended the session by summarizing what people seemed to be saying: that while they suffered from deficits of proper attention, they anticipated being rejected, and so retreated, surrendering agency. However, I realized that there was more to what had occurred. *Each person had insisted on being visible.* Not one merely capitulated, no matter the consequences. Ben spoke for the group: "I don't want to stop...I can't stop"—raising and lowering hopes, antagonizing everyone, and displeasing himself. Each person had found ways to be "dramatic," "harsh," and "formidable." Each participated in a self-defeating interpersonal process involving provocation and withdrawal, which represented enduring strategies of getting attention.

Let us identify some of the self-defeating AGMs of the major players, their etiologies, and their jarring effects on other members and on group process. Shaun did not speak the language of his immigrant parents or of the group; he reminded us as well as demonstrated. While his unsolicited opinions, off-centered remarks, and tedious excuses predictably drew the group's ire, they were also partially successful as bids for attention, and Shaun continued undeterred. Dwight exhibited little control of the reactive feelings and behaviors, first directed towards his uncompromising mother, even when aware that he was becoming "too much, too angry." Dwight's explosive AGMs, while momentarily relieving, made him sorrowful and apologetic, and hence they were self-defeating. Dorit reported "often feel invisible [in group]…like with my father who ignored me." She justified and explained away her self-defeating AGMs, expressed by a contemptuous tone and frigid gestures, which she misidentified merely as "withdrawing," despite contrary testimonies regarding their intimidating power. Like the "seething" Josh, who also reported a history of parental self-centeredness and neglect, Dorit could be "a downer," "mopey," "scary," and "hostile."

Notice how phonotypical patterns (APA, 2013) played out. In reference to gender, three of the four men present (Shaun, Dwight, and Ben) displayed the *disinhibited/social* style in our sessions and in their reports of outside behavior, while Josh and the three of the women (Dorit, the psychosomatic Katherine, and Jenna, who described herself as a shutout/shut-in) tended to the *inhibited/withdrawn* style. But regardless of gender or location on the introversive–extroversive continuum, they all remained troubled by childhood feelings of loneliness and isolation. Like the self-impoverishing Ben, who declared himself still "the wild child, doing what I wanted," no one seemed to be in any rush to alter self-defeating modes of seeking attention, whether met with care, curiosity, thoughtful challenge, interpretation, hurt, fear, disapproval, or disregard.

I had left that session with lingering dissatisfaction. Despite my efforts, the members had neglected to address their own aggression and ignored the unresolved tensions in the room. The members had attempted to deal with each other with no immediate success and I felt I did no better.

I had concluded the first session expanding on a member's quip: "So Ben isn't the only one suffering from an 'attention deficit,'" which I believed was effective for summary and closure. However, my dynamic formulation that proceeded it proved to be insufficient: "You don't want to be visible, if you're going to be displeasing and shut out." A fuller elucidation, more to the core of the group enactments and the underlying motivations of the participants, evolved after a period of self-exploration and literature review. Being shut-out does not extinguish desires to be visible; rather, it *activates* urges, mechanisms, and behaviors to become visible, pleasing or not.

My therapeutic desires thwarted, I too had felt invisible, and likely, feelings of neglect and disregard spurred my closing summary, which, I suspect, had vestiges of a self-defeating AGM. How much attention do I still need? Apparently, a lot! Not for the first time, I left a session wishing I had said less, or said more better. Still, these interpretive efforts directed me towards the better. "The truth rebels," Lacan (1967/2002, p. 267) reminds us. "However inexact it might be one has all the same tickled something."

Jammed within a *nodule* of unremembered memories and "unthought knowns" (Bollas, 1989), I had been tickled unpleasantly and achieved no relief by my words and actions. Two remarks from group haunted my mind: Shaun's "I think you are a performer. You love to dramatize!" and Ben's sardonic "I had an attention disorder." I cannot pinpoint when and if I consciously thought of my father, or its moment, but a *nuclear idea* coalesced. I had found a concept: self-defeating AGMs, and how they played out in the drama of our group, everywhere, and for all of us. Several months later, another group session occurred—replete with self-defeating AGMs—that provided opportunity for further elucidation. Even in situations in which individuals knowingly and intentionally behave in ways that have negative outcomes or are likely to fail and bring harm, there are trade-offs (Baumeister & Scher, 1988). Now I could more fully understand—and begin to explore with the group—the nature of the benefits wished for, the goals achieved, and the unfulfilled desires that continue for us all. I had formulated a motivational trilogy of relief, retribution, and reparation.

A segment from a group session several months later

Jenna: I need to start. My very best friend in Connecticut has cancer. I feel I have to drive out every weekend to see her. I'm exhausted already from my mother. I absolutely have to be there for her [the elderly mother] even though she's never happy with me—or for me. You all say I'm crazy, but I couldn't live with myself.

> Katherine ventured, tentatively to intercede, without clarifying whether she was referring to mother or friend:
>> You must resent her. [Jenna shudders] I know this is hard to hear, maybe from me who likes to be supportive and not contradict. I'd rather accommodate and be upset—literally, I can't eat sometimes. Hello... my childhood as a "perfect child," with lots of stomachaches.

> "No, it's not [hard to hear]," Jenna replied sharply, rebuking Katherine with an air of moral superiority the *PDM-2* (Lingiardi & McWilliams, 2017) ascribes to those individuals exhibiting a *masochistic (self-defeating) personality style.* "I'm just trembling, so upset with everything. I don't resent my friend, just her being sick. But I know I'm full of resentment, even though I always try to do the right thing." And then, partially relenting, "Ok maybe [I try] too much and don't take care of myself."

> Katherine, shaken and quieted, made eye contact with Dorit, in a bid for reassurance despite Jenna's halfhearted repair. Substantiating both women, Dorit confessed not only to resentment but also to hateful feelings and behaviors:
>> It took me a long time to admit how I can hate my own son sometimes—not only my husband. I can freeze him [the husband] out. But I'm so guilty if I don't give in to my son's demands, so I do, but not nicely.

Dwight: I'm in a similar bind. I make recommendations at work—I can plead or have a fit—it lands on me to stay late to clean up other people's messes. Same in my marriage—she wouldn't listen to me, I felt like an idiot, working hard, bailing us out, and then she tried to take everything in our divorce. And I was ready to do it. I become psychotic—"You're a fucking idiot"—I hear it over and over as a real voice. But I give in and I know it's the wrong thing to.

"*I'm* the fucking idiot," Ben blurted, with a not unfamiliar histrionic flair. "I lost a lot of money in the market again."

SHAUN: Does your wife know?

The question (or questioner) set Ben off: "Listen, *I* have to make money. *I'm* the one, not my wife—she has a nice life, does what she wants, makes $30,000 with a part time job, no Social Security or pension. *I* take care of it, for my wife, my employees, my children, all of them fuckers.

Ben's outburst brought the members into silence until Shaun resumed his questioning: "Did you sell, or are you talking of paper losses?"

"No, no! Don't go there!" Ben cautioned. He put his fingers in his ears and started humming.

"Let me finish!" Shaun demanded, ignoring interpersonal danger signals once again.

Ben began to sing loudly, and others rushed in to explain to Shaun what was going on.

"I have the floor!" Shaun leaned menacingly towards Ben. "Fuck you! Go fuck yourself! You're being very rude and immature. I care for you and want to help. I can't believe that you called your children "fuckers."

"Fuck you too!" Ben replied, but without rancor, as if charmed by Shaun's adaptation of his expletive language. "I know you were trying to help, and I was actually trying to help you [by humming], to alert you to what you were doing."

"What a way of being helpful!" several exclaimed, which Ben acknowledged sheepishly. The group turned to Shaun: "I didn't know so much anger was in you." "You behave this way elsewhere?" "Do you think you could have talked to Ben, rather than push back?"

"Not really," Shaun insisted. "What else could I do? Either take it or tell him to go to hell."

Shaun's rhetorical question allowed me access to an analogous situation that Shaun had brought up in an individual session. "Didn't you just 'fuck up' pushing back?"

Shaun registered blank. I registered my own therapeutic exasperation.

SHAUN: You mean with my wife?

The group waited expectantly until he continued.

"My wife brushed against me with so much force I lost balance. I fell and she called me a 'klutz.' I got up and pushed her: 'See how this feels.' It wasn't very hard, but she said 'you hurt me' and charged with fists. I grabbed them, and held her against the wall. I was furious. I turned white, shaking and let her go."

Shaun assured the disapproving group: "I had never done anything like that before. She has, and *I* have been the one with bruises. But we're good now, ever since our [marital] session with Rich, we're talking again. She's being nice to me."

Shaun's self-justifying narrative dismayed the members: "Happy ever after?" "Did you apologize?" "You could own your own behavior if she won't—all the more reason to." Once again Shaun had misrepresented himself and brought on the group's negative attention. In actuality, we had addressed the mutual violence in the marital session, and Shaun had done just what the group had implored.

I suggested that Shaun's predicament with his wife and in group with Ben was hardly his alone. "Everyone wants to show those fuckers who brush against us with force and disregard." Thinking of my own history of persistent self-defeating AGMs, I reflected, not too sympathetically: "You all have been saying this: 'take it or push back.'" The irony was not lost; the tension dissipated, and members took the advice offered to Shaun and directed themselves to their own behavior. Silently, I shared their resolutions to do better.

Review of the second session

Observe the sequence of narratives and enactments involving self-defeating AGMs. Attempting to break out of her introversive pattern, Katherine interrupted Jenna's chronicle of self-sacrifice to suggest underlying resentment. As if proving the point, Jenna took umbrage, sending Katherine into retreat. Coming to Katherine's rescue—itself often a self-defeating AGM—Dorit connected her resentment to insurmountable aggression (freezing husband) and ostensible submission (to her "hated" son). Dwight's tortured account of workplace and marital compliance followed; turning hatred and contempt inward, he declared himself psychotic, a fucking idiot. "No," Ben insisted, *he* is the fucking idiot, being the resentful caretaker of his "fuckers." Self-defeating AGMs reached a crescendo in the Ben-Shaun pushbacks, bringing the group to its vociferous climax and therapeutic denouement.

"I have the floor!" Shaun had insisted. I could not but wonder whether the members, in empathically volunteering their own stories, as well as in their enactive displays, were also competing for floor, one-upping each other with self-defeating AGMs of ever-increasing intensity and brooking no interference. It is the essence of the self-defeating AGM to activate others to respond affectively and with self-defeating AGM counter-display. This was my opportunity to call attention to individual as well as group dynamics.

When individuals are confronted with their own contribution to their recurrent difficulties, and whether delivered gingerly (as the timorous

Katherine to Jenna), aggressively (as in the Ben and Shaun exchange), educationally (as in advice giving), or interpretively (by several members and the therapist), the group must cope with denial, rationalization, and outright hostility. Dwight had addressed Shaun in the first session: "It's like you're oblivious! You don't listen but carry out your own agenda." In actuality, all the participants told about and carried out their own characteristic self-defeating AGM agenda with self-relieving mindlessness. The partial list included monopolizing, spacing out, seething, moping, guilt-tripping, dramatizing, withdrawing, intellectualizing, bellowing, and bullying. Whether conspicuously introversive or extroversive, everyone found a way to express "fuck you" and "fuck you too"—to brush against each other with some violence to connective links, mental and interpersonal. However, by their very public displays, members were also trying to be "helpful," as Ben and Shaun declared, to "show" what harm has been committed and to seek recognition and repair.

Relief, retribution, and reparation: further discussion of the two sessions

Originating and continuing as expressions of helplessness and frustration, self-defeating AGMs mutate into antagonistic instruments of relief, retribution, and reparation. No longer merely targeting the offending originator, but its transferential group representatives, self-defeating AGMs avenge the impingements, assaults, and rejections of childhood. They are also fraught attempts to be understood and attended to. Shaun spoke to the retributive core of self-defeating AGMs: "What else could I do? Either take it or tell him to go to hell." Accommodate, internalize the hurt and angry feelings towards figures who should help us, or push back, triumphantly (if only momentarily) relieving pent-up anxieties, seething tensions, and rage. Some short-term goals are thus achieved. However, like the "exhausted" Jenna, "regretful" Dwight, or the digestively impaired Katherine, and whether adopting an ostentatiously introversive or extroversive behavioral path, one remains guilt-ridden, depleted, and disconnected.

Individuals get caught in their *nodules* and can be left behind, therapists too. I had been irritated by the irruptions in the first session, and attempted, unsuccessfully, to quell myself with a hastily conceived interpretation. Despite the turmoil of the later session and the momentary threat of violence between two members, I found myself relaxed by what I had come to understand about self-defeating AGMs. I had attended to me, and knowing more, I felt no press to do or say anything. A group such as ours expects irruptions and interpersonal conflict, and we have lived through them before (and since). A *nuclear idea*, self-defeating AGM, went unnamed but provided an empathic lens through which I could protect targets and potential scapegoats by universalizing their words, narratives, and group and subgroup enactments. "Everyone wants to show those fuckers who brush against us with force and disregard." By implication, I included myself.

For reparation to occur, individuals need to feel invited back into relationships and attended to. In our group, whether affirmed or confronted, all were invited and all accepted the invitation. At times obstinate and contentious, no one was proud of such behavior, and no one left the sessions unduly angry, or without underlying mutual affection and an unstated wish to do better and be more mature. In subsequent sessions, the members, increasingly familiar with each other's self-defeating AGMs and less reactive, could more skillfully function as curative agents, reflecting on the relational disruptions and less induced to join in.

These sessions captured some of the complexity and developmental origins of the individualized maladaptive patterns represented in the efforts of all of us to be seen and heard. Some interactions engulfed the group in conflict and self-defeating AGM counter-displays; other interactions moved the group in the direction of understanding; and many did both. Self-defeating AGMs were not unidirectional, but multidirectional, interactive, and reciprocal—as were the reparative efforts.

Giving attention to self-defeating AGMs

Our focus must be on how a person seeks attention and seeks solutions to "attention deficits." Some members seem to take their share, bringing in narratives and relating thoughtfully. They genuinely enjoy being part of the process and giving of themselves. However, by their habitual conformity to surface group norms, attention-getting needs remain dissociated, hidden from others and themselves. Seen and heard, "well-behaved" group citizens such as Katherine risk remaining unrecognized. Other individuals such as Ben may be more interested in airing their problems than solving them. In seizing attention via a self-defeating AGM, a member may be rebuffed, punished, condemned, or ignored. Since there seems to be a direct correlation between social exclusion and self-defeating behaviors (Baker & Baumeister, 2017), group process must address rather than merely repeat traumatogenic responses to such behaviors.

At times, therapists and group members unintentionally respond with moral overtones or undertones— thereby censuring emotional communication or exacerbating hurts. Conversely, a sympathy-infused approach may reinforce the conviction that suffering brings connection and unwittingly invite more of the same behavior. While the therapist's intervention might be necessary to cool down overheated interactions and monitor appropriate boundaries, education and interpretation alone will fail. The person must live through the process of expressing self-defeating AGMs and the group must live with that person too. Here lay opportunities to play out and reconfigure old patterns. To feel vindicated, one needs to feel that the other—actual and in absentia—feels, or could have felt, pain and sorrow. Consequently, as our tolerance and empathy for those who have hurt us increases, wounds begin to heal.

In group, as in life, no one is recognized exactly in the way one has wished, and no member is immediately fulfilled, and never fully. In giving attention to the felt deficits in receiving attention, and in giving attention to displays of self-defeating AGMs, there is redress, deeply felt, and more authentic than explanations, apologies, or profusions of love.

Situating the therapist

It has occurred to me that I am one of the fuckers that my patients have to deal with—and that they serve that role for me. We disappoint in fantasy, and at times fail in actuality, stimulating attention deficits sometimes at the very moments we attempt to satisfy genuine needs. We shun expressions of love (Jacobs, 2001) and retaliate rather than empathically understand the frustrated desire that hides behind ultimatums of hate. We feel captive by demands and schedules: some are imposed by the exigencies of work and personal life, but many are prisons of our creations. Unwarranted sacrifices may be requested only in our own minds. Through the arrangements we volunteer or agree to, we become victims, saviors, and bullies.

As therapists, we promote ourselves by the ideas that we offer and how we offer them (sometimes by silence), and we cannot be sure that they are not self-defeating. Our subjective reactions cannot be put aside, and they affect clinical assessment and decision-making. Although I understand cognitively that as therapist, I am always a center of attention and attention-seeking, I may not feel it. It is not difficult for me to feel frustrated, misunderstood, shut out, or invisible. Like Jenna, I need to be needed and can try too hard. I mope and seethe inwardly and contemptuously like Josh, and become harsh and formidable like Dwight and Dorit, dramatic like Ben, and off-point and insistent like Shaun. Urges to express self-defeating AGMs, similar to the narratives and actions of the group members, reverberated in these sessions, I suspect in every session, and regularly throughout my day. Likely I am not the best judge of what I do about them.

Our self-defeating AGMs contribute to therapeutic insufficiency, to errors of omission and commission, to momentary and longer lasting interpersonal ruptures, clinical impasses, stalemates, and outright failures. Some may be brought to our clinical awareness, but none can be fully understood or conclusively assessed. Still, we learn from them, and as we adjust our communications, we demonstrate the essential therapeutic motive: to attend, and to attend better, to meet and repair attention deficits in others and in ourselves too.

Concluding remarks

Ferenczi (1919) suggested that neurosis represents spontaneous attempts at self-healing. I suggest that self-defeating AGMs are antagonizing attempts at alerting the Other to heal us. Ben addressed Shaun: "I know you were trying to help, and I was actually trying to help you [by humming and covering his ears], to alert you to what you were doing [in your attempt to help me]." "What a way of being helpful!" members rebuked Ben. I have been similarly rebuked on other occasions.

In doing our work, we strain to hear the music in the cacophonic rhythms that call attention to hurt, anger, and need. Not only judgments regarding "badness" (Baumeister et al., 2001), but *all* judgments from others constrain freedom, individuality, and communion. Our most beloved figures become our "fuckers." Ben's obscenity captured an emotional truth no less effectively than Sartre's (1946/1989) famous "Hell is the Other." The self-defeating attention-seeker speaks to the therapist, other group members collectively and specifically, and to the other Others, the figures of the unconscious who have failed to adequately attend, provide options, and adequately repair. A presence real and imaginary, radiating bad judgments and good, it is the beloved Other who imprisons and alienates self from oneself. The unreachable Other is the source of our desire and our distress (Lacan, 1967/2002). We rage and turn against the Other and against ourselves, becoming "exhausted," "crazy," "fucking idiots" in our submissions and rebellions. Nothing can extinguish the hope that our "fuckers" will recognize our needs, absolve our guilt, and fulfill our wishes. Humming, glaring, seething, yelling, cursing, complying, or rebelling—ostentatious or surreptitious—self-defeating AGMs sing to the Other.

Epilogue

Richard M. Billow

> You shall no longer take things at second or third hand, nor look through
> the eyes of the dead, nor feed on the spectres in books,
> You shall not look through my eyes either, nor take things from me,
> You shall listen to all sides and filter them from your self.
>
> [Walt Whitman, *Song of Myself*]

The maestro, Toscanini, declared: "Every time I conduct the same piece, I think how stupid I was the last time I did it" (Gottlieb, 2017, p. 20). Our discipline, too, is inspired and limited by stupidity: how we utilize our ignorance according to theory, craft, personality, and let's face it, inherent talent. Raised in the Dark Ages of classical psychoanalysis and ego psychology, I was taught: "When in doubt, shut up." Never the most obedient of students, I tended to follow the reverse, and still do. Doubt makes me anxious, but I treasure doubt, offer doubt, and make efforts to instill doubt in others.

Each leader deals with uncertainty and misdirection. No way to circumvent stupidity. No way to avoid being blindsided by assigned roles and configurations, false notes that we bring, and those thrust upon us while we do our work. We struggle to escape a confined mindset: speaking a voice not wholly our own, enacting scenarios directed by "spectres in books"—idealized versions of whoever we have read and guides us. With apologies to Walt Whitman, it is impossible "to filter them from yourself."

The unconscious is the leader of any clinical hour, we may agree, but whose unconscious? It is *your* unconscious, in mental contact with Freud's, Klein's, Winnicott's, perhaps Bion's and Foulkes's too, resonating with the collective unconsciousness of all those who have exposed you to human wisdom and clinical work. If Lacan is correct in advising the analyst to guard against being "the subject supposed to know," and if Foulkes (1964/2018) is correct that the group's desire to be led is the greatest resistance to overcome, we greatly resist too. We are attached to our leaders, love them, fight them, and fight those who challenge our attachments.

In making efforts to filter, we *need* to speak, to right (write) ourselves out of our idealized theories and theorists, trusting ourselves to develop our own versions of psychic reality. If we minimize our clinical interactions and let others do the work, how do we participate in our own working through? How do we develop our creative capacities? When I say "it is all about 'me,'" it is to emphasize ironically that creativity concentrates on what we do not know about ourselves, less so on whatever is going on with others. *Psychic truth is always in rehearsal*: perspectival and revisable. Our interventions, derived from subjective experience and *participation* in social relations, allows for learning. Opting out of expressing subjectivity diminishes opportunities for getting it better, for feedback and discourse, and for revision.

While socially induced forces ("G") push us towards a therapeutic attitude facile and self-protective, they can push us in the opposite direction too. For those of you young enough, and with strong stomachs and stamina, try leading groups of challenging adolescents. I did. I came to enjoy being called stupid—and worse. "A four-eyed, dickless wonder" remains among my favorites. Dr. Billow's stupidity was a rallying cry around which angry and truant adolescents could organize. "Yes, stupid, but not dumb enough not to take your parents money," I harmonized. They found an adequately antisocial leader. In truth, I *was* stupid, until they wormed into my guts and informed my therapeutic core. (This is what Winnicott meant by saying that the baby raises the family.)

The old joke goes like this. The tourist asks: "How do I get to Carnegie Hall?" The New Yorker answers: "Practice, practice, practice." We practice what we preach by turning inward, attending as best we can to the discordant and concordant notes of our emotional involvement, tolerating the oscillations of paranoid-schizoid and depressive pleasure and pain. Turning outward, we try to absorb, understand, and respond to the music of other players—their themes of meaning and varying rhythms, and the effects of our mutual presence.

I try to do nothing without forethought, yet preserve a freedom to be spontaneous, appreciating that what I observe, say, and omit have elements of what Bion referred to as "0": the not-known and can never be known. Indeed, it is important not to know, and not convey knowing too much (Ogden, 2018; Winnicott, 1965). I alter the mode of my communications and their nature to address shifting interests, led by my own ignorance, which seeks to be informed. In attending to processes of resistance, rebellion, and refusal—which arise continually in the course of every therapeutic alliance, no matter its cohesiveness, duration, and sophistication—I vary what, and if, I say and when. To move others, we must be moved by what we hear (Wachtel, 2011). Our own voice is moving too, when it connects to an authentic self that drives it.

We have, then, opportunity in stupid. The vague ambiguities of reverberation and repercussion offer direction as to how to think about what is happening and what *could* happen. To reach psychic truth, we search for depth, for meaningful resonance. Each gesture is collaboration and waits to play fresh. "Every time an analyst sees something freshly, everything that he has considered becomes worthy of re-consideration" (Bion, 1974, p. 205). It is up to us—*and not the individual patient or group*—to make sure that happens. Minds "meet" (Aron, 1996); the meetings are never without risk, without doubt. Minds *change* when something shakes up confining relationships—mental and actual—that every person is liable to fall into.

We are all "little nodal points" in social networks (Foulkes, 1948/1983, p. 14). Not all of one size and shape, however. People differ in power and influence, the therapist most of all. To the extent that he or she is equipped with a deep understanding of developmental and unconscious roots of character and behavior—*learned from the inside out*—the therapist especially is attuned to hidden dimensions of personality. He or she must be capable and willing to approach interactions with an unwavering attitude to help individuals—oneself included—to claim potentials.

Individuals enter, trust, and adapt to our norms at different times and to different degrees, arriving at different nodal points in our own development. They stay, prosper, and leave; we continue. An accumulating history of learning and practice expresses itself in who we are and what we do. Hopefully, professional and personal development brings to the lone figure of the aging therapist wisdom and savoir faire—good luck with that. The most consistent finding in all psychotherapy studies is that patient retention, acquiescence, and satisfaction in treatment depends on the quality of the individual's relationship with the therapist. I remind you of our responsibility without diminishing the importance of the other players. So, no less than with an orchestra or jazz combo, and whether is called analysis, individual psychotherapy, counseling, or group—it carries the spirit of your name and the actuality of your influence.

Experienced therapists, like seasoned practitioners of any discipline, are more alike than different, no matter our professed theories, institutional affiliations, and technical orientation. Within the frame of talk therapy, we assess what a person is capable of hearing and how best to say it. This is the essence of the art of therapy—of any activity between individuals involving learning. We greet, we listen, we speak. We open and close the clinical hour. Our actions vary in the degree and type of verbal activity: ambiguity and play (testing reality), clarifications (reality testing), empathic communications (holding, mirroring), translation (containing), whole group, interpersonal, and intrapsychic focus, accommodation, confrontation, reconstruction, interpretation, and so forth.

But we tend to have a larger, not smaller, *presence*, being more relaxed and available. We know more, and knowledge allows us to hold onto knowledge less, to express more, not less of ourselves over time. Like all activity and inactivity by the therapist, we infringe on *and* free up each person's dependence and independence. Each session impinges on the last, and each session is a rehearsal for the next, a place that may exist only in thought, but endures, somewhere in mind. No matter where we are in our own or another's development, we both contribute to and interfere with the collaborative enterprise. Isn't this true in all interpersonal relationships?

To such terms and metaphors as doctor, analyst, therapist, participant-observer, group facilitator, guide, dynamic administrator, leader, conductor, counselor, convener, dance partner, let's add ski instructor—please substitute your favorite sport. I am describing an embodied thinker in motion, performing with unique rhythm and talent. Speaking personally, on and off the slopes I want to be with somebody who is damned good. Not merely to aid me in solving my problems but to demonstrate, encourage, and nudge—to push me into growth, to grapple with problems that I didn't even know existed. All of us are capable of reaching an understanding of dynamics, but it is not so easy to do something useful with it. Typical of learning, we tend to pick up new bad habits while shucking off old ones. For the therapist, what better opportunity for practice than combined individual-group psychotherapy, wherein all eyes instruct, and the instructor him- or herself is scrutinized.

Whatever our modality of treatment: individual, group, or my preference of combined individual-group, we offer ideas to those who have their own mores, modes of interaction, and myths. Necessarily, we confront intellectual and cultural loyalties, as well as habitual ways of thinking and doing. To be damned good, we must serve as a "very impertinent" Other (Lacan, 1953/1977, p. 213), disrupting preverbal and symbiotic relationships to those other Others, the looming heroes and villains of transference and countertransference. The challenge remains *to think*. To embrace the clinical experience in its disquieting and yet soothing fullness opens our own mind to change.

"I am trying to get it right," a patient concedes, momentarily, "of course, that's partly defined by what you like."

"You don't want me to express my opinions?"

"You might as well, I know you have them."

The clinical hour abounds with opinions about what is right and how to best proceed. Why attempt to hide opinions from mutual scrutiny? The search for meaning is inherent; hence our communal love of truth. I can relax and rely on the libidinal pull of curiosity. I put trust in the power of ideas. When ideas hit the right notes, they draw people together, establish relationships, and advance discourse, no matter how seemingly contentious.

For me, this is the core of being relational: friendly to one's own mind and the minds of others.

This turns me with gratitude to the suitably impertinent, opining Dr. Tzachi Slonim. Therapists need "a certain amount of cruelty" and shouldn't be "too nice" (Carl Jung, in Atlas & Aron, 2018, p. 117). So do damned good editors, who must have the courage and confidence to subject a writer's precious words and ideas to scrutiny, and offer one's own opinions. Not easy to break through predispositions for mutually idealizing scenarios between a respected elder and a younger colleague eager to learn. Dr. Slonim broke through with incisive thinking, lucid writing, and creative ideas (including the subtitle of this volume).

A writer—not unlike a therapist—has to take responsibility to make a presence known. Studied screens, whether of silence or active participation, analytic or otherwise, produce therapeutic artifacts and may even be iatrogenic (Gill, 1994). Rereading my earlier writings, I take solace in being a consistent presence, and I have not discovered anything to recant. I would say some things differently, yet there is much that I could not say as well today. I have been told that I write better, and that I have "mellowed" as a person and practitioner. Something has not changed, however, which I insist has to do with stupidity—a desire to wait until I can say something that takes me past what I can understand. My words make an implicit invitation to others: to supplement, to object, to correct.

Inviting you, the reader, I have asserted my own leadership. My opinions about the nature of our work and how to do it are more and less right, more and less compatible, tolerable, and welcomed. "It all depends," as we clinicians like to say regarding decisions: therapeutic, aesthetic, and otherwise. It depends on your opinions too. Can we agree that every clinical hour, satisfying or not, provides opportunities for a growth experience for all participants? I trust that this volume addresses a basic need—to learn, discover, create. It has served that need in me.

Bibliography

Agassi, J., & Meidan, A. (2008). *Philosophy from a skeptical perspective*. New York: Cambridge University Press.

Agazarian, Y. M. (2012). Systems-centered group psychotherapy: A theory of living human systems and its systems-centered practice. *Group, 36*(1), 19–36.

American Psychiatric Association. (2013). *Diagnostic and statistical manual of mental disorders, fifth edition (DSM-5)*. Washington, DC: American Psychiatric Publishing.

Aron, L. (1991). The patient's experience of the analyst's subjectivity. *Psychoanalytic Dialogues, 1*, 29–51.

Aron, L. (1996). *A meeting of minds*. Hillsdale, NJ: Analytic Press.

Aron, L. (1999). Clinical choices and the relational matrix. *Psychoanalytic Dialogues, 9*, 1–29.

Atlas, G., & Aron, L. (2018). *Dramatic dialogue: Contemporary clinical practice*. New York: Routledge.

Austin, H. (1962). *How to do things with words*. Oxford: Clarendon Press.

Bach, S. (2016). *Chimeras and other writings*. New York: IPBooks.

Baker, L., & Baumeister, R. (2017). Alone and impulsive: Self-regulatory capacity mediates and moderates the implications of exclusion. In K. Williams & S. Nida, *Ostracism, exclusion, and rejection* (pp. 29–45). New York: Routledge.

Balint, M. (1965). *Primary love and psychoanalytic technique*. New York: Liveright.

Baranger, M., Baranger, W., & Mom, J. (1983). Process and non-process in analytic work. *IJP, 64*, 1–15.

Barrows, S. B. (1986, September 10). 'Mayflower Madam' Tells All. (M. Christy, Interviewer), *Boston Globe*.

Barthes, R. (1967). *The death of the author* (A. Leavers, Trans.). New York: Smith and Hill.

Baumeister, R., Bratslavsky, E., Finkenauer, C., & Vohs, K. D. (2001). Bad is stronger than good. *Review of General Psychology, 5*, 323–370.

Baumeister, R., & Scher, S. (1988). Self-defeating behavior patterns among normal individuals: Review and analysis of common self-destructive tendencies. *Psychological Bulletin, 104*, 3–22.

Beebe, B., & Stern, D. N. (1977). Engagement-disengagement and early object experiences. In N. Freedman & S. Grand, *Communicative structures and psychic structures* (pp. 35–55). New York: Plenum Press.

Benjamin, J. (1990). An outline of intersubjectivity: The development of recognition. *Psychoanalytic Psychology, 7*, 33–46.

Benjamin, J. (2018). *Beyond doer and done to. Recognition theory, intersubjectivity, and the third.* New York: Routledge.

Bennis, W. G., & Shepard, H. A. (1956). A theory of group development. *Human Relations, 9*, 415–437.

Bernstein, J. (2007). On criticism and being criticized: Some considerations. *Modern Psychoanalysis, 32*(1), 11–19.

de Bianchedi, E. (1997). From objects to links: Discovering relatedness. *Melanie Klein and Object Relations, 15*, 227–233.

Billow, R. M. (1997). Entitlement and counter entitlement in group therapy. *IJGP, 47*, 459–474.

Billow, R. M. (1998). Entitlement and the presence of absence. *Melanie Klein and Object Relations, 16*, 537–554.

Billow, R. M. (1999). An intersubjective approach to entitlement. *Psychoanalytic Quarterly, 68*, 441–461.

Billow, R. M. (2000). From countertransference to "passion". *Psychoanalytic Quarterly, 69*(1), 93–119.

Billow, R. M. (2003a). Rebellion in group. *IJGP, 53*, 331–351.

Billow, R. M. (2003b). *Relational group psychotherapy: From basic assumptions to passion.* London: Jessica Kingsley Publishers.

Billow, R. M. (2005). The two faces of the group therapist. *IJGP, 55*, 167–187.

Billow, R. M. (2007). On refusal. *IJGP, 57*(4), 419–449.

Billow, R. M. (2009). The radical nature of combined psychotherapy. *IJGP, 59*(1), 1–28.

Billow, R. M. (2010a). On resistance. *IJGP, 60*(3), 313–346.

Billow, R. M. (2010b). Resistance, rebellion and refusal in groups: The 3 Rs. London: Karnac.

Billow, R. M. (2012). On hostage taking (A psychoanalytic object). *IJGP, 62*(1), 45–66.

Billow, R. M. (2013a). Appreciation "Le Non/Nom". *Group Analysis, 46*, 33–47.

Billow, R. M. (2013b). Sense and sensibility in group psychotherapy. *IJGP, 63*, 474–501.

Billow, R. M. (2013c). The invited presenter: Outrageousness and outrage. *IJGP, 63*, 317–345.

Billow, R. M. (2015). *Developing nuclear ideas: Relational group psychotherapy.* London: Karnac.

Billow, R. M. (2016). Psychic nodules and therapeutic impasses. *IJGP, 66*, 1–19.

Billow, R. M., & Mendelsohn, R. (1990). The interviewer's "presenting problems" in the initial interview. *Bulletin of the Menninger Clinic, 54*, 391–397.

Bion, W. R. (1959). Attacks on linking. *IJP, 40*, 308–315.

Bion, W. R. (1961). *Experiences in groups.* London: Tavistock.

Bion, W. R. (1962). *Learning from experience.* London: Heinemann.

Bion, W. R. (1963). *Elements of psychoanalysis.* London: Heinemann.

Bion, W. R. (1965). *Transformations.* London: Heinemann.

Bion, W. R. (1967a). Notes on memory and desire. *Psychoanalytic Forum, 2*, 271–280.

Bion, W. R. (1967b). *Second thoughts.* London: Heinemann.

Bion, W. R. (1970). *Attention and interpretation*. London: Tavistock.

Bion, W. R. (1973). *Bion's Brazilian lectures 1: São Paulo*. Rio de Janeiro: Imago Editora.

Bion, W. R. (1974). *Bion's Brazilian lectures 2: Rio/São Paulo*. Rio de Janeiro: Imago Editora.

Bion, W. R. (1977). *Seven servants*. New York: Aronson.

Bird, B. (1972). Notes on transference: universal phenomenon and hardest part of analysis. *Journal of American Psychoanalytic Association, 20*, 267–301.

Birksted-Breen, D. (2016). Bi-Ocularity, the functioning mind of the psychoanalyst. *IJP, 97*, 25–40.

Blechner, M. J. (1987). Panel II entitlement and narcissism: Paradise sought. *Contemporary Psychoanalysis, 23*, 244–254.

Bleandonu, G. (1994). *Wilfred Bion: His life and works, 1897–1979*. New York: Other Press.

Blos, P. (1963). The concept of acting out in relation to the adolescent process. *Journal of Academic Child Psychiatry, 2*, 118–136.

Blos, P. (1979). Adolescent concretization. In *The adolescent passage*. New York: International University Press.

Boesky, D. (2000). Affect, language, and communication. *IJP, 81*, 257–262.

Bollas, C. (1984). Moods and the conservative process. *IJP, 65*, 203–212.

Bollas, C. (1989). *The shadow of the object: Psychoanalysis of the unthought known*. London: Free Associations Books.

Bollas, C. (2011). *The Christopher Bollas reader*. New York: Routledge.

Bradbury, R. (1992). *Zen in the art of writing*. New York: Bantum Books.

Bromberg, P. M. (1983). The mirror and the mask: On narcissism and psychoanalytic growth. In A. P. Morrison (Ed.), *Essential papers on narcissism* (pp. 438–466). New York: New York University Press.

Bromberg, P. M. (2006). *Awakening the dreamer: Clinical journeys*. Mahwah, NJ: The Atlantic Press.

Bromberg, P. M. (2009). Multiple self-states, the relational mind, and dissociation: A psychoanalytic perspective. In P. F. Dell & J. A. O'Neill (Eds.), *Dissociation and dissociative disorders: DSM and beyond* (pp. 637–652). New York: Routledge.

Butler, S. (1912/1951). *Samuel Butler's notebooks*. New York: Dutton.

Caper, R. (1997). A mind of one's own. *IJP, 78*, 265–278.

Chused, J. (1992). The patient's perception of the analyst. *Psychoanalytic Quarterly, 63*, 161–184.

Coen, S. J. (1988). Superego aspects of entitlement (In rigid characters). *JAPA, 36*, 409–427.

Cohen, L. (1992). *Anthem. On the future*. New York: Columbia Records Albums.

Cohen, B., & Schermer, V. (2002). On scapegoating in therapy groups: A social constructivist and intersubjective outlook. *IJGP, 52*, 89–109.

Davies, J. (1999). Dissociation, therapeutic enactment and transference-countertransference process. *Gender and Psychoanalysis, 2*, 241–259.

Dell, P., & O'Neil, J. (Eds.). (2009). *Dissociation and the dissociative disorders: DSM and beyond*. New York: Routledge.

Derrida, J. (2005). *Writing and difference*. London: Routledge.

Dickinson, E. (1960). Tell all the trutrh but tell it slant. In T. H. Johnson (Ed.), *The complete poems of Emily Dickinson.* Boston, MA: Little, Brown.

Dijksterhuis, A., & Aarts, H. (2010). Goals, attention and (un)consciousness. *Annual Review of Psychology, 61,* 467–490.

Diplomacy. (2018, August 6). Retrieved from Oxford Dictionaries: https://en.oxforddictionaries.com/definition/diplomacy

Durkin, H. E. (1964). *The group in depth.* New York: International Universities Press.

Drayton, M. (1594/1896). Idea (poem). In M. F. Crow (Ed.), *Elizabethan sonnet-cycles* (pp. 211–276). London: Kegan, Paul, Trench, Trubner & Co.

Dreikurs, R., & Solz, R. (1964). *Children: The challenge.* New York: Hawthorn/Dutton.

Eigen, M. (1985). Between catastrophe and faith. In A. Phillips (Ed.), *The electrified tightrope* (pp. 211–255). Northvale, NJ: Aronson.

Erikson, E. H. (1950/1993). *Childhood and society.* New York: Norton.

Erikson, E. H. (1962). Reality and actuality-an address. *JAPA, 10,* 451–474.

Ezquerro, A. (2010). Cohesion and coherency in group analysis. *Group Analysis, 43,* 496–504.

Ezriel, H. (1950). A psycho-analytic approach to the treatment of patients in groups. *British Journal of Psychiatry, 96,* 774–779.

Faimberg, H. (1996). Listening to listening. *IJP, 77,* 667–677.

Faimberg, H. (2005). *The telescoping of generations: Listening to the narcissistic links between generations.* New York: Routledge.

Ferenczi, S. (1919). *Further considerations to the technique of psycho-analysis.* London: Hogarth.

Foucault, M. (2001). *The hermeneutics of the subject.* (F. Ewald, A. Fontana, Eds., & G. Burchell, Trans.). New York: Picador.

Foulkes, S. H. (1948/1983). *Introduction to group analytic psychotherapy.* London: Karnac.

Foulkes, S. H. (1964/2018). *Therapeutic group analysis.* New York: Routledge.

Foulkes, S. H., & Anthony, E. J. (1964). *Therapeutic group analysis.* London: George Allen and Unwin.

Foulkes, S. H., & Anthony, E. J. (1965). *Group psychotherapy: The psychoanalytic approach.* Baltimore, MD: Penguin.

Frank, K. (1997). The role of the analyst's inadvertent self–revelations. *Psychoanalytic Dialogues, 7,* 281–314.

Freud, S. (1894). The neuro-psychoses of defence. In J. Strachey (Ed.). *The standard edition* (J. Strachey, Trans., Vol. 3, pp. 41–61). London: Hogarth Press.

Freud, S. (1895). Project for a scientific psychology. In J. Strachey (Ed.). *The standard edition.* London, UK: Hogarth.

Freud, S. (1896). Letter 52 from extracts from the Fliess papers. In J. Strachey (Ed.). *The standard edition* (J. Strachey, Trans., pp. 233–239). London: Hogarth.

Freud, S. (1900). The interpretation of dreams. In J. Strachey (Ed.). *The standard edition* (J. Strachey, Trans., Vols. 4–5, pp. 1–625). London: Hogarth.

Freud, S. (1905). Three essays on the theory of sexuality. In J. Strachey (Ed.), *The standard edition* (J. Strachey, Trans., Vol. 7, pp. 123–244). London: Hogarth.

Freud, S. (1912). Recommendations to physicians practicing psycho-analysis. In J. Strachey (Ed.). *The standard edition* (J. Strachey, Trans., Vol. 12, pp. 109–120). London: Hogarth.

Freud, S. (1913). Totem and taboo. In J. Strachey (Ed.). *The standard edition* (J. Strachey, Trans., Vol. 13, pp. vii–162). London: Hogarth.

Freud, S. (1914). On the history of the psychoanalytic movement. In J. Strachey (Ed.). *The standard edition* (J. Strachey, Trans.). London: Hogarth.

Freud, S. (1915). The unconscious. In J. Strachey (Ed.). *The standard edition* (J. Strachey, Trans., Vol. 14, pp. 166–214). London: Hogarth.

Freud, S. (1916). Some character-types met with in psycho-analytic work. In J. Strachey (Ed.). *The standard edition* (J. Strachey, Trans., pp. 309–333). London: Hogarth.

Freud, S. (1917a). A metapsychological supplement to the theory of dreams. In J. Strachey (Ed.). *The standard edition* (J. Strachey, Trans., Vol. 14, pp. 217–235). London: Hogarth.

Freud, S. (1917b). Mourning and melancholia. In J. Strachey (Ed.). *The standard edition* (J. Strachey, Trans., Vol. 14, pp. 243–258). London: Hogarth.

Freud, S. (1921). Group psychology and the analysis of the ego. In J. Strachey (Ed.). *The standard edition* (J. Strachey, Trans., Vol. 18, pp. 67–143). London: Hogarth.

Freud, S. (1923). The ego and the id. In J. Strachey (Ed.). *The standard edition* (J. Strachey, Trans., Vol. 19, pp. 3–66). London, UK: Hogarth.

Freud, S. (1930). Civilization and its discontent. In J. Strachey (Ed.), *The standard edition* (J. Strachey, Trans., Vol. 21, pp. 57–145). London: Hogarth.

Freud, S. (1938). An outline of psychoanalysis. In J. Strachey (Ed.). *The standard edition* (J. Strachey, Trans., Vol. 23, pp. 144–207). London: Hogarth.

Gabbard, G. O. (1997). A reconsideration of objectivity in the analyst. *IJP, 78*, 15–26.

Gans, J. (2016). Demonstration of a mature psychotherapy group: A new member joins. Retrieved from http://www.gapdallas.com/newmember

Gans, J. (2006, Winter). My abiding therapeutic core: Its emergence over time. *Voices*, 14–29.

Ganzarian, R. (1989). *Object relations group psychotherapy*. Madison, WI: International University Press.

Gediman, H. K., & Wolkenfeld, F. (1980). The parallelism phenomenon in psychoanalysis and supervision: Its reconsideration as a triadic system. *Psychoanalytic Quarterly, 49*, 234–255.

Gedo, J. E. (1977). Notes on the psychoanalytic management of archaic transferences. *JAPA, 25*, 787–803.

Gewitz, J. (1956). A factor analysis of some attention-seeking behaviors of young children. *Child Development, 27*, 17–36.

Ghent, M. (1990). Masochism, submission, surrender—Masochism as a perversion of surrender. *Contemporary Psychoanalysis, 26*, 108–136.

Gide, A. (1902/1996). *The immoralist*. (R. Howard, Trans.) New York: Vintage Books.

Gill, M. M. (1994). *Psychoanalysis in transition*. Hillsdale, NJ: Analytic Press.

Goffman, E. (1972). *Presentation of self in everyday life*. New York: Doubleday.

Goldman, D. (2017). *A beholder's share*. New York: Routledge.

Gottlieb, R. (2017, July 2). *Allegro Con Brio*. Book review of Harvey Sachs, Toscanini: Musician of Conscience. New York Times Book Review.

Greenberg, J. (1995). Self-disclosure: Is it psychoanalytic? *Contemporary Psychoanalysis, 31*, 193–205.

Greenson, R. R. (1967). *The technique and practice of psychoanalysis*. New York: International Universities Press.

Grey, A. (1987). Entitlement: An interactional defense of self-esteem. *Contemporary Psychoanalysis, 23,* 255–262.

Grossmark, R. (2007). The edge of chaos: Enactment, disruption, and emergence in group psychotherapy. *Psychoanalytic Dialogues, 17,* 479–499.

Grossmark, R. (2010). Review of Phillip Bromberg's awakening the dreamer. *Psychoanalytic Psychology, 27,* 85–93.

Grotstein, J. S. (1995). American view of the British psychoanalytic experience: Psychoanalysis in counterpoint. *Fort Da, 1,* 4–10.

Grotstein, J. S. (1999). Projective identification reassessed. *Psychoanalytic Dialogues, 9,* 187–203.

Harper, E., & Rowan, A. (1999). Group subversion as subjective necessity—Towards a Lacanian orientation to psychoanalysis in group settings. In C. Oakley (Ed.), *What is a group? A New look at theory in practice* (pp. 168–203). London: Rebus.

Herman, J. L. (1997). *Trauma and recovery.* New York: Basic Books.

Hoffman, I. Z. (1991). Discussion: Towards a social-constructivist view of the psychoanalytic situation. *Psychoanalytic Dialogues, 1,* 74–105.

Hoffman, I. Z. (1992). Expressive participation and psychoanalytic discipline. *Contemporary Psychoanalysis, 2,* 1–14.

Hopper, E. (2001). Difficult patients in group analysis: The personification of (ba) I:A/M. *Group, 25,* 139–171.

Horowitz, L. (1983). Projective identification in dyads and groups. *IJGP, 33,* 259–279.

Hullah, P. (2016). *We found her hidden: The remarkable poetry of Christina Rossetti.* Singapore: Partridge Publishing.

Jacobs, T. J. (1993). The inner experiences of the analyst: Their contribution to the analytic process. *IJP, 74,* 7–14.

Jacobs, T. J. (1999). On the question of self-disclosure by the analyst. *Psychoanalytic Quarterly, 68*(2), 159–183.

Jacobs, T. J. (2001). On misreading and misleading patients. *IJP, 82,* 653–669.

Janis, I. (1963). Group identification under conditions of external danger. *British Journal of Medical Psychology, 36,* 227–238.

Johnson, S. (1759/1985). *The history of Rasselas, prince of Abissinia.* London: Penguin Classics.

Karen, R. (2001). *The forgiving self.* New York: Doubleday.

Karen, R. (2012). Beckoning: The analyst's growth as a therapeutic agent. *Contemporary Psychoanalysis, 48*(3), 301–328.

Kelly, K. V. (1997). Classics revisited: Heinrich Racker's transference and countertransference. *JAPA, 45,* 1253–1259.

Kernberg, O. F. (1975). *Borderline conditions and pathological narcissism.* New York: Aronson.

Klein, M. (1935). A contribution to the psychogenesis of manic-depressive states. *IJP, 16,* 145–174.

Klein, M. (1940). Mourning and its relation to manic depressive states. *IJP, 21,* 125–153.

Klein, M. (1952). Some theoretical conclusions regarding the emotional life of the infant. In R. Money-Kyrle (Ed.). *Envy and gratitude* (pp. 61–93). New York: Delacorte Press.

Klein, M. (1975). *Love, guilt and reparation.* New York: Delacorte Press.

Klein, R., & Schermer, V. (Eds.). (2000). *Group psychotherapy for psychological trauma*. New York: Guilford.

Kohut, H. (1971). *The analysis of the self: A systematic approach to the psychoanalytic treatment of narcissistic personality disorders*. New York: International University Press.

Kohut, H. (1976). Creativeness, charisma and group psychology. In J. E. Gedo & G. E. Pollock (Eds.), *Freud: The fusion of science and humanism* (pp. 793–843). New York: International Universities Press.

Lacan, J. (1953/1977). The function and field of speech and language in psychoanalysis. In *Écrits: A selection* (A. Sheridan, Trans., pp. 179–225). New York: Norton.

Lacan, J. (1967/2002). *The seminar of Jacques Lacan. Book XIV: The logic of phantasy*. London: Karnac.

Ladan, A. (1992). On the secret fantasy of being an exception. *IJP, 73*, 29–38.

Laing, R. D. (1970). *Knots*. New York: Vintage.

Laplanche, J. (1999). *Essays on otherness* (J. Fletcher, Ed.). London: Routledge.

Laplanche, J., & Pontalis, J. B. (1973). *The language of psychoanalysis*. New York: Norton.

Lennon, J. (1980). *Beautiful boy. On Double fantasy stripped down*. Geffen Records.

Levi, P. (1958). *Survival in Auschwitz: The Nazi assault on humanity*. New York: Orion Press.

Levin, S. (1970). On the psychoanalysis of attitudes of entitlement. *Bulletin of the Philosophical Association of Psychoanalysis, 20,* 1–10.

Levine, H. (2012). The analyst's theory in the analyst's mind. *Psychoanalytic Inquiry, 32*, 18–32.

Levenson, E. (1996). Aspects of self-revelation and self-disclosure. *Contemporary Psychoanalysis, 32*, 237–248.

Lingiardi, V., & McWilliams, N. (2017). *Psychodynamic diagnostic manual, second edition (PDM-2)*. New York: Guilford Press.

Lipin, T. (1992). Dr. Otto Isakower's analyzing instrument: Reflections three decades later. *Journal of Clinical Psychoanalysis, 1*, 227–228.

Margolin, A. (2005). *Drunk from the bitter truth: The poems of Anna Margolin*. (S. Kumove, Trans.) Albany, New York: SUNY Press.

McLaughlin, J. (1991). Clinical and theoretical aspects of enactment. *JAPA, 29*, 595–614.

Meissner, W. (1976). Schreber and the paranoid process. *Annual of Psychoanalysis, 4*, 3–40.

Meltzer, D. (1978). *The Kleinian development part III: The clinical significance of the work of Bion*. Perthshire: Clunie Press.

Michels, R. (1988). The psychology of rights. In V. D. Volkan & T. C. Rodgers (Eds.), *Attitudes of entitlement: Theoretical and clinical issues* (pp. 53–62). Charlottesville: University Press of Virginia.

Migliorati, P. (1989). The image in group relationships. *Group Analysis, 22*, 189–199.

Mills, J. (2005). A critique of relational psychoanalysis. *Psychoanalytic Psychology, 22*, 144–188.

Mirtani, J. L. (1996). *A framework for the imaginary*. Northvale, NJ: Aronson.

Mitchell, S. (1993). *Hope and dread in psychoanalysis*. New York: Basic Books.

Modell, A. (1984). *Psychoanalysis in a new context*. New York: International Universities Press.

Montaigne, M. (1685/1958). *The complete essays of Montaigne* (D. M. Frame, Trans.). Stanford: Stanford University Press.

Nelson, M. (2011). *The art of cruelty*. New York: Norton.

Nitsun, M. (1996). *The anti-group: Destructive forces and their creative potentials*. London: Routledge.

Nitsun, M. (2015). *Beyond the anti-group*. London: Routledge.

Ogden, T. H. (1994). The analytic third: Working with intersubjective clinical facts. *IJP, 75*, 3–19.

Ogden, T. H. (1997). Some thoughts on the use of language in psychoanalysis. *Psychoanalytic Dialogues, 7*, 1–21.

Ogden, T. H. (2003). On not being able to dream. *IJP, 84*, 17–30.

Ogden, T. H. (2011). Reading Susan Isaacs: Toward a radically revised theory of thinking. *IJP, 92*, 925–942.

Ogden, T. H. (2018). The feeling of real: On Winnicott's "Communicating and not communicating leading to a study of certain opposites". *IJP, 99*(6), 1288–1304.

Ormont, L. R. (1992). *The group therapy experience*. New York: St. Martins.

Orwell, G. (1946/1981). Reflections on Gandhi. In *George Orwell: A collection of essays* (pp. 171–180). New York: Harcourt.

Orwell, G. (1971). *The collected essays, journalism and letters of George Orwell*, Volume 4, 1945–1950. First Edition. In front of your nose. Boston, MA: Mariner Books.

Orwell, G. (2008). *All art is propaganda*. New York: Mariner Books.

Perelberg, R. (2015). On excess, trauma and helplessness: Repetition and transformations. *IJP, 96*, 1453–1476.

Pines, M. (1985). Psychic development and the group analytic situation. *Group, 9*(1), 24–37.

Poland, W. (2000). The analyst's witnessing and otherness. *JAPA, 48*, 17–34.

Racker, H. (1968). *Transference and countertransference*. Madison, CT: International Universities Press.

Rappoport, P. (2017). Combined therapy as a clinical tool: Special focus on difficult patients. In R. Friedman & Y. Doron (Eds.), *Group analysis in the land of milk and honey* (pp. 149–162). London: Karnac.

Reis, B. (2009). Performative and enactive features of psychoanalytic witnessing: The transference as the scene of address. *IJP, 90*, 1359–1372.

Renik, O. (1993). Analytic interaction: Conceptualizing technique in light of the analyst's irreducible subjectivity. *Psychoanalytic Quarterly, 62*, 553–571.

Renik, O. (1995). The ideal of the anonymous analyst and the problem of self-disclosure. *Psychoanalytic Quarterly, 64*, 466–495.

Renik, O. (1996). The analyst's self-discovery. *Psychoanalytic Inquiry, 16*, 390–400.

Russell, B. (1927/1970). *An outline of philosophy*. London: Allen & Unwin.

Sandler, J. (1976). Countertransference and role responsiveness. *International Review of Psychoanalysis, 3*, 43–47.

Sartre, J. P. (1946/1989). No exit. In J. P. Sartre (Ed.), *No exit and three other plays* (pp. 3–47). New York: Vintage International Edition.

Schafer, R. (1970). The psychoanalytic vision of reality. *IJP, 51*, 279–297.

Searles, H. (1979). *Countertransference and related subjects*. New York: International Universities Press.

Searles, H. (1968–1969). Roles and paradigms in psychotherapy. *Psychoanalytic Review, 55*(4), 697–700. Marie Coleman Nelson (Ed.), Benjamin Nelson, Murray H. Sherman, and Herbert S. Strean. New York and London: Grune & Stratton, 1968, ix+373 pp.

Segal, H. (1957). Notes on symbol formation. *IJP, 78*, 43–52.

Scheidlinger, S. (1964). Identification: The sense of belonging and of identity in small groups. *IJGP, 14*, 291–306.

Scheidlinger, S. (1974). On the concept of "mother-group". *IJGP, 24*, 417–428.

Shabad, P. (1993). Paradox and the repetitive search for the real: Reply to Ghent, Lachmann, and Russell. *Psychoanalytic Dialogues, 3*, 523–533.

Shakespeare, W. (1603/1961). The tragedy of Hamlet, prince of Denmark. In *The complete works*. New York: Harcourt.

Shay, J. J. (2017). Contemporary models of group psychotherapy: Where are we today? *IJGP, 67*, 7–12.

Simons, P. (1992). Women in frames. The gaze, the eye, the profile in Renaissance portraiture. In N. Broude & M. Garrard (Eds.), *The expanding discourse. Feminism and art history* (pp. 39–57). New York: Westview Press.

Smith, H. (2000). Countertransference, conflictual listening, and the analytic object relationship. *JAPA, 48*, 95–128.

Sondheim, S. (1984). *Sunday in the park with George*.

Spence, D. (1982). *Narrative truth and historical truth. Meaning and interpretation in psychoanalysis*. New York: W. W. Norton.

Spock, B. (1946). *The common sense book of baby and child care*. New York: Duell, Sloan and Pearce.

Stark, M. (1994). *A primer on working with resistance*. Northvale, NJ: Aronson.

Steiner, J. (1985). Turning a blind eye: the cover-up for Oedipus. *International Review of Psychoanalysis, 12*, 161–172.

Steiner, J. (1994). *Psychic retreats*. London: Routledge.

Stern, D. B. (2009). *Partners in thought: Working with unformulated experience, dissociation, and enactment*. New York: Routledge.

Stolorow, R. D. (1997). Principles of dynamic systems, intersubjectivity, and the obsolete distinction between one-person and two-person psychologies. *Psychoanalytic Dialogues, 23*, 859–868.

Symington, N. (1983). The analyst's act of freedom as an agent of therapeutic change. *International Review of Psychoanalysis, 10*, 783–792.

Thiele, A., & Bellgrove, M. A. (2018). Neuromodulation of attention. *Neuron, 97*, 769–785.

Thomas, D. (1954). *A child's christmas in Wales*. New York: New Directions.

Thucydides. (c. 460 BC–400 BC). *History of the Peloponnesian war*. (R. Warner, Trans.) Penguin Classics.

Trilling, L. (1972). *Sincerity and authenticity*. Cambridge: Harvard University Press.

Tulving, E. (2002). Episodic memory: From mind to brain. *Annual Review of Psychology, 53*, 1–25.

Wachtel, P. L. (2011). *Therapeutic communication. Knowing what to say when* (2nd ed.). New York: Guilford Press.

Wellek, R., & Warren, A. (1956). *Theory of literature.* New York: Harcourt, Brace & World.

Whitaker, D. (1989). Group focal conflict theory: Description, illustration and evaluation. *Group, 13,* 225–251.

Whitaker, D., & Lieberman, M. (1964). *Psychotherapy through the group process.* Chicago: Aldine.

Whitman, W. (2004). Song of myself. In F. Murphy (Ed.), *The complete poems.* London: Penguin Classics.

Williams, P. (2010). *Invasive objects: Minds under siege.* New York: Routledge.

Winnicott, D. W. (1949). Hate in the countertransference. *IJP, 30,* 69–74.

Winnicott, D. W. (1965). *Maturational processes and the facilitating environment.* London: Hogarth Press.

Winnicott, D. W. (1971). *Playing and reality.* London: Pelican.

Yalom, I. D. (1995). *The theory and practice of group psychotherapy (fourth edition).* New York: Basic Books.

Yalom, I. D., & Leszcz, M. (2005). *The theory and practice of group psychotherapy (fifth edition).* New York: Basic Books.

Index

Note: Page numbers followed by "n" denote endnotes.

Taylor & Francis Group
an **informa** business

Taylor & Francis eBooks

www.taylorfrancis.com

A single destination for eBooks from Taylor & Francis
with increased functionality and an improved user
experience to meet the needs of our customers.

90,000+ eBooks of award-winning academic content in
Humanities, Social Science, Science, Technology, Engineering,
and Medical written by a global network of editors and authors.

TAYLOR & FRANCIS EBOOKS OFFERS:

A streamlined
experience for
our library
customers

A single point
of discovery
for all of our
eBook content

Improved
search and
discovery of
content at both
book and
chapter level

REQUEST A FREE TRIAL
support@taylorfrancis.com

R Routledge
Taylor & Francis Group

CRC CRC Press
Taylor & Francis Group